Fat-Storing Cells and Liver Fibrosis

FALK SYMPOSIUM 71

Fat-Storing Cells and Liver Fibrosis

EDITED BY

C. Surrenti
Unità di Gastroenterologia
Dipartimento di Fisiopatologia Clinica
Università di Firenze,
Viale Morgagni, 85
I-50134 Firenze, Italy

A. Casini
Unità di Gastroenterologia
Dipartimento di Fisiopatologia Clinica
Università di Firenze,
Viale Morgagni, 85
I-50134 Firenze, Italy

S. Milani
Unità di Gastroenterologia
Dipartimento di Fisiopatologia Clinica
Università di Firenze,
Viale Morgagni, 85
I-50134 Firenze, Italy

M. Pinzani
Centro Interuniversitario di Fisiopatologia
Epatica
Istituto di Clinica Medica II
Università di Firenze
Viale Morgagni, 85
I-50134 Firenze, Italy

Proceedings of the 71st Falk Symposium held in Florence, Italy,
July 1–3, 1993

KLUWER ACADEMIC PUBLISHERS
DORDRECHT / BOSTON / LONDON

Distributors

for the United States and Canada: Kluwer Academic Publishers, PO Box 358, Accord Station, Hingham, MA 02018-0358, USA
for all other countries: Kluwer Academic Publishers Group, Distribution Center, PO Box 322, 3300 AH Dordrecht, The Netherlands

A catalogue record for this book is available from the British Library.

ISBN 0-7923-8842-9

Published in the United Kingdom by Kluwer Academic Publishers, PO Box 55, Lancaster, UK.

Kluwer Academic Publishers BV incorporates the publishing programmes of D. Reidel, Martinus Nijhoff, Dr W. Junk and MTP Press.

Typeset by Lasertext Ltd., Stretford, Manchester
Printed in Great Britain by Hartnolls Ltd., Bodmin, Cornwall

Contents

CONTENTS

Preface

C. SURRENTI

In the past 10 years our understanding of the pathophysiology of liver fibrosis has enormously increased. The development and application of cell biology, molecular biology and protein biochemistry has led to the discovery of a complex network of interactions among cells, extracellular matrix, and soluble factors which are involved in the development and maintenance of tissue architecture and function. The modification of these interrelationships is today believed to be responsible for the development of liver fibrosis.

The deposition of extracellular matrix in the liver is a common response to a variety of hepatic injuries, such as virus infection, intoxication by xenobiotics, autoimmune mechanisms, and genetic disorders. Although the formation of a scar can be considered a physiological response to an acute injury, the perpetuation of the damage in the liver may lead to a progressive accumulation of extracellular matrix exceeding the capacity for removal. This excess of fibrotic tissue may itself be responsible for important dysfunctions of the organ. From a dynamic viewpoint, hepatic fibrosis can be considered as the result of an imbalance among synthesis, secretion, deposition, and degradation of extracellular matrix components. The altered regulation of this metabolic process determines the accumulation of collagens, non-collagenous glycoproteins, proteoglycans and glycosaminoglycans in the extracellular spaces.

In spite of substantial progress in the understanding of the mechanisms leading to the development of hepatic fibrosis, there are still many questions in need of definite answers.

Many soluble and insoluble factors are known to influence extracellular matrix metabolism, and *in vitro* studies are yielding information on the possible role of some of them in the pathophysiology of hepatic fibrosis. Among others, special attention has been paid to soluble factors which modulate extracellular matrix synthesis and degradation such as transforming growth factor beta, tumour necrosis factor alpha, interleukin 1, and to those which stimulate mesenchymal cell proliferation, such as platelet-derived growth factor. However, we know that some of these molecules may have opposite effects, either by inhibition of synthesis or stimulation of matrix degradation. In addition, their effect may be modulated by the matrix itself, by specific adhesion to some of its components. Therefore, the first question to be addressed is which factors do actually regulate *in vivo* extracellular matrix metabolism in normal and fibrotic liver and, which is the interplay among different factors *in vivo*, in the regulation of the metabolism of hepatic extracellular matrix?

Studies *in vivo* and *in vitro*, employing morphological, immunological, biochemical, and molecular biological methods have shown that fat-storing cells, myofibroblasts, fibroblasts, and to a lesser extent endothelial cells, are likely to be the major source of extracellular matrix components in normal and fibrotic liver. The role of hepatocytes in this context is still controversial; we still have to clarify how they contribute to hepatic fibrogenesis.

The clinical management of patients with fibrotic liver disease is still unsatisfactory. One major point in the management of these patients is the follow-up of the progression of hepatic fibrosis. Serum markers of fibrogenesis and fibrolysis have been proposed and evaluated to assess the metabolism of extracellular matrix. The question emerging from the analysis of the studies using this test is: do we really have simple, sensitive, and specific serum markers of fibrogenesis or fibrolysis to assess the clinical evolution of chronic liver disease?

One of the most important aims of basic research in hepatic fibrosis is to help develop therapies for its treatment. Various therapeutic strategies have recently been suggested for the treatment of hepatic fibrosis, and some clinical trials have already been reported. On the basis of these experiences, can we say that we can treat hepatic fibrosis with safe and effective therapies?

We hope that this meeting will help to establish a basis to find an answer to these questions.

We express our gratitude to all speakers and participants, and in particular to Dr Herbert Falk and his Foundation who provided fundamental support in the organization of this symposium.

Poll on naming of fat-storing cells

Speakers and attendees at the Falk Symposium 71 were asked to choose the name they would prefer for 'fat-storing cells'.

One hundred and twenty people responded; the results were as follows:

Ito cell	42
Perisinusoidal stellate cell	25
Fat-storing cell	24
Lipocyte	1
Liver-specific pericyte	7
Others	4
Vitamin A-storing cell	2

List of Principal Authors

M. J. P. Arthur
University Medicine, Level D, South
  Block
Southampton General Hospital
Tremona Road
Southampton SO9 4XY
UK

S. Bellentani
Cattedra di Gastroenterologia
Policlinico
Via del Pozzo 71
I-41100 Moderna
Italy

G. Bray
Chelsea and Westminster Hospital
369 Fulham Road
London SW10 9NH
UK

G. Budillon
Cattedra di Gastroenterologia II
Facoltà di Medicine
Università di Napoli
Federico II
I-80131 Napoli
Italy

J. Caballería
Liver Unit
Hospital Clinic i Provincial
Villaroel 170
08036 Barcelona
Spain

A. Casini
Unità di Gastroenterologia
Dipartimento di Fisiopatologia Clinica
Università di Firenze
Viale Morgagni 85
I-50134 Firenze
Italy

B. Clément
INSERM U-49
Unité de Recherches Héptaologiques
Hopital de Ponchaillou
F-35033 Rennes Cedex
France

B. H. Davis
Gastroenterology Section
Department of Medicine
University of Chicago
Chicago, Illinois
USA

V. J. Desmet
Universitaire Ziekenhuis Sint Rafael
Laboratorium voor Histochemie en
  Cytochemie
Minderbroederstraat 12
B-3000 Leuven
Belgium

A. Floreani
Cattedra di Gastroenterologia
Università di Padova Policlinico
Via Guistiniani 2
I-35100 Padova
Italy

S. L. Friedman
Liver Center Laboratory, Building 40
Room 4102, San Francisco General
  Hospital
University of California
San Francisco, CA 94110
USA

P. Gentilini
1st Clinica Medica Generale e
  Terapia Medica II
Università di Firenze
Viale Morgagni 85
I-50134 Firenze
Italy

A. Gressner
Abteilung Klinische Chemie und
  Zentrallaboratorien
Klinikum der Phillips-Universität
Baldingerstrasse
D-35033 Marburg
Germany

E. G. Hahn
Medizinische Klinik I mit Poliklinik der
  Friedrich-Alexander-Universität
Krankenhausstr. 12
D-91054 Erlangen
Germany

H. Herbst
Institute of Pathology
Klinikum Steglitz
Free University Berlin
D-12200 Berlin
Germany

A. M. Jezequel
Institute of Experimental Pathology
  and Department of
  Gastroenterology
University of Ancona
CP 538
I-60100 Ancona
Italy

C. S. Lieber
Alcohol Research and Treatment
  Center
Liver Disease and Nutrition Section
Bronx VA Medical Center
130 West Kingsbridge Rd
Bronx
New York, NY 10468
USA

J. J. Maher
Liver Center Laboratory, Bldg 40,
  Rm 4102
San Francisco General Hospital
1001 Potrero Avenue
San Francisco, CA 94110
USA

K. M. Mak
Alcohol Research and Treatment
  Center
Bronx VA Medical Center
130 West Kingsbridge Road
Bronx
New York, NY 10468
USA

F. Marra
Department of Medicine
University of Texas Health Science
  Center
7703 Floyd Curl Drive
San Antonio, TX 78284-7882
USA

J. M. Mato
Instituto de Investigaciones
  Biomedicas
CSIC
Arturo Duperier no-4
28029 Madrid
Spain

S. Milani
Unità di Gastroenterologia
Dipartimento di Fisiopatologia Clinica
Università di Firenze
Viale Morgagni 85
I-50134 Firenze
Italy

M. Odenthal
Department of Pathology
University of Mainz
Langenbeckstr. 1
D-55101 Mainz
Germany

G. Paumgartner
Medizinische Klinik II
Klinikum Großhadern
Universität München
Marchioninistr. 15
D-8000 München 70
Germany

A. Pietrangelo
Clinica Medicale Generale e Terapia
  Medica III
Via del Pozzo 71
I-41100 Modena
Italy

M. Pinzani
Istituto di Clinica Medica II
Università di Firenze
Viale Morgagni 85
I-50134 Firenze
Italy

LIST OF PRINCIPAL AUTHORS

G. Ramadori
Department of Internal Medicine
Section of Gastroenterology and
 Endocrinology
University of Göttingen
Robert-Koch-Str 40
D-37027 Göttingen
Germany

E. Roda
Cattedra di Gastroenterologia
Università di Bologna
Policlinico S. Orsola
Via Massarenti 9
I-40138 Bologna
Italy

C. Surrenti
Unità di Gastroenterologia
Dipartimento di Fisiopatologia Clinica
Università di Firenze
Viale Morgagni 85
I-50134 Firenze
Italy

H. Tsukamoto
Division of Gastroenterology and
 Hepatology
Metrohealth Medical Center
2500 MetroHealth Drive
Cleveland, OH 44109-1998
USA

K. Wake
Department of Anatomy
Faculty of Medicine
Tokyo Medical and Dental University
Yushima 1-5-45, Bunkyo-ku
Tokyo 113
Japan

M. A. Zern
Jefferson Medical College
Department of Medicine
Division of Gastroenterology
1025 Walnut Street, College 901
Philadelphia, PA 19107
USA

1
Perisinusoidal fat-storing cells of the liver

K. WAKE

INTRODUCTION

The perisinusoidal fat-storing cells (stellate cells; lipocytes) of the liver are mesenchymal cells with unusual long branching cytoplasmic processes which encompass the sinusoid, prominent vitamin A lipid droplets, and synthetic activity of collagens and other extracellular matrix. Various splanchnic organs in vertebrate bodies contain a similar population of the cells. In mammalian species, however, we can see the most typical type of the cells in the perisinusoidal lesion of the hepatic parenchyma. In this narrow site the stellate cells share characteristic features of structure and function, being interconnected or intercommunicated with other sinusoidal cells and parenchymal cells. Clear features of the morphology of these cells and a stellate cell lineage are emerging and are reviewed here for better understanding of the cell and molecular biology, and the pathology of these cells. More detailed reviews on many topics of these cells have been written by Wake[1,2], Blomhoff and Wake[3], Gressner[4] and Ramodori[5].

HISTORICAL BACKGROUND

The perisinusoidal cells in the liver were first observed in 1876 by von Kupffer[6], using the gold chloride method (Figs 1 and 2). These cells were called '*Sternzellen* (stellate cells)'. By the same method, Rothe (1882)[7] observed clear inclusions in their cytoplasm. He considered these inclusions as the small nuclei. These inclusions are now known to be vitamin-A-containing lipid droplets[8]. The gold reaction occurs at the surface of the lipid droplets containing vitamin A, and then the reaction product diffuses to the cytoplasm of the cell body and thick processes[9]. In the interval since the initial report the elements located perisinusoidally in the liver have come to be described by several investigators. The new level of morphology of these cells was achieved by the exercise of technical procedures. Zimmermann[10] described

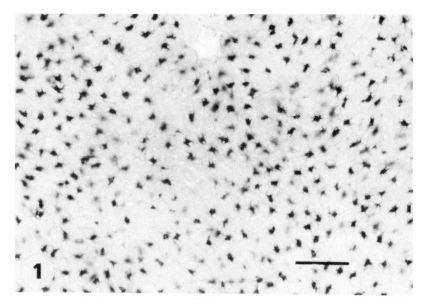

Fig. 1 Low magnification view of gold chloride preparation of rat liver. Sternzellen (stellate cells; fat-storing cells) are distributed regularly in hepatic lobules. Kupffer's gold chloride method. (bar = 100 μm)

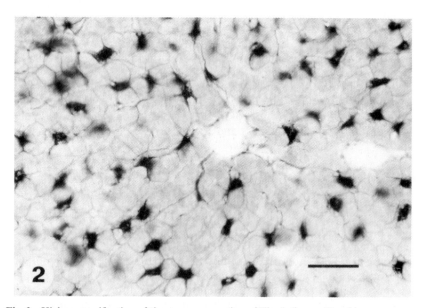

Fig. 2 Higher magnification of the same preparation of Fig. 1. (bar = 50 μm)

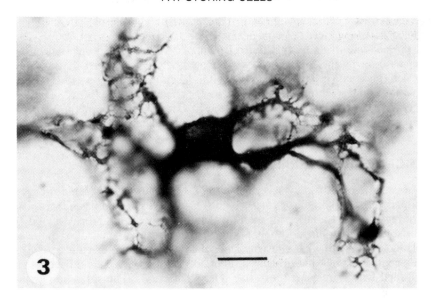

Fig. 3 A pericyte (stellate cells; fat-storing cells) in rat liver. Perisinusoidal processes studded with thorn-like microprojections (spines; hepatocyte-contacting processes) surround sinusoids. Golgi's silver method. (bar = $10\,\mu$m)

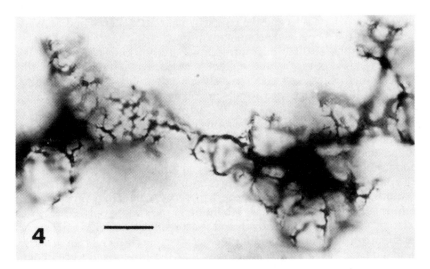

Fig. 4 Two stellate cells encompass a sinusoid uninterruptedly. Golgi's silver method. (bar = $10\,\mu$m)

the dendritic cells in the hepatic lobule using the Camilo Golgi silver method (Figs 3 and 4). These dendritic cells were designated 'pericytes in the liver', because these cells extended long cytoplasmic processes surrounding capillaries similar to those of pericytes in other organs. Ito[11] observed the perisinusoidal cells storing lipid droplets in the cytoplasm. The cells were called 'fat-storing cells'. Yamagishi[12], in an early electron microscope study, examined fine structures of these cells. Suzuki[13] documented their autonomic innervation by the Bielschowsky silver method. Wake proved that a variety of cell types which have been described independently using various staining methods and techniques are the same perisinusoidal cells[1,2,8]. Different methods show different faces of the cell. Over 20 names in the literature given to this cell indicate the stellate cell's complicated history[1].

LOCATION AND THREE-DIMENSIONAL STRUCTURE

The stellate cells display several long and branching cytoplasmic processes extended from a spindle or corn cell body. Two types of cytoplasmic processes are recognized: the intersinusoidal or interhepatocellular processes and the perisinusoidal or subendothelial processes. The former penetrate hepatic cell plates and extend to the nearby sinusoids, while the latter emit a series of adjacent periodic side-branches subendothelially, whose lateral edges are studded with numerous thorn-like microprojections. The spreading area of individual stellate cells can amount to a length of 120 μm in rabbit liver[2].

Thorn-like microprojections or spines are one of the most characteristic structures of these cells[14,15] (Figs 3–5). They are commonly found in the stellate cells of various vertebrates[2]. These minute projections face the microvillous facet of the parenchymal cells and establish intercellular contacts between the stellate cells and the parenchymal cells[16] (Figs 4 and 5). We call these spines the 'hepatocyte-contacting processes' of the stellate cells.

The functions of these microprojections are not known; however, these processes might serve as the epithelio-mesenchymal interaction for cell differentiation. Close cell contacts between odontoblast processes and the epithelial cells are suggested to play a role in the differentiation of amelo-blasts[17]. Electron microscopically the extracellular matrix at the interface between the tip of the microprojections and the hepatocyte cell membrane is mainly composed of the basal lamina. It has been suggested that the basal lamina guides the differentiation of mesenchymal cells[18]. Hepatocytes added to sinusoidal cells in culture reconstitute cell trabeculae and the parenchymal cell cords establish numerous contacts with well-spread sinusoidal cells[19].

Another possible function of the hepatocyte-contacting processes is to perform a mechanism of contact inhibition of the stellate cells. Gressner and Lahme[20] showed that the growth and functional activity of the stellate cells are suppressed *in vitro* by adding the hepatocyte cell membrane. Based on these data they proposed a hypothesis that the loss of cell-to-cell contact between stellate cells and hepatocytes might play an important role in the proliferation and transformation to the myofibroblasts of the stellate cells in consequence of hepatocellular damage.

Figs 5 and 6 Scanning electron micrographs showing perisinusoidal processes (PS) of stellate cells in the rat liver fractured after maceration with 6 mol NaOH. Tips of the hepatocyte-contacting processes (arrows) make contact with hepatocyte (H). E, Endothelial cell; S, sinusoid; SD, space of Disse. (bar = 3 μm (Fig. 5); 1 μm (Fig. 6))

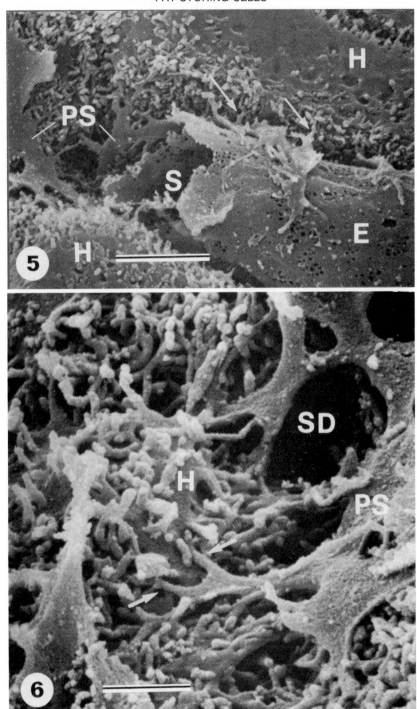

INTRALOBULAR HETEROGENEITY

The three-dimensional structure and size of the stellate cells differ from zone to zone[21]. When the lobular parenchymal mass of the porcine liver was divided into 10 zones of equal width, called zones 1–10, extending from the periphery to the centre of the lobules, in the most peripheral zone (zone 1), these cells are small and possess short, smoothly contoured perisinusoidal processes which only occasionally exhibit branchings and hepatocyte-contacting processes. The stellate cells in zones 2–4 are larger and endowed with better-developed processes than those of cells located in zone 1. Since the sinusoids become wider in zones 5–8 the processes of stellate cells elongate, bearing conspicuous branchings and numerous hepatocyte-contacting processes. In zones 9 and 10 these cells display several thick processes studded with long hepatocyte-contacting processes.

The intralobular heterogeneity of stellate cells is also evidenced by the intensity of the immunoreaction against desmin. The immunoreaction is more intense in the periportal area than in the centrilobular area in the rat liver[22]. In the pig liver the immunoreactivity is moderate in zone 1, strong in zones 2–4, becomes weaker in zones 5–8, and almost disappears in zones 9 and 10[21].

The volume of vitamin A-lipid droplets of the stellate cells in the pig liver also differs among zones along the sinusoidal axis[21]. The mean volume is small in zone 1 and increases by zone 4 and then decreases gradually to zone 10. Some stellate cells in zones 9 and 10 contain no lipid droplets.

In summary, stellate cells in zone 1 are small and contain minute vitamin A-lipid droplets. The cells in zones 2–4 store abundant vitamin A and extend encompassing processes that show intense desmin immunoreaction. In zones 5–8 the cells are conspicuously dendritic in appearance, each process being more elongated and attenuated with numerous hepatocyte-contacting processes, whereas their desmin immunoreactivity and vitamin A storage are reduced. In zones 9 and 10 the stellate cells have an irregular branching pattern and few or no lipid droplets.

POSTNATAL DEVELOPMENT

Cytoplasmic processes of the stellate cells develop rapidly after birth[16]. The cells are round with scanty processes in 1-day-old rats. At weeks 1–2 the cell body becomes fusiform in shape and thick primary processes extend longitudinally and branch out laterally. These secondary processes are studded with a limited number of hepatocyte-contacting processes. At weeks 2 and 3 the processes elongate and embrace the sinusoid. Some processes look membranous with perforations at several sites. These defects seem to enlarge gradually and fuse together, leaving free ends of thin cytoplasmic strands. Lipid droplets increase in size and number during the first few weeks postnatally. The retinyl palmitate content in the liver and the labelling of retinol on the lipid droplets increase rapidly in the liver of neonates after commencement of suckling[23]. Stellate cell growth continues up to 5–7 weeks.

That the rapid postnatal growth of the dendritic processes of stellate cells

6

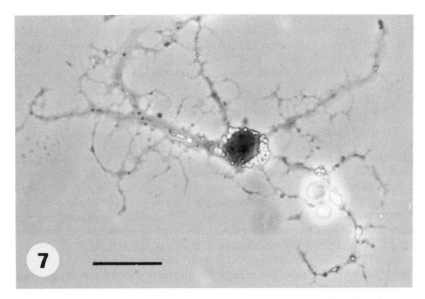

Fig. 7 A cultured stellate cell of rat liver 24 h after seeding. Dendritic branches with thorn-like microprojections develop. Vitamin A-lipid droplets (clear spots) are distributed in the cell body, some of which are seen in the processes. (bar = 20 μm)

might be under the influence of Kupffer cell activation after birth is suggested by data obtained by the following *in vitro* experiments.

MORPHOLOGY OF THE CELLS *IN VITRO*

The isolated stellate cells change their shape continuously in culture. After seeding on plastic, stellate cells extend thin fan-shaped membranous processes around the nucleus. As these processes expand further, their appearances become dendritic from their proximal portions[24]. These dendritic processes of cultured stellate cells are also studded with thorn-like microprojections similar to those of the stellate cells *in vivo* (Fig. 7). A number of vitamin A-lipid droplets are distributed in the rounded cell body and along their dendritic processes.

In our culture system the cells change their shapes gradually from dendritic to membranous 2 days after seeding. The cell bodies and their nuclei become flat, and cell organelles and vitamin A-lipid droplets, which become smaller, are disseminated widely in the membranous processes. The cellular edge becomes smooth, losing its thorn-like microprojections. After 4 days the cells show a fibroblast-like appearance and prominent stress fibres in the cytoplasm, losing vitamin A-lipid droplets.

When Kupffer-cell-conditioned medium (KCCM) is added to the culture medium 2–3 days after seeding, membranous processes of the stellate cells change to dendritic with the formation of many thorn-like microprojections[24]. This change begins as early as 5 min and reaches a maximum within 60 min after adding the KCCM, and the cells recover within 60 min after removing the KCCM. Since a similar change is observed after adding prostaglandin E_2 (PGE_2)[25], one of the potential mediators in the KCCM stimulating spine formation is considered to be PGE_2. Friedman et al.[26] also demonstrated that the processes of the stellate cells develop significantly after adding the KCCM.

A STELLATE CELL LINEAGE

The most striking difference between the stellate cells of lower vertebrates and those of mammals is their distribution in the liver. The 'fibroblasts' in the hepatic interstitial connective tissue of the fibrous capsule, the perivascular interstitium and the hilar formation of the lamprey, myxinoids and eels have vitamin A-lipid droplets in the cytoplasm[27,28]. There is, in these species, no differentiation between the interstitial 'fibroblasts' and the perisinusoidal stellate cells in the liver. Fundamentally, both cell types comprise a common system of connective tissue in the liver. In a case of liver fibrosis without hepatocyte injury, which is induced by pig serum, both cell types play a major role in the formation of septum formation[29]. Location of the stellate cells of lamprey and eel[27] differs from that of the mammalian perisinusoidal stellate cells. In these fishes thick collagen bundles distribute not only between the stellate cells and hepatocytes, as observed in mammalian livers, but also between the endothelial cells and stellate cells. Some of these stellate cells attach to the endothelial cells, while some cells adhere strongly to the collagen fibres which distribute independently from the sinusoidal wall. These stellate cell conditions are also observed in a case of hepatic fibrosis in mammalian livers. During phylogeny the stellate cells dislocate nearer to the sinusoid.

The pillar cells in the lamprey gill filaments are curious cells; they are endothelial lining cells of the blood lacunae and share vitamin A storage[30]. Furthermore these cells are contractile to regulate blood flow in the gill filaments. It is suggested that the pillar cells originated from mesenchymal cells and did not differentiate along any one of the three different paths to become capillary endothelial cells, perivascular vitamin A-storing cells, or vascular smooth muscle cells, thus retaining several morphological and functional features in common among the three cell types. Evidence is growing that the stellate cells and their related cells, as defined morphologically and by a distinct group of cytoskeletal markers such as desmin[31], and α-smooth muscle actin[32], are part of a connected system. Thus the idea of an 'endothelial–smooth muscle cells axis' has been tentatively proffered[30]. In the same way as the perisinusoidal stellate cells, the pericytes and the myofibroblasts are positioned in this spectrum. From this view it is natural that regulation of blood flow in the sinusoids by contraction and relaxation of the perisinusoidal stellate cells has been shown to be one of the new strategies of stellate cell investigation[33].

References

1. Wake K. Perisinusoidal stellate cells (fat-storing cells, interstitial cells, lipocytes), their related structure in and around the liver sinusoids, and vitamin A-storing cells in extrahepatic organs. Int Rev Cytol. 1980;66:303–53.
2. Wake K. Liver perivascular cells revealed by gold- and silver-impregnation methods and electron microscopy. In: Motta PM, editor. Biopathology of the liver. An ultrastructural approach. Dordrecht: Kluwer; 1988:23–36.
3. Blomhoff R, Wake K. Perisinusoidal stellate cells of the liver: important roles in retinol metabolism and fibrosis. FASEB J. 1991;5:271–7.
4. Gressner AM. Major topics of fibrosis research: 1990 update. In: Wisse E, Knook DL, McCuskey RS, editors. Cells of the hepatic sinusoid, Vol 3. Leiden: Kupffer Cell Foundation; 1991:136–44.
5. Ramadori G. The stellate cell (Ito cell, fat-storing cell, lipocyte, perisinusoidal cell) of the liver. New insights into pathophysiology of an intriguing cell. Virchows Arch B Cell Pathol. 1991;61:147–58.
6. Kupffer C von. Ueber Stenzellen der Leber. Briefliche Mitteilung an Prof. Waldeyer. Arch Mikr Anat. 1876;12:353–8.
7. Rothe P. Ueber die Sternzellen der Leber. Inaugural dissertation, Munich University, 1882.
8. Wake K. 'Sternzellen' in the liver: perisinusoidal cells with special reference to storage of vitamin A. Am J Anat. 1971;132:429–62.
9. Wake K, Motomatsu K, Senoo H et al. Improved Kupffer's gold chloride method for demonstrating the stellate cells storing retinol (vitamin A) in the liver and extrahepatic organs of vertebrates. Stain Technol. 1986;61:193–200.
10. Zimmermann KW. Der feinere Bau der Blutcapillaren. Z Anat. 1923;68:29–109.
11. Ito T. Cytological studies on stellate cells of Kupffer and fat storing cells in the capillary wall of the human liver. Acta Anat Nippon. 1951;26:2.
12. Yamagishi M. Electron microscope studies on the fine structure of the sinusoidal wall and fat-storing cells of rabbit liver. Arch Histol Jpn. 1959;18:223–61.
13. Suzuki K. The end apparatus of the vegetative nervous system. In: Proceedings of the sixteenth General Assembly of the Japan Medical Congress, Osaka, 1963;4:13–28.
14. Takahashi-Iwanaga H, Fujita T. Application of an NaOH maceration method to a scanning electron microscopic observation of Ito cells in the rat liver. Arch Histol Jpn. 1986;49:349–57.
15. Wake K. Vitamin A-storing cells. Electron-Microscopy. 1986;21:74–80.
16. Wake K, Motomatsu K, Ekataksin W. Postnatal development of the perisinusoidal stellate cells in the rat liver. In: Wisse E, Knook DL, McCuskey RS, editors. Cells of the hepatic sinusoid, Vol 3. Leiden: Kupffer Cell Foundation; 1991:269–75.
17. Slavkin HC, Bringas P. Epithelial–mesenchyme interactions during odontogenesis. IV. Morphological evidence for direct heterotypic cell-cell contacts. Devel Biol. 1976;50:428–42.
18. Slavkin HC. Embryonic tooth formation. A tool for developmental biology. Oral Sci Rev. 1974;4:1–136.
19. Wanson JC, Mosselmans R. Coculture of adult rat hepatocytes and sinusoidal cells: a new experimental model for the study of ultrastructural and functional properties of liver cells. In: Popper H, Bianchi L, Gudat F, Reutter W, editors. Communications of liver cells. Lancaster: MTP Press; 1980:239–51.
20. Gressner AM, Lahme B. Inhibitory actions of hepatocyte plasma membranes on proliferation, protein- and proteoglycan synthesis of cultured rat fat storing cells. In: Wisse E, Knook DL, McCuskey RS, editors. Cells of the hepatic sinusoid, Vol 3. Leiden: Kupffer Cell Foundation; 1991:237–54.
21. Wake K, Sato T. Intralobular heterogeneity of perisinusoidal stellate cells in porcine liver. Cell Tissue Res. 1993;273:227–37.
22. Geerts A, Lazou JM, De Bleser P et al. Tissue distribution and proliferation kinetics of fat-storing cells in CCl4 injured rat liver. In: Wisse E, Knook DL, McCuskey RS, editors. Cells of the hepatic sinusoid, Vol 3. Leiden: Kupffer Cell Foundation; 1991:233–6.
23. Matsuomoto E, Hirosawa K, Abe K et al. Development of the vitamin A-storing cell in mouse liver during late fetal and neonatal periods. Anat Embryol. 1984;169:249–59.

24. Wake K, Kishiye T, Yamamoto H *et al.* Kupffer cells modulate the configuration of perisinusoidal stellate cells. In: Wisse E, Knook DL, editors. Cells of the hepatic sinusoid, Vol. 4. Leiden: Kupffer Cell Foundation; 1993 (in press).

25. Wake K, Kishiye T, Yamamoto H *et al.* Sinusoidal cell function life under the microscope. In: Gressner AM, Ramadori G, editors. Molecular and cell biology of liver fibrogenesis. Dordrecht: Kluwer; 1992:45–51.

26. Friedman SL, McGuire RF. PDGF-dependent stimulation of rat hepatic lipocyte proliferation by human Kupffer cell medium. In: Wisse E, Knook DL, McCuskey RS, editors. Cells of the hepatic sinusoid, Vol 3. Leiden: Kupffer Cell Foundation; 1991:230–2.

27. Wake K. The Sternzellen of von Kupffer – after 106 years. In: Knook DL, Wisse E, editors. Sinusoidal liver cells. Amsterdam: Elsevier; 1982:1–12.

28. Wake K, Motomatsu K, Senoo H. Stellate cells storing retinol in the liver of adult lamprey, *Lampetra japonica.* Cell Tissue Res. 1987;249:289–99.

29. Bhunchet E, Wake K. Role of mesenchymal cell populations in porcine serum-induced rat liver fibrosis. Hepatology. 1992;16:1452–73.

30. Wake K, Sato T, Ekataksin W *et al.* Pillar cells in gill filaments of the lamprey, *Lampetra japonica.* Biomed Res. 1989;10(Suppl 3):597–605.

31. Yokoi Y, Namihisa T, Kuroda H *et al.* Immunohistochemical detection of desmin in fat-storing cells (Ito cell). Hepatology. 1984;4:709–14.

32. Ramadori G, Veit T, Schwogler S *et al.* Expression of the gene of the alpha-smooth muscle-actin isoform in rat liver and in rat fat-storing (ITO) cells. Virchows Arch B Cell Pathol. 1990;59:349–57.

33. Kawada N, Klein H, Decker K. Eicosanoid-mediated contractility of hepatic stellate cells. Biochem J. 1992;285:367–71.

Section I
Cellular sources of extracellular matrix

2
Role of hepatocytes and Ito cells in the synthesis and deposition of extracellular matrix

B. CLEMENT, F. LEVAVASSEUR, O. LOREAL, J. LIETARD, A. L'HELGOUALC'H and A. GUILLOUZO

INTRODUCTION

Extracellular matrices consist of pericellular macromolecules organized in either interstitial or basement membrane structures that interact with most cells in multicellular organisms. They provide mechanical cohesiveness for cells and, consequently, play a major role in tissue architecture. In addition, extracellular matrix (ECM) components induce specific signals either directly by interacting with cell membranes through specific receptors or indirectly as reservoirs for various soluble factors, e.g. cytokines and growth factors. The normal liver contains several specialized cells that interact with a heterogeneous ECM[1]. Unlike most epithelia, hepatocytes interact with a loose ECM consisting of interstitial collagens (types I, III, V and VI), fibronectin and proteoglycans, and small quantities of basement membrane components, i.e. laminin and collagen IV, as well as perlecan, a heparan sulphate proteoglycan, continuously deposited in the space of Disse[2-9]. Changes in matrix distribution and composition occur in several physiological and pathological situations, such as development, regeneration, fibrosis and carcinogenesis. Thus, ECM formation appears to be a dynamic process that depends on the physiological state of liver cells. Accordingly, in many respects one may consider fibrogenesis as a normal response for cells to an altered environment. During the past 10 years the origin of the ECM has been extensively investigated. It has been concluded that, in the normal adult, non-parenchymal cells, particularly Ito cells – also called fat-storing cells, are the major source of ECM. A more recent field of investigation concerns the interactions between cells and ECM and the role of cell–cell cooperation in matrix deposition both in normal and pathological situations.

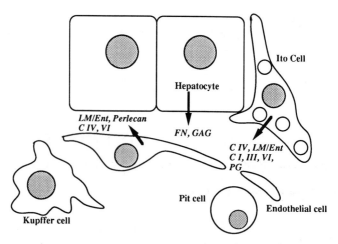

Fig. 1 Cellular origin of the main extracellular matrix components located in the space of Disse. LM/Ent: laminin/entactin complex; FN: fibronectin; GAG: glycosaminoglycans; PG: proteoglycans; CI, III, IV, VI: collagens I, III, IV and VI. (Taken from refs 5, 7, 8, 10, 11, 13 and 23)

NON-PARENCHYMAL CELLS ARE THE MAJOR SOURCES OF MATRIX PROTEINS

A variety of approaches have been used by several laboratories for identifying the cellular sources of ECM components in the liver, including *in-vivo* labelling, immunoelectron microscopy, and detection of specific matrix mRNAs by *in-situ* hybridization and their quantitation in purified liver cell populations (reviewed in ref. 10). Although some controversies remain, it has become clear during the past few years that non-parenchymal cells are major producers of ECM components in normal adult liver. In portal spaces, vascular endothelial cells and bile duct cells are probably the main sources of basement membrane components. In the lobule, both endothelial cells and Ito cells actively participate in the synthesis of the loose ECM interacting with parenchymal cells (Fig. 1). Endothelial cells express most ECM components, particularly basement membrane components. Interestingly, this cell type is probably the main source of perlecan that interacts with hepatocyte microvilli[4,5]. Ito cells contain precursors of collagens I, III, IV and VI, fibronectin, laminin and entactin, and their corresponding mRNAs[10–14]. Surprisingly, Ito cells were found to express a variant form of the classical laminin initially characterized from the Engelbreth–Holm–Swarm mouse sarcoma tumour. Indeed, only laminin B2 chain mRNAs were readily detectable by northern blot in freshly isolated Ito cells, but neither A nor B1 chain mRNA[13].

Following a variety of chronic injuries the liver may become fibrotic, leading to the formation of cirrhosis. During this process dramatic changes occur in both the amount and distribution of ECM components. Fibroblast-like cells are recruited in injured areas while Ito cells undergo phenotypic change towards a myofibroblastic appearance. Immunoelectron microscopy studies, and more recently *in-situ* hybridization, have shown that these cells produce both interstitial and basement membrane components, and are probably a major source of fibrosis[8,10,15-17]. Quantitatively these cells appear to produce higher levels of matrix mRNAs in experimental models of hepatic fibrosis compared with their normal adult counterparts. Indeed, increases of the steady state levels of α_1(I) and α_1(III) procollagen mRNAs were respectively 30- and 5-fold the normal levels in freshly isolated Ito cells following experimental fibrosis in rat[18]. Another important source of fibrotic material is biliary cells. In an experimental model of extrahepatic cholestasis induced in the rat by bile-duct ligation, it has been shown that proliferating biliary cells contained high levels of various ECM components, particularly the basement membrane components laminin and collagen IV, and probably produced tenascin[19,20].

HEPATOCYTES MAY EXPRESS ECM COMPONENTS

Whether ECM components other than fibronectin may originate from hepatocytes has been a matter of debate. Early studies with primary hepatocyte cultures have led to the conclusion that parenchymal cells could be an important source of collagens[21,22]. Careful re-examination of a putative role of hepatocytes in matrix formation by immunoelectron microscopy enabled several investigators to visualize only minute amounts of collagen precursors in these cells in normal adult rat and human livers (reviewed in ref. 10). In addition, recent *in-situ* hybridization studies failed to detect significant quantities of collagen mRNA in hepatocytes[12]. Thus it has been concluded that, in normal adult liver, parenchymal cells may not express collagens at high levels. Other matrix components are probably produced by these cells, including various glycosaminoglycans, e.g. heparan sulphate, and high levels of plasma fibronectin which may remain trapped in the space of Disse[11].

The ability of hepatocytes to express ECM components depending on their state of differentiation has been investigated in fetal and perinatal livers, in humans and in the rat[23,24]. Immunoelectron microscopy studies and northern-blot analyses have shown that immature hepatocytes may express basement membrane components, e.g. laminin and collagen IV, in the fetus. This capacity is lost during their maturation, since hepatocytes in newborn livers contain only small amounts of laminin. It is noteworthy that, in parallel, a decrease in staining intensity for laminin located in the space of Disse is observed during this period. The fact that highly specialized epithelial cells such as hepatocytes lose their ability to express basement membrane components during the differentiation process is in agreement with similar observations in other tissues. Interestingly, recent studies on the formation of rat intestinal basement membrane showed that laminin mRNAs are enriched in crypt enterocytes, and that the steady-state level of these transcripts decreases in the superficial villus enterocyte fraction, thus suggesting that laminin chain genes are transcribed at different rates as the enterocyte differentiates[25].

Following carbon tetrachloride administration in adult rats, laminin and collagen IV have been detected by immunohistochemistry in both sinusoidal endothelial cells and Ito cells, collagens I and III being detectable in hepatocytes[26,27]. *In-vivo* labelling also suggested that hepatocytes might be an important source of collagen after carbon tetrachloride treatment[28]. On the other hand, *in-situ* hybridization in fibrotic human and rat livers has shown that $\alpha_1(I)$, $\alpha_1(III)$, $\alpha_1(IV)$ and laminin B2 mRNAs were preferentially located in non-parenchymal cells[16,17]. These studies confirm previous immunoelectron studies in alcoholic human livers showing that sinusoidal endothelial cells, Ito cells and fibroblastic-like cells are the major sites of formation of the ECM components in fibrotic and cirrhotic human livers[7,8]. Moreover, in some cases hepatocytes appeared also to be involved in the production of some, but not all, ECM components, particularly basement membrane components during the capillarization process, in alcoholic fibrotic livers and in hepatocarcinoma[23,29]. These findings were supported by the recent demonstration of a faint intracellular labelling for matrix proteins in some hepatocytes located close to altered areas, in bile-duct ligated rat livers[19].

HEPATOCYTES INTERACT WITH ECM COMPONENTS THROUGH SPECIFIC RECEPTORS

Adhesion molecules mediate interactions between cells and the extracellular milieu. Among these molecules, specific receptors allow cells to recognize ECM proteins. During the past few years the molecular mechanisms by which hepatocytes interact with ECM located in the space of Disse have been investigated (reviewed in ref. 30). First lines of evidence showing that hepatocytes specifically bind individual extracellular matrix proteins came from *in-vitro* studies[31,32]. After their isolation from rat liver, hepatocytes can be set up on various substrata made of purified ECM components. Interestingly, the most efficient matrix molecules for attachment and spreading appear to be the less effective for maintenance of liver-specific functions, i.e. fibronectin and collagens vs laminin. These findings suggest that specific membrane proteins mediate hepatocyte interaction to distinct components of the hepatic ECM.

Integrins are heterodimers consisting of non-covalently associated α and β subunits that mediate both cell–substratum and cell–cell adhesion[1]. The integrin family is divided into at least three groups according to their common β chain. Most of integrins interacting with extracellular matrix components belong to the $\beta 1$ – or VLA – subfamily. β_1 integrins serve as receptors for fibronectin ($\alpha_1\beta_1$; $\alpha_3\beta_1$; $\alpha_5\beta_1$; $\alpha_v\beta_1$), collagens ($\alpha_1\beta_1$; $\alpha_2\beta_1$; $\alpha_3\beta_1$), and laminin ($\alpha_1\beta_1$; $\alpha_2\beta_1$; $\alpha_3\beta_1$; $\alpha_6\beta_1$). In addition, other integrins from the $\beta 3$ (e.g. $\alpha_v\beta_3$) β_4 (e.g. $\alpha_6\beta_4$) and β_5 subfamilies (e.g. $\alpha_v\beta_5$) have been shown to interact with matrix proteins. Since integrins were found to be present in every tissue or cell so far studied, it was expected integrins would be found in the liver. Recently, Volpes et al.[33] have studied by immunohistochemistry the distribution of the β_1 chain and the variable α chain – 1 to 6 – of the

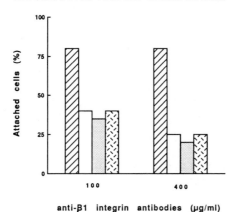

Fig. 2 Inhibition of hepatocyte attachment by anti-β_1 integrin antibodies. Hepatocytes were incubated with specific anti-β_1 integrin antibodies immediately after their isolation prior to seeding onto perlecan (□), laminin/nidogen complex (▧) or recombinant nidogen (▨) (2 µg per 0.32 cm² well). Attachment assay was carried out after 30 min. The amounts of attached cells are given as the percentage of cells that attached to dishes coated with Lm/Nd without antibodies. Each assay was carried out in duplicate in two independent experiments (▨: normal IgG). (Taken from ref. 5 and Levavasseur et al., submitted)

VLA subfamily in normal, inflammatory and cholestatic human livers. The common β_1 chain was always detected in portal spaces and in the sinusoids, while the pattern of staining for the α chains was different according to the structure analysed and/or the pathological state of the liver. Specifically, only α_1 and α_5 chains were evidenced on both hepatocytes and sinusoidal cells in normal livers. By contrast, hepatocytes became positive for α_2, α_3, α_5 and α_6 chains in inflammatory and/or cholestatic livers. Another strategy to identify integrins is to isolate these proteins from purified cell populations. The first identified integrin in hepatocytes was the fibronectin receptor. Johansson et al.[34], have isolated a fibronectin receptor which specifically bound cell-binding fibronectin domain in a R-G-D-dependent manner. It appeared to consist of a β_1 chain associated with an α chain distinct from that in fibroblastic cell lines. β_1 integrins are also involved in the interactions of hepatocytes with perlecan[5], entactin/nidogen (Levavasseur et al., submitted) and laminin, particularly the $\alpha_1\beta_1$, $\alpha_3\beta_1$ and $\alpha_6\beta_1$ integrins[35] (Fig. 2).

ECM binding proteins that do not belong to the integrin family have also been identified in hepatocytes. Rubin et al.[31] have isolated rat liver glycoproteins with affinity for collagen I. More recently, a $M_r = 80\,000$ protein on the surface of hepatocytes was found to bind collagen IV and also other basement membrane components, including laminin and perlecan[36]. The core protein of perlecan has been shown to interact directly with freshly isolated rat hepatocytes through $M_r = 36\,000/38\,000$ cell surface-associated proteins[37]. Laminin binding protein(s) can also be isolated from cell membranes by affinity chromatography on laminin–Sepharose[38]. Northern-blot analysis revealed that hepatocytes contain 1.1 kb mRNA species for a 32 kDa laminin binding protein (LBP-32)[26]. Interestingly, the steady-state LBP-32 mRNA level was much higher in fetal and neoplastic hepatocytes, as well as in hepatoma cell lines, than in the normal adult liver[39]. In addition, this overexpression paralleled the expression of B_1 and/or B_2 laminin chains.

Taken together, these findings suggest that hepatocytes express a complex set of receptors for ECM components that varies depending on the phenotype and/or the pericellular environment. This led to the hypothesis that hepatocytes might play a critical role in matrix deposition within the space of Disse.

ARE LIVER CELL CULTURES RELEVANT MODEL SYSTEMS OF HEPATIC FIBROGENESIS?

It has been shown that most liver cells, except Kupffer cells, produce ECM components *in vitro*. Early studies demonstrated that fibroblast-like cells derived from tissue explants and rat liver epithelial cells (RLEC) express high levels of all the matrix components so far studied. Sinusoidal and parenchymal cells in primary cultures may express various matrix components depending on the duration of culture. Whether ECM expression by these cells is related to disruption of cell–cell interactions, loss of specific soluble factors, adaptation to an artificial environment, i.e. plastic surface, or whether they correspond to an actual *in-vivo* situation(s) is questionable.

It is currently hypothesized that phenotypic changes undergone by Ito cells after a few days in culture correspond to an 'activated' state of these cells in fibrotic livers. Thus, after 5–6 days, Ito cells gradually lose lipid droplets, express smooth muscle α-actin and desmin and start to proliferate[40]. In parallel they express more interstitial matrix components than their 'quiescent' counterparts, i.e. during the first days in culture, that produce predominantly basement membrane components, e.g. laminin and collagen IV. Surprisingly, most neosynthesized matrix components remain soluble in cell media and are poorly associated with cell layer when maintained in standard medium conditions.

Hepatocytes also exhibit phenotypic changes in primary culture[41]. Immediately after cell isolation a dramatic decline of the transcription of liver-specific genes occurs, that results in the loss of most adult liver-specific functions after a few days, and a shift towards a fetal-like state. Interestingly, a rapid transient overexpression of c-fos in hepatocytes is found after liver disruption, and c-myc is maintained in long-term culture of normal adult rat hepatocytes[42]. Moreover, sequential activation of the proto-oncogenes, c-fos, c-myc, jun family and c-Ki-ras were described in growth-stimulated hepatocyte cultures. This cascade of events is similar to that occurring during liver regeneration after two-thirds partial hepatectomy. Normal adult hepatocytes which are not major matrix producers *in vivo* become able to express various basement membrane components, including laminin, particularly the B_2 chain, perlecan and collagen IV after a few days in culture[10].

Interestingly, hepatoma cell lines also express these components at high levels. We have recently investigated the molecular mechanisms involved in the transcriptional activation of laminin B_2 gene (Levavasseur et al., unpublished). Transfection of deletion mutants of the 5'-flanking region of murine laminin B_2 gene in hepatoma cells indicated that a segment covering the -224 to -94 bp region contained potential regulatory elements. This segment included three GC boxes, a sequence interacting with the EGR family, and a CCCTCCCATCT-containing motif which bound nuclear factors from both hepatoma cells and normal hepatocytes in footprinting analyses. Gel shift retardation assays showed that two different complexes, Y and Z, were formed with CCCTCCCATCT and nuclear factors from hepatoma cells. Interestingly, the CTC-containing motif is present in the 5'-flanking region of various genes coding for ECM proteins, housekeeping genes and proto-oncogenes that are all overexpressed in hepatoma cell lines and in normal hepatocytes during liver disruption by collagenase perfusion and in primary cultures. This motif might constitute functionally significant regulatory elements for growth-related genes.

In both conventional primary culture of Ito cells and hepatocytes, immunolocalization and immunoprecipitation of matrix proteins from both media and cell layers revealed that most secreted matrix proteins are present in soluble form and do not assemble in a complex meshwork around cells. In contrast, if both cell types are associated in co-culture an abundant and complex ECM is deposited around hepatocyte cords[43]. Reticulin fibres can easily be visualized between both cell populations and over hepatocyte cords, but not in conventional pure cultures (Fig. 3). Components of the ECM present in co-culture are similar to those found in vivo, including fibronectin, laminin/entactin and collagens proIII and IV. It is noteworthy that matrix deposition occurs only in areas in which both cell types form intimate contact. Interestingly, this process is correlated with the expression of ZO1, a specific tight-junction-associated protein, in co-cultured hepatocytes only. Matrix deposition could result from a cooperation between a major matrix-producing cell, i.e. an Ito cell, and a cell that is capable of modulating matrix deposition, i.e. a hepatocyte. The molecular mechanisms involved in such a process are likely complex, and might include synthesis of structurally intact molecules, synthesis of specific cytokines, inhibition of matrix degradation, and expression of specific matrix receptors.

CONCLUSION

Hepatic fibrosis is now clearly described as a dynamic process that involves synthesis, degradation and deposition of ECM components. Major breakthroughs have been made in identifying the cell types responsible for the synthesis and/or degradation of the main ECM components in both normal and fibrotic livers. Studying the molecular mechanisms involved in the regulation of these complex processes would require a re-evaluation of liver cell culture conditions. Indeed, that liver cells in culture undergo prompt phenotypic changes after their isolation in parallel with an increase in extracellular matrix synthesis, suggests caution in the interpretation of molecular events involved in this process. In addition, recent data indicate

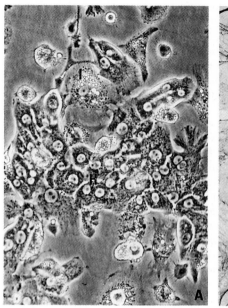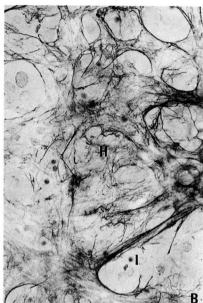

Fig. 3 Co-culture of Ito cells and hepatocytes. Phase-contrast microscopy (**A**) and reticulin staining (**B**) of 4-day-old co-cultures. Both cells form close contacts and reticulin fibres are located on hepatocyte cords and between Ito cells (I) and hepatocytes (H) ($\times$ 675). (Taken from ref. 43)

that there might be important discrepancies between synthesis and deposition of ECM components. Hepatocyte/Ito cell co-culture appears to be a potent model system for studying fibrogenesis *in vitro* since, unlike in conventional pure cultures, ECM is deposited between the two cell types. Since hepatic fibrosis is a net accumulation of ECM in the intercellular spaces, the molecular mechanisms involved in matrix deposition may be considered as main targets for potential therapeutic strategies.

Acknowledgements

The authors were supported by the Institut National de la Santé et de la Recherche Médicale (INSERM) and grants from the Association pour la Recherche contre le Cancer. F. Levavasseur was a recipient of a fellowship from La Ligue Nationale contre le Cancer.

References

1. Schuppan D, Somasundaram R, Just M. The extracellular matrix: a major signal transduction network. In: Clément B, Guillouzo A, editors. Cellular and molecular aspects of cirrhosis. Paris: Les Editions INSERM–John Libbey; 1992:115–34.

2. Hahn E, Wick G, Pencev D et al. Distribution of basement membrane proteins in normal and fibrotic liver: collagen type IV, laminin and fibronectin. Gut. 1982;21:63–71.
3. Martinez-Hernandez A. The hepatic extracellular matrix. I. Electron immunohistochemical studies in normal liver. Lab Invest. 1984;51:57–74.
4. Geerts A, Geuze HJ, Slot JW et al. Immunogold localization of procollagen I, fibronectin and heparan sulfate proteoglycan on ultrathin frozen sections of the normal rat liver. Histochemistry. 1986;84:355–62.
5. Rescan PY, Loréal O, Hassell JR et al. Distribution and origin of the basement membrane component perlecan in rat liver and hepatocyte primary culture. Am J Pathol. 1993;142: 199–208.
6. Grimaud JA, Druguet M, Peyrol S et al. Collagen immunotyping in human liver. Light and electron microscope study. J Histochem Cytochem. 1980;28:1145–56.
7. Clément B, Rescan PY, Baffet G et al. Hepatocytes may produce laminin in fibrotic liver and in primary culture. Hepatology. 1988;8:794–803.
8. Clément B, Grimaud JA, Campion JP et al. Cell types involved in collagen and fibronectin production in normal and fibrotic human liver. Hepatology. 1986;6:225–34.
9. Maher JJ, Friedman SL, Roll FJ et al. Immunolocalization of laminin in normal rat liver and biosynthesis of laminin by hepatic lipocytes in primary culture. Gastroenterology. 1988;94:1053–62.
10. Clément B, Loréal O, Rescan PY et al. Cellular origin of the hepatic extracellular matrix. In: Gressner AM, Ramadori G, editors. Molecular and cellular biology of liver fibrogenesis. Lancaster: Kluwer; 1992:85–98.
11. Clément B, Emonard H, Rissel M et al. Cellular origin of collagen and fibronectin in the liver. Cell Mol Biol. 1984;30:489–96.
12. Milani S, Herbst H, Schuppan D et al. In situ hybridization for procollagens types I, III and IV mRNA in normal and fibrotic rat liver: evidence for predominant expression in nonparenchymal liver cells. Hepatology. 1989;10:84–92.
13. Loréal O, Levavasseur F, Rescan PY et al. Differential expression of laminin chains in hepatic lipocytes. FEBS Lett. 1991;290:9–12.
14. Geerts A, Greenwel P, Cunningham M et al. Identification of collagen, fibronectin and laminin gene transcripts in freshly isolated liver cells. In: Clément B, Guillouzo A, editors. Cellular and molecular aspects of cirrhosis. Paris: Les Editions INSERM–John Libbey; 1992:215–18.
15. Takahara T, Kojima T, Miyabayashi C et al. Collagen production in fat-storing cells after carbon tetrachloride intoxication in the rat. Immunoelectron microscopic observation of type I, type III collagens, and prolyl hydroxylase. Lab Invest. 1988;59:509–21.
16. Nakatsukasa H, Nagy P, Everts RP et al. Cellular distribution of transforming growth factor-β_1 and procollagen type I, III and IV transcripts in carbon tetrachloride-induced rat liver fibrosis. J Clin Invest. 1990;85:1833–43.
17. Milani S, Herbst H, Schuppan D et al. Procollagen expression by nonparenchymal rat liver cells in experimental biliary fibrosis. Gastroenterology. 1990;98:175–84.
18. Maher J, McGuire R. Extracellular matrix gene expression increases preferentially in rat lipocytes and sinusoidal endothelial cells during hepatic fibrosis in vivo. J Clin Invest. 1990;86:1641–8.
19. Abdel-Aziz G, Rescan PY, Clément B et al. Cellular sources of matrix proteins in experimentally induced cholestatic rat liver. J Pathol. 1991;164:167–74.
20. Miyazaki H, Eyken PV, Roskams T et al. Transient expression of tenascin in experimentally induced cholestatic fibrosis in rat liver: an immunohistochemical study. In: Gressner AM, Ramadori G, editors. Molecular and cellular biology of liver fibrogenesis. Lancaster: Kluwer; 1992:176–80.
21. Sakakibara K, Saito M, Umeda M et al. Native collagen formation by liver parenchymal cells in culture. Nature. 1976;262:316–18.
22. Tseng SCG, Lee PC, Ells PF et al. Collagen synthesis by rat hepatocytes and sinusoidal cells in primary monolayer culture. Hepatology. 1982;2:13–18.
23. Rescan PY, Clément B, Yamada Y et al. Differential expression of laminin chains and receptor (LBP-32) in fetal and neoplastic hepatocytes compared to normal adult hepatocytes in vivo and in culture. Am J Pathol. 1990;137:701–9.
24. Rescan PY, Clément B, Grimaud JA et al. Participation of hepatocytes in the production

21

of basement membrane components in human and rat liver during the perinatal period. Cell Diff Develop. 1989;26:131–44.

25. Weiser MM, Sykes DE, Killen PD. Rat intestinal basement membrane synthesis. Epithelial versus non-epithelial contributions. Lab Invest. 1990;62:325–30.

26. Sakakibara KS, Igarashi S, Hatahara T. Localization of type III procollagen aminopeptide antigenicity in hepatocytes from cirrhotic human liver. Virchows Arch A Pathol Anat Histol. 1985;408:219–28.

27. Martinez-Hernandez A. The hepatic extracellular matrix. II. Electron immunohistochemical studies in rats with CCl₄-induced cirrhosis. Lab Invest. 1985;53:166–86.

28. Chojkier M, Lyche KD, Filip M. Increased production of collagen in vivo by hepatocytes and nonparenchymal cells in rats with carbon tetrachloride-induced hepatic fibrosis. Hepatology. 1988;8:803–14.

29. Albrechsten R, Wewer UM, Thorgeirsson SS. De novo deposition of laminin-positive basement membrane in vitro by normal hepatocytes and during hepatocarcinogenesis. Hepatology. 1988;8:538–46.

30. Clément B, Rescan PY, Loréal O et al. Hepatocyte–matrix interactions. In: Clément B, Guillouzo A, editors. Cellular and molecular aspects of cirrhosis. Paris: Les Editions INSERM–John Libbey; 1992:177–86.

31. Rubin K, Hook M, Obrink B et al. Substrate adhesion of rat hepatocytes: mechanisms of attachment to collagen substrates. Cell. 1981;24:463–70.

32. Bissell DM, Stamatoglou SC, Nermut MV et al. Interactions of hepatocytes with type IV collagen, fibronectin and laminin matrices. Distinct matrix-controlled modes of attachment and spreading. Eur J Cell Biol. 1986;40:72–8.

33. Volpes R, Van Den Oord JJ, Desmet VJ. Distribution of the VLA family of integrins in normal and pathological human liver tissue. Gastroenterology. 1991;101:200–6.

34. Johansson S, Forsberg E, Lundgren B. Comparison of fibronectin receptors from rat hepatocytes and fibroblasts. J Biol Chem. 1987;262:7819–24.

35. Forsberg E, Paulsson M, Timpl R et al. Characterization of a laminin receptor on rat hepatocytes. J Biol Chem. 1990;265:6376–81.

36. Clément B, Yamada Y. A 80 kDa protein is a major receptor for basement membrane on the surface of hepatocytes. Exp Cell Res. 990;187:320–3.

37. Clément B, Segui-Real B, Hassell JR et al. Identification of a cell surface binding protein for the core protein of basement membrane proteoglycan. J Biol Chem. 1989;264:12467–71.

38. Clément B, Segui-Real B, Savagner P et al. Hepatocyte attachment to laminin is mediated through multiple receptors. J Cell Biol. 1990;110:185–92.

39. Rescan PY, Clément B, Yamada Y et al. Expression of laminin and its receptor LBP-32 in human and rat hepatoma cells. Hepatology. 1991;13:289–96.

40. Gressner AM, Bachem MG. Cellular sources of noncollagenous matrix proteins: role of fat-storing cells in fibrogenesis. Sem Liver Dis. 1990;10:304–46.

41. Guguen-Guillouzo C, Guillouzo A. Modulation of functional activities in cultured rat hepatocytes. Mol Cell Biochem. 1983;53/54:35–56.

42. Etienne PL, Baffet G, Desvergne B et al. Transient expression of c-fos and constant expression of c-myc in freshly isolated and cultured normal adult rat hepatocytes. Oncogene Res. 1988;3:255–62.

43. Loréal O, Levavasseur F, Fromager C et al. Cooperation of Ito cells and hepatocytes in the deposition of an extracellular matrix in vitro. Am J Pathol. 1993;143:538–44.

3
Fat-storing cells as major producers of collagens and laminin

J. J. MAHER

Fat-storing cells have been implicated as producers of extracellular matrix proteins for several years. Histochemical studies were the first to link these cells with hepatic fibrosis, pointing out their proximity to collagen fibrils and their association with fibrous scars[1-3]; with the subsequent development of techniques to isolate and culture fat-storing cells from intact liver, numerous additional studies have confirmed their matrix-synthetic capacity[4-7]. Fat-storing cells produce a wide variety of extracellular matrix proteins, including collagens I, II and IV[6,7]; the glycoproteins fibronectin[8], laminin[9], entactin[10], tenascin[11] and undulin[12]; heparan sulphate proteoglycan[13,14]; and the proteoglycan core proteins biglycan and decorin[15]. Fat-storing cells are not, however, the sole matrix-producing cells in liver (see contributions by other authors in this volume); sinusoidal endothelial cells, biliary ductular cells, and in some instances hepatocytes also contribute to extracellular matrix synthesis.

One issue of extreme interest to researchers in the field of hepatic fibrogenesis is whether fat-storing cells represent the major extracellular matrix-producing cells in liver. If so, therapeutic interventions designed to prevent or arrest hepatic fibrosis can be targeted specifically to these cells. Research in our laboratory has addressed the relative contributions of hepatocytes, sinusoidal endothelial cells and fat-storing cells to the production of collagens and laminin in culture and *in vivo*. Our findings support the notion that fat-storing cells are indeed the major effectors of hepatic fibrogenesis.

COLLAGEN AND LAMININ PRODUCTION BY FAT-STORING CELLS IN CULTURE

Friedman and colleagues were the first in our laboratory to compare collagen synthesis in parenchymal and non-parenchymal cells in culture[6]. At 5 days after plating on uncoated tissue-culture plastic, fat-storing cells produced at least 6 times more collagen than either sinusoidal endothelial cells or hepatocytes at 2 days of primary culture. Type I collagen was the predominant species synthesized by fat-storing cells under the above culture conditions; the majority of the collagen produced was secreted into the culture medium. Cell-associated collagen represented approximately 30% of the total collagen produced by fat-storing cells in primary culture. Immunostaining of cell layers with an anti-type I collagen, however, demonstrated that much of this collagen was deposited in the form of an extracellular matrix.

The finding that fat-storing cells far exceeded hepatocytes in their capacity to produce collagen had to be reconciled with previous reports that hepatocytes produce abundant collagen in culture[16-19]. Of note in these earlier studies was that hepatocytes produced little collagen in early primary culture, but acquired this capacity after several days. We recognized that hepatocyte isolates, even after several cycles of washing and centrifugation, are contaminated by fat-storing cells[20]. We postulated that fat-storing cells, rather than hepatocytes, were probably the collagen-producing cells in hepatocyte cultures, particularly if they proliferate as the cultures mature. We performed experiments in which hepatocyte isolates were prepared by three separate methods: (a) low-speed centrifugation, (b) centrifugal elutriation, and (c) centrifugal elutriation followed by density-gradient centrifugation. We plated hepatocytes from each isolate in primary culture, and assessed the degree of fat-storing cell contamination by staining them with immunohistochemical markers specific for fat-storing cells. Hepatocyte cultures prepared by low-speed centrifugation contained an average of 10% fat-storing cells at 48 h after plating. When these cultures were re-examined at 8 days after plating, fat-storing cells comprised 75% of the total. Hepatocyte cultures prepared with cells purified by either centrifugal elutriation or centrifugal elutriation/density-gradient centrifugation had $\leq 2\%$ fat-storing cells; at 8 days, contamination remained $< 10\%$. We monitored collagen synthesis in hepatocyte cultures prepared by all three methods over a period of 8 days (Fig. 1). Hepatocytes prepared by low-speed centrifugation, which had the largest proportion of fat-storing cells, had the highest level of collagen synthesis. Indeed, collagen production in hepatocyte cultures correlated linearly with the degree of contamination by fat-storing cells. These findings confirmed our hypothesis that fat-storing cells far exceed hepatocytes in their ability to produce collagen, even at late intervals of primary culture.

We subsequently addressed whether fat-storing cells were the major producers of laminin in primary culture[9]. Using fat-storing cells, sinusoidal endothelial cells and hepatocytes all at 4 days after plating, we examined each cell population for laminin by immunocytochemistry. Fat-storing cells exhibited intense laminin staining in primary culture; hepatocytes, by contrast, exhibited no specific staining. Endothelial cells were largely negative for laminin but exhibited greater background staining than did hepatocytes. That fat-storing cells actually synthesize laminin in primary culture was confirmed by immunoprecipitation of radiolabelled laminin from cells metabolically labelled with [^{35}S]methionine (Fig. 2). The laminin produced by fat-storing cells in culture migrates as two bands of molecular weights 324 and 200 kDa. The 200-kDa band is presumed to represent both the B1

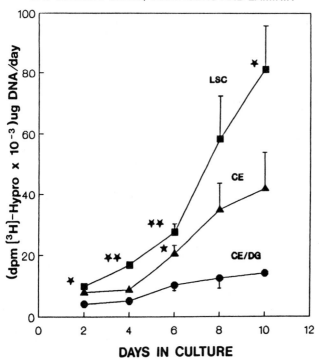

Fig. 1 Collagen produced in hepatocyte cultures prepared by three different methods. Graph illustrates the incorporation of radioactive proline into peptide-bound [^{3}H]hydroxyproline, by cells purified either by low-speed centrifugation (LSC), centrifugal elutritation (CE) or centrifugal elutriation plus density gradient centrifugation (CE/DG). *$p < 0.05$; **$p < 0.01$ vs CE/DG. (Reprinted from the *Journal of Clinical Investigation*, 1988;82:450–9, by copyright permission of the American Society for Clinical Investigation)

and B2 chains, which are similar in size; the 324-kDa peptide, however, is smaller than its counterpart in EHS laminin (the A subunit, which migrates at ~440 kDa). This raises the question whether lipocytes produce a variant of EHS laminin, substituting the A subunit with a smaller analogue. Three A-subunit variants have been described to date in mammalian tissues: A', produced by 3T3 adipocytes, which migrates at 230–250 kDa[21]; M, produced by Schwann cells, muscle and placenta, which migrates as two bands at 300 and 80 kDa[22]; and K, which has been identified in skin and has a molecular weight of 190 kDa[23]. Ongoing studies are under way to determine whether lipocyte-derived laminin contains one of these variant subunits.

COLLAGEN AND LAMININ PRODUCTION BY FAT-STORING CELLS *IN VIVO*

Having implicated fat-storing cells as the major producers of collagen and laminin in liver cell culture, we wished to determine whether fat-storing cells were also the predominant source of extracellular matrix during hepatic

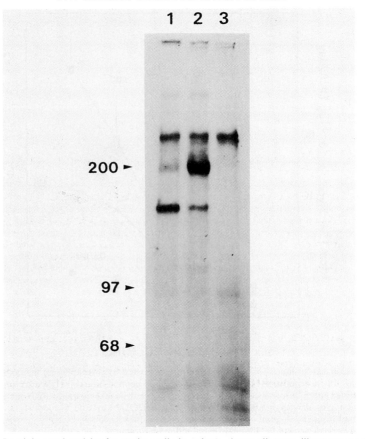

Fig. 2 Laminin produced by fat-storing cells in culture. Autoradiogram illustrates proteins immunoprecipitated from fat-storing cell culture medium using either antilaminin antibodies (lanes 1 and 2) or a non-specific IgG (lane 3). Antilaminin antibodies precipitate peptides with molecular weights 324, 200, and 155 kDa. The larger two peptides represent laminin; the smallest represents entactin, which co-precipitates with laminin. The band above 200 kDa is non-specific. (Reprinted from ref. 9, with permission)

fibrogenesis *in vivo*. To address this question[24] we provoked fibrotic liver injury in rats by either common bile duct ligation or administration of CCl_4. At a time when fibrogenesis was active we isolated hepatocytes, sinusoidal endothelial cells and fat-storing cells and examined extracellular matrix mRNA levels in each; extracellular matrix gene expression, rather than synthesis, was measured in these experiments in order to provide an assessment of matrix phenotype as it exists *in vivo*. Matrix synthesis cannot be measured without placing liver cells in primary culture, which may alter their behaviour relative to that in the intact organ.

In normal liver there was little or no expression of mRNA encoding type I collagen in either hepatocytes, endothelial cells or fat-storing cells. This is in keeping with the notion that even fat-storing cells are 'quiescent' in a

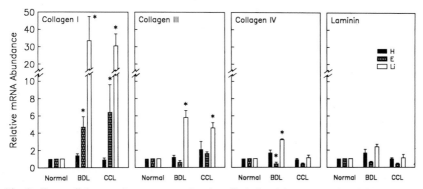

Fig. 3 Extracellular matrix gene expression in cells isolated from normal and fibrotic liver. Graph illustrates the relative abundance of mRNAs encoding collagen types I, III and IV and laminin (B2) in normal, bile duct-ligated (BDL) and carbon tetrachloride-treated (CCL) liver. mRNA signals were quantitated in hepatocytes (H), endothelial cells (E) and lipocytes (Li); bars represent the relative abundance of mRNA in each cell population as compared to its counterpart in normal liver (arbitrarily set at 1.0). Note that mRNA for collagen types I, III and IV all increase significantly in lipocytes during hepatic fibrogenesis *in vivo*. *$p < 0.05$ vs normal liver. (Reprinted from the *Journal of Clinical Investigation*, 1990;86:1641–8, by copyright permission of the American Society for Clinical Investigation)

healthy adult organ. mRNAs encoding types III and IV collagen were present in both sinusoidal endothelial cells and fat-storing cells from normal liver; laminin mRNA (B2 subunit) was visible in sinusoidal endothelial cells and fat-storing cells, and faintly in hepatocytes. After bile duct ligation and CCl₄ administration, expression of type I collagen mRNA increased dramatically in non-parenchymal cells. In lipocytes, expression increased as much as 30-fold (Fig. 3); in endothelial cells, type I collagen mRNA increased approximately 6-fold. In neither of the two models of fibrosis was type I collagen gene expression induced in hepatocytes.

mRNAs encoding collagen types I, III and IV all increased significantly in fat-storing cells during hepatic fibrogenesis *in vivo* (Fig. 3). Up-regulation of extracellular matrix gene expression was not observed in endothelial cells (with the exception of type I collagen as noted above) or hepatocytes, suggesting that these two cell populations are not the ones affected by fibrogenic stimuli *in vivo*. We conclude from these experiments that fat-storing cells are the major effectors of hepatic fibrogenesis *in vivo*. The data suggest that therapy for fibrotic liver disease may be effective if targeted specifically to fat-storing cells.

References

1. Kent G, Gay S, Inouye T *et al.* Vitamin A-containing lipocytes and formation of type III collagen in liver injury. Proc Natl Acad Sci USA. 1976;73:3719–22.
2. Minato Y, Hasumura Y, Takeuchi J. The role of fat-storing cells in Disse space fibrogenesis in alcoholic liver disease. Hepatology. 1983;3:559–66.
3. Horn R, Junge J, Christofferson P. Early alcoholic liver injury: activation of lipocytes in

acinar zone 3 and correlation to degree of collagen formation in the Disse space. J Hepatol. 1986;3:333–40.

4. Senoo H, Hata R-I, Nagai Y *et al.* Stellate cells (vitamin A-storing cells) are the primary site of collagen synthesis in non-parenchymal cells in the liver. Biomed Res. 1984;5:541–8.
5. Kawase T, Shiratori Y, Sugimoto T. Collagen production by rat liver fat-storing cells in primary culture. Exp Cell Res. 1986;54:183–92.
6. Friedman SL, Roll FJ, Boyles J *et al.* Hepatic lipocytes: the principal collagen-producing cells of normal rat liver. Proc Natl Acad Sci USA. 1985;82:8681–5.
7. Geerts A, Vrijsen R, Rauterberg J *et al. In vitro* differentiation of fat-storing cells parallels marked increase of collagen synthesis and secretion. J Hepatol. 1989;9:59–68.
8. Ramadori G, Knottel T, Odenthal M *et al.* Synthesis of cellular fibronectin by rat liver fat-storing (Ito) cells; regulation by cytokines. Gastroenterology. 1992;103:1313–21.
9. Maher JJ, Friedman SL, Roll FJ *et al.* Immunolocalization of laminin in normal rat liver and biosynthesis of laminin by hepatic lipocytes in primary culture. Gastroenterology. 1988;94:1053–62.
10. Ramadori G. Pathogenesis of liver fibrosis. Synthesis of collagen and non-collagen proteins in cell culture and in vivo. Z Gastroenterol. 1992;Suppl 1:17–20.
11. Ramadori G, Schwogler S, Veit T *et al.* Rat tenascin gene expression in rat liver and in rat liver cells. In vivo and in vitro studies. Virchows Arch B Cell Pathol. 1991;60:145–53.
12. Knittel T, Armbrust T, Schwogler S *et al.* Distribution and cellular origin of undulin in rat liver. Lab Invest. 1992;67:779–87.
13. Schafer S, Zerbe O, Gressner AM. The synthesis of proteoglycans in fat storing cells of rat liver. Hepatology. 1987;7:680–7.
14. Arenson DM, Friedman SL, Bissell DM. Formation of extracellular matrix in normal rat liver: lipocytes as a major source of proteoglycan. Gastroenterology. 1988;95:441–7.
15. Meyer DH, Krull N, Dreher KL *et al.* Biglycan and decorin gene expression in normal and fibrotic rat liver: cellular localization and regulatory factors. Hepatology. 1992;16:204–16.
16. Tseng SCG, Lee PC, Ells PF *et al.* Collagen production by rat hepatocytes and sinusoidal cells in primary monolayer culture. Hepatology. 1982;2:13–18.
17. Tseng SCG, Smuckler EA, Stern R. Types of collagen synthesized by normal rat liver hepatocytes in primary culture. Hepatology. 1983;3:955–63.
18. Diegelmann RF, Guzelian PS. Collagen formation by the hepatocyte in primary monolayer culture and *in vivo.* Science. 1983;219:1343–5.
19. Hata R-I, Ninomaya Y, Sano J *et al.* Activation of collagen synthesis in primary culture of rat liver parenchymal cells (hepatocytes). J Cell Phys. 1985;122:333–42.
20. Maher JJ, Bissell DM, Friedman SL *et al.* Collagen measured in primary cultures of normal rat hepatocytes derives from lipocytes within the monolayer. J Clin Invest. 1988;82:450–9.
21. Aratani Y, Kitagawa Y. Enhanced synthesis and secretion of type IV collagen and entactin during adipose conversion of 3T3-L1 cells and production of unorthodox laminin complex. J Biol Chem. 1988;263:16163–9.
22. Ehrig K, Leivo I, Argraves WS *et al.* Merosin, a tissue-specific basement membrane protein, is a laminin-like protein. Proc Natl Acad Sci USA. 1990;87:3264–8.
23. Marinkovich MP, Lunstrum GP, Keene DR *et al.* The dermal-epidermal junction of human skin contains a novel laminin variant. J Cell Biol. 1992;119:695–703.
24. Maher JJ, McGuire RF. Extracellular matrix gene expression increases preferentially in rat lipocytes and sinusoidal endothelial cells during hepatic fibrosis in vivo. J Clin Invest. 1990;86:1641–8.

4
Expression of non-collagenous matrix glycoproteins and protease inhibitors in rat liver and rat liver cells

G. RAMADORI and S. SCHWÖGLER

INTRODUCTION

Liver fibrosis as the consequence of repeated cell damage, caused by a variety of different events, is characterized by massive changes in the molecular structure of the extracellular matrix. A great part of our recent studies concentrated on distribution and cellular origin of different glycoproteins identified as components of the extracellular matrix and on protease inhibitors involved in matrix turnover. Gene expression and its modulation by cytokines was also studied in fat-storing cells (FSC), which are playing a dominant role in the development of liver fibrosis.

In normal liver, typical basement membranes occur around bile ducts, blood and lymphatic vessels, but they are absent in the perisinusoidal space. In these locations, basement-membrane-like matrices of unusual low density are present. The development of continuous basement membrane structures in liver sinusoids during fibrogenesis[1] attracted attention to typical components of this kind of extracellular matrix, such as laminin and entactin. Laminin forms the periphery of basement membranes and is exclusively present in this kind of extracellular matrix[2]. Entactin is a sulphated glycoprotein with binding sites for laminin, collagen type IV, fibronectin and cell surfaces[3], and might therefore play an important role in the organization of the matrix network. We studied entactin distribution in normal and fibrotic rat liver and gene expression of entactin and laminin in cell cultures of different rat liver cells.

Fibronectins are multifunctional glycoproteins which are found in association with cell surfaces and extracellular matrices, but also as free circulating plasma proteins in blood and other body fluids. This protein family is thought to play a pacemaker function in liver fibrosis as fibronectin

29

accumulation precedes the increased deposition of other matrix components. Fibronectin is synthesized by most liver cell populations such as hepatocytes, endothelial cells, Kupffer cells and FSC. However, cellular synthesis sites and the type (plasma or cellular) of deposited fibronectin during fibrosis are still a matter of debate. The heterogeneity of these proteins is due to the mechanism of alternative splicing, since different mRNA types originate from a transcript of a single gene[4]. Splicing of the fibronectin pre-mRNA at various exons coding for distinct type III domains (ED1, ED2 and V) creates at least 10 different polypeptides. Expression of these different fibronectin species seems to be dependent on the cell type or the tissue[5]. cDNAs or specific antisera directed against the alternatively spliced regions permit the differentiation between plasma and cellular fibronectin. Using these tools we examined distribution and gene expression of cellular fibronectin in dependence on the degree of liver damage, as well as fibronectin gene expression in cultured liver cells.

Tenascin is a large six-arm-shaped protein of the extracellular matrix which is mostly transiently expressed in developing tissues and tumours. *In vitro*, tenascin binds to a variety of cell types influencing the adherence to the substratum and the migration of the cells[6]. The sparse distribution of tenascin in normal skin shows a predominant association with basal membranes[7]. As the protein was also thought to play an important role in wound healing[8], a process showing parallels to fibrosis, we investigated whether tenascin is expressed in normal as well as in damaged rat liver, and which cell types are able to express the tenascin gene.

Another member of the fibronectin–tenascin superfamily is undulin, a recently described component[9] of the connective tissue with a molecular mass of about 1000 kDa. Light and ultrastructural patterns suggest that undulin could be responsible for supramolecular organization by interconnecting collagen fibrils to fibril bundles[9]. Suspecting a role of this protein during fibrogenesis we examined the distribution of this protein in the liver, and its synthesis in isolated liver cells.

Fibrinogen, a plasma glycoprotein consisting of three polypeptide chains, is involved in the final step of blood coagulation. Thrombin-induced cleavage of α and β chains results in a conversion of the soluble protein into fibrin monomers[10] forming a preliminary matrix in wounds. We examined whether possible participation of fibrinogen in liver fibrogenesis represents another similarity between wound healing and liver fibrosis.

Pathobiochemical changes of liver fibrosis are not exclusively characterized by alterations of the synthesis of matrix-forming components; the gene expression of proteins which could be indirectly involved in matrix turnover also has to be taken into consideration. Synthesis and secretion of α_2-macroglobulin (α_2-M) and C1-esterase-inhibitor (C1-INH), both representing important serum protease inhibitors, as well as the influence of cytokines on gene expression of these proteins, were examined.

METHODS

Acute and chronic liver damage was induced by oral administration of CCl_4 in maize oil (50%, v/v) according to the methods of Yokoi *et al.*[11] and

Proctor and Chatamatra[12] as described earlier[13]. Control animals were treated with maize oil alone. Cryostat sections of rat livers were incubated with specific antisera against cellular fibronectin, fibrinogen, tenascin, undulin, entactin and laminin. Antigen–antibody complexes were detected by FITC-labelled antibodies. Hepatocytes, FSC, Kupffer cells and endothelial cells were isolated and cultured from female Wistar rats according to standard techniques. Gene expression was studied in total RNA extracted from liver tissue or from isolated cells by means of Northern blot hybridization using specific cDNA probes. *In situ* hybridization studies were performed on liver sections and on isolated cells. Examination of protein synthesis and secretion was performed by biosynthetic labelling of isolated and cultured cells of rat liver, smooth muscle tissue and skin, followed by immunoprecipitation, SDS-PAGE analysis and autoradiography. Cells were further examined by immunocytochemistry using specific antisera.

RESULTS

By immunohistochemistry we could determine tenascin[14], laminin[15] and undulin[16] as structural proteins of the normal rat liver. Cellular fibronectin was detectable only in trace amounts[17]. Tenascin exhibited a fibre-like distribution along the sinusoids, whereas only a slight unspecific staining was found around the portal fields and the central veins, and no positivity was detected in the vessels. Laminin was present in the vessel walls of the portal tract and of the central vein, but it was also positive in a linear pattern along the sinusoidal lining. Incubation of normal liver with an undulin-specific antiserum revealed a positive staining of extracellular, densely packed fibrils in the portal stroma and thin rims around the central veins. Along the space of Disse, undulin showed discontinuous undulating fibres. Localization of entactin in normal liver was more difficult. Entactin showed distinct deposits in the vessel walls, whereas in the parenchyma a spot-like pattern outside the hepatocytes seemed to indicate a localization in single cells[15]. Cellular fibronectin was detected in small amounts in a pattern similar to that of total fibronectin at the vessel walls and along the sinusoids. The walls of the portal tract and of the central veins, as well as the sinusoidal space, were immunostained by the antiserum directed against fibrinogen. Double-staining against fibrinogen and marker proteins specific for endothelial cells, FSC, or Kupffer cells revealed that fibrinogen deposits were localized in the vicinity of non-parenchymal cells[18].

In acutely damaged liver, tenascin-specific staining increased in the areas of necrosis and along the sinusoids. Laminin exhibited a stronger staining in the vessels, too, and increased staining along the sinusoids indicated growth of extracellular matrix. In the parenchyma, positivity and number of entactin-staining cells, as well as the positivity in the vessels, increased. Deposits of undulin, as well as those of cellular fibronectin, significantly accumulated in the necrotic fields of acutely damaged livers. Even 12 h post-intoxication a significant accumulation of fibrinogen/fibrin in the areas of necrosis could be observed, reaching a maximum after 48 h. After the second CCl_4 administration fibrinogen exhibited a fibre-like positivity to an extent similar to that of fibronectin.

In chronically damaged rat liver, tenascin showed a strong positivity in the fibrous septa and along the sinusoids. The staining pattern was distinctly different from that obtained from normal liver, possibly indicating the incorporation of the protein into the extracellular matrix. Positivity of the spot-like entactin pattern and the laminin staining along the sinusoids increased distinctly in chronically damaged liver, and was found in and around the cells of the fibrous septa connecting portal area and central vein or two portal areas, or around a pseudolobule. The septa and sinusoids of fibrotic liver stained distinctly positive for undulin, resembling the pattern of fibronectin. Immunodetection of fibrinogen/fibrin revealed a fibre-like positivity within the septa which was also similar to the pattern of fibronectin. Cellular fibronectin exhibited an overall distribution, but was mainly deposited in the necrotic pericentral areas of acutely damaged liver and later accumulated in the fibrotic septa of chronically damaged liver. By double-staining, the deposition patterns of tenascin, laminin, entactin, undulin and cellular fibronectin were completely identical to, or almost identical to the staining pattern of specific markers for mesenchymal cells, e.g. desmin. In contrast, production of fibrin/fibrinogen could be detected by immunostaining of cultured liver cell exclusively in hepatocyte cultures.

After *in situ* hybridization of normal liver a few entactin-positive cells were detectable in the vessel walls and scattered along the sinusoids, whereas no transcripts specific for cellular fibronectin were found and a moderate amount of signals specific for fibrinogen was distributed over the whole parenchyma. In acutely damaged liver, significantly elevated amounts of entactin-specific transcripts were detectable in the vessel walls and scattered along the sinusoids. Single cells distributed over the parenchyma were positive for cellular fibronectin. In acutely damaged livers, fibrinogen-specific transcripts were only localized in hepatocytes in the vicinity of necrotic areas. Chronically damaged liver showed distinct entactin-positive cells in the fibrous septa, whereas cells expressing cellular fibronectin were mostly detected at the margins of the septa, and fibrinogen-positive signals were localized in the hepatocytes outside the fibrous septa.

Using specific antisera for immunoprecipitation from cell lysates and supernatants of isolated and cultured cells of rat liver, FSC were identified as the major cellular source of tenascin, entactin, laminin, undulin and cellular fibronectin. However, endothelial cells could also contribute to the synthesis of entactin and undulin, whereas gene expression of these matrix glycoproteins in Kupffer cells and hepatocytes could be ruled out. Increasing time of cultivation, known to effect an 'activation' process in FSC similar to that of FSC in fibrotic liver, caused increasing synthesis and secretion rates of these proteins, whereas in endothelial cells no comparable augmentation, or a decrease, was observed during cultivation. Increase during cultivation also applied to the gene expression of α_2-M and C1-INH in FSC, both important serum protease inhibitors with a wide range of activity. Incubation of FSC with dexamethasone caused a distinct, dose-dependent increase of the spontaneous α_2-M synthesis, whereas gene expression of fibronectin remained unaffected[19]. A similar stimulating effect was observed for C1-INH synthesis after treatment of the cells with interferon γ (IFN-γ). Incubation of FSC with transforming growth factor-β (TGF-β) caused a distinct inhibition of C1-INH synthesis in dependence on the concentration[20]. The influence of IFN-γ and TGF-β on the synthesis of cellular fibronectin in cultured FSC was opposite to that of C1-INH. Synthesis of fibrinogen was detectable only in hepatocyte cultures. Examination of the mRNA in cell cultures by Northern blot or *in situ* hybridization using specific cDNA probes confirmed the results obtained at the protein level.

DISCUSSION

Fibronectin, fibrinogen, tenascin, undulin, entactin and laminin were found to represent non-collagenous components of the accumulating extracellular matrix in fibrotic liver. Gene expression of fibrinogen was detected exclusively in hepatocytes, whereas deposition of cellular fibronectin, tenascin, undulin, entactin and laminin could be attributed to local synthesis of these proteins in mesenchymal cells. The results obtained from studies performed on isolated and cultured liver cells demonstrated that these mesenchymal cells might be predominantly represented by FSC. As FSC in culture show the same characteristics of 'activation' observed *in vivo* during fibrogenesis, i.e. an enhanced proliferation[21], depletion of lipid vacuoles, expression of cytoskeletal protein smooth-muscle-α-actin[13] and increased protein synthesis[20,22-24], this assumption was confirmed by examining the time-course of protein synthesis in dependence on culture age of the cells: synthesis and secretion of each protein showed a distinct increase. However, as gene expression of tenascin, entactin, undulin, and fibronectin was also detectable in endothelial cells, although to a lesser extent, this cell type might also contribute to enhanced matrix deposition during fibrogenesis. As exclusively the production of fibrinogen could not be detected in the areas of necrosis in fibrotic liver, we assume that fibrinogen/fibrin deposits derive from plasma fibrinogen and the fibrinogen stores in platelets. Therefore, fibrinogen, and probably plasma fibronectin, might be the only components of accumulating extracellular matrix in fibrotic liver which are not produced locally.

Increasing deposition of fibrinogen, cellular fibronectin and tenascin, known to play important roles in wound healing, stresses the similarity of wound healing and fibrosis in damaged liver. Fibrinogen as well as tenascin have been suggested as contributing to the formation of matrices on which fibroblasts migrate into the wound area[8,25]. Fibronectin is deposited before the accumulation of other biomatrix components as collagen occurs[26], indicating a template function of fibronectin for collagen deposition during fibrogenesis.

Though the Disse-space of normal liver shows no continuous basement membrane, basement membrane components such as fibronectin, collagen IV and proteoglycans are prevalent. Laminin also seems to be present, though there is lack of consensus concerning its distribution[27]. Therefore, increasing gene expression of entactin during fibrogenesis could be responsible for the connection of these components, and thus initiate the formation of basement-membrane-like structures observed in fibrotic livers[1]. As recently reported[28], interstitial collagenase, 92 kDa gelatinase and especially matrilysin are very potent in cleaving the entactin molecule. Susceptibility of entactin to degradation by endogenous proteases with cleavage sites occurring at both ends of the polypeptide chain has been demonstrated[29,30]. These results indicate that the remodelling process of the extracellular matrix during liver fibrosis could be initiated by the cleavage of this protein.

Little is known about the functions of undulin. The protein has been found in association with collagen type I fibrils; therefore a possible role in the supramolecular organization of the extracellular matrix was considered. However, as the interaction of undulin is mediated through a domain in the α_2-chain which is susceptible for collagenase[31], undulin could also participate in the regulation of collagen degradation.

Binding affinities of entactin to laminin[32], collagen type IV, cell surfaces[33], fibronectin[34] and fibrin(ogen)[35] signify that interactions between cells, collagens and other non-collagenous matrix proteins take place in a very complex way during the fibrogenic remodelling process of the extracellular matrix.

The synthesis of protease inhibitors by FSC[20,24], as well as their release of proteases such as type IV collagenase–gelatinase[36] might also contribute to alterations of the connective tissue. Although the dominant participation of FSC in matrix accumulation is well accepted, little information is provided concerning a possible role of this cell type in matrix degradation, as this process in general is poorly investigated[37,38]. α_2-M modifies the activity of proteolytic enzymes. Enhancement of α_2-M synthesis in FSC by pharmacological doses of dexamethasone might therefore indicate that corticosteroids inhibit fibrosis through a direct influence on the gene expression in these cells. TGF-β, known to support matrix accumulation by stimulating the gene expression of matrix proteins and protease inhibitors, showed a contrary, inhibiting effect on the gene expression of C1-INH. It was speculated that activation of TGF-β could be initiated by plasmin[39], which is inhibited by C1-INH. C1-INH would therefore represent an antagonist of TGF-β, which might explain the down-regulation of C1-INH synthesis by TGF-β. On the other hand, stimulation of C1-INH gene expression and inhibition of cellular fibronectin synthesis in FSC by IFN-γ would support the antifibrogenic effects of this cytokine, which is currently being considered as a potential pharmaceutical agent for therapy in hepatic fibrosis[40].

Acknowledgement

This work was supported by grants from the Deutsche Forschungs-Gesellschaft (SFB 311/17 and Ra 362/5-3).

References

1. Hahn E, Wick G, Pencen D *et al.* Distribution of basement membrane proteins in normal and fibrotic liver: Collagen type IV, laminin, fibronectin. Gut. 1980;21:63–71.
2. Sage H, Prizl P, Bornstein P. Characterisation of cell matrix associated collagens synthesized by aortic endothelial cells in culture. Biochemistry. 1981;20:436–42.
3. Mann K, Deutzmann R, Timpl R. Characterization of proteolytic fragments of the laminin-nidogen complex and their activity in ligand-binding assays. Eur J Biochem. 1989;178: 71–80.
4. Kornblihtt K, Vibe-Pedersen, Baralle FE. Human fibronectin: molecular cloning evidence for two mRNA species differing by an internal segment coding for a structural domain. EMBO J. 1984;3:221–6.
5. Gutman A, Kornblihtt AR. Identification of a third region of cell-specific alternative splicing in human fibronectin mRNA. Proc Natl Acad Sci. 1987;84:7179–82.
6. Chiquet-Ehrismann R, Kalla P, Pearson CA *et al.* Tenascin interferes with fibronectin action. Cell. 1988;53:383–90.
7. Lightner VA, Gumkowski F, Bigner DD *et al.* Tenascin hexabrachion in human skin: biochemical identification and localization by light and electron microscopy. J Cell Biol. 1989;108:2483–93.
8. Mackie EJ, Halfter D, Liverani D. Induction of tenascin in healing wounds. J Cell Biol. 1988;107:2757–67.
9. Schuppan D, Cantaluppi MC, Becker J *et al.* Undulin, an extracellular matrix glycoprotein associated with collagen fibrils. J Biol Chem. 1990;265:8823–32.
10. Fuller G. Synthesis and secretion of fibrinogen. In: Glaumann H, Peters T, Redman JR, eds. Plasma protein secretion by the liver. London and New York: Academic Press; 1983:405–22.
11. Yokoi Y, Namishia T, Matszaki K *et al.* Distribution of Ito-cells in experimental hepatic fibrosis. Liver. 1988;8:42–52.
12. Proctor E, Chatamra K. High yield micronodular cirrhosis in the rat. Gastroenterology. 1982;83:1183–90.
13. Ramadori G, Veit T, Schwögler S *et al.* Expression of the gene of the α smooth muscle-actin isoform in rat liver and in rat fat-storing (ITO) cells. Virchows Arch B Cell Pathol. 1990;59:349–57.
14. Ramadori G, Schwögler S, Veit Th *et al.* Tenascin gene expression in rat liver and rat liver cells: *in vivo* and *in vitro* studies. Virchows Arch B Cell Pathol. 1990;60:145–53.
15. Schwögler S, Neubauer K, Knittel T *et al.* Entactin gene expression in normal and fibrotic rat liver and in rat liver cells. (Submitted.)
16. Knittel T, Armbrust T, Schwögler S *et al.* Distribution and cellular origin of undulin in rat liver. Lab Invest. 1992;67:779–87.
17. Odenthal M, Neubauer K, Meyer zum Büschenfelde KH *et al.* Localization and mRNA steady state level of cellular fibronectin in rat liver undergoing a CCl$_4$-induced acute damage or fibrosis. Biochem Biophys Acta. 1993;1181:266–72.
18. Neubauer K, Armbrust T, Knittel T *et al.* Fibrinogen-gene-expression in normal and damaged rat liver: comparison with fibronectin. (Submitted.)
19. Ramadori G, Knittel T, Schwögler S *et al.* Dexamethasone modulates α$_2$-macroglobulin and apolipoprotein E gene expression in cultured rat liver fat storing (Ito) cells. Hepatology. 1991;14:875–82.
20. Schwögler S, Odenthal M, Knittel T *et al.* Fat storing cells (FSC) of the rat liver synthesize and secrete C1-esterase-inhibitor; modulation by cytokines. Hepatology. 1992;16:794–802.
21. De Leeuw AM, McCarthy SB, Geerts A *et al.* Purified rat liver fat storing cells in culture divide and contain collagen. Hepatology. 1984;4:392–403.
22. Ramadori G, Rieder H, Knittel T *et al.* Fat storing cells (FSC) of rat liver synthesize and secrete fibronectin. Comparison with hepatocytes. J Hepatol. 1987;4:190–7.
23. Ramadori G, Rieder H, Theiss F *et al.* Fat storing (Ito) cells of rat liver synthesize and secrete apolipoproteins. Comparison with hepatocytes. Gastroenterology. 1989;97:163–73.
24. Andus T, Ramadori G, Heinrich PC *et al.* Cultured Ito cells of the rat liver express the alpha-2-macroglobulin-gene. Eur J Biochem. 1987;168:641–6.
25. Grinnell F, Feld M, Minter D. Fibroblast adhesion to fibrinogen and fibrin substrata:

requirement for cold insoluble globulin (plasma fibronectin). Cell. 1980;19:517–25.
26. Martinez-Hernandez A. The hepatic extracellular matrix: II. Electron immunohistochemical studies in rats with CCl$_4$-induced cirrhosis. Lab Invest. 1985;53:166–86.
27. Martinez-Hernandez A, Martinez Delgado F, Amenta PS. The extracellular matrix in hepatic regeneration: localization of collagen types I, III, IV, laminin and fibronectin. Lab Invest. 1991;64:157–66.
28. Sires UI, Griffin GL, Broekelmann TJ et al. Degradation of entactin by matrix metalloproteinases. J Biol Chem. 1993;268:2069–74.
29. Paulsson M, Dziadek M, Suchaner C et al. Nature of sulphated macromolecules in mouse Reichert's membrane. Evidence for tyrosine O-sulphate in basement membrane proteins. Biochem J. 1985;231:571–9.
30. Dziadek M, Paulsson M, Timpl R. Identification and interaction repertoire of large forms of the basement membrane protein nidogen. EMBO J. 1985;4:2513–18.
31. Schuppan D, Schmid R, Ackermann R et al. The interaction of undulin with type I collagen is mediated through a domain in the carboxy terminal region of the α2(I) chain. J Cell Biol. 1990;111:394a (abstract).
32. Mann K, Deutzmann R, Timpl R. Characterization of proteolytic fragments of the laminin-nidogen complex and their activity in ligand-binding assays. Eur J Biochem. 1989;178:71–80.
33. Mann K, Deutzmann R, Aumailley M et al. Amino acid sequence of mouse nidogen, a multidomain basement membrane protein with binding activity for laminin, collagen IV, and cells. EMBO J. 1989;8:65–72.
34. Wu C, Reing J, Chung AE. Entactin forms a complex with fibronectin and co-localizes in the extracellular matrix of the embryonal carcinoma-derived 4CQ cell line. Biophys Biochem Res Commun. 1991;178:1219–25.
35. Wu C, Chung AE. Potential role of entactin in hemostasis. Specific interaction of entactin with fibrinogen A alpha and B beta chains. J Biol Chem. 1991;266:18802–7.
36. Arthur MJP, Friedman SL, Roll FJ et al. Lipocytes from normal rat liver release a neutral metalloproteinase that degrades basement membrane (type IV) collagen. J Clin Invest. 1989;84:1045–9.
37. Arthur MJP, Friedman SL, Bissel DM. Gelatinase secretion by hepatic lipocytes. In Wisse E, Knook DL, Decker K, editors. Cells of the hepatic sinusoid, Vol. 2. Rijswijk, Netherlands: Kupffer Cell Foundation; 1989:57–60.
38. Arthur MJP. Matrix degradation in the liver. In: Bissel DM, editor. Connective tissue metabolism and hepatic fibrosis. Semin Liver Dis. 1990;10:47–55.
39. Lyons RM, Gentry LE, Purchio AF et al. Mechanism of activation of latent recombinant transforming growth factor β1 by plasmin. J Cell Biol. 1990;110:1361–7.
40. Brenner DA, Alcorn JM. Therapy for hepatic fibrosis. Semin Liver Dis. 1990;10:75–83.

5
Expression of extracellular matrix components in normal and fibrotic liver

S. MILANI

INTRODUCTION

In the past decade advances in cell biology and molecular biology techniques have dramatically changed our concepts about the biological significance of the extracellular matrix (ECM) in normal and fibrotic liver. As mentioned in other chapters of this book, the ECM is not only necessary to confer mechanical coherence to multicellular tissues, but it is also endowed with essential biological functions influencing cell proliferation, differentiation, migration, and gene expression by interaction with cell membrane receptors and binding of biomolecules in their active or inactive forms (reviewed in ref. 1). Therefore, the hepatic ECM is not only the glue filling spaces among cells or the end-product of a dysregulated healing process leading to fibrosis, but also an essential source of information which may modulate cell–cell and cell–matrix interactions.

These properties result from complex interactions among individual ECM components locally assembled to meet the needs of the cells with which they are in contact (reviewed in ref. 2). The variable composition of ECM implies the existence of specialized matrices which may change their biological properties in different physiological and pathological conditions.

In normal adult liver the amount and composition of ECM are constant, being regulated by finely tuned mechanisms aiming at the maintenance of homeostasis. However, in various physiological conditions such as tissue development and growth, and in pathological processes such as regeneration, repair or fibrosis, they may undergo important alterations which may modify the structure and function of the organ.

The application of biochemical and gene expression analysis methods to liver-derived cell cultures has increased our knowledge about the possible regulatory pathways of hepatic ECM components. Electron microscopy, immunohistology and *in-situ* hybridization methods have allowed a more precise interpretation of the relationship existing between expression of individual ECM components and local modulation of cell function or tissue repair mechanism in the liver.

This chapter will focus on the distribution and gene expression of major ECM components in normal and fibrotic human liver, as they can be appreciated by immunohistological methods and *in-situ* hybridization techniques. Data obtained from animal models will also be mentioned. The nature and functions of individual ECM molecules, as well as the expression and distribution of proteoglycans and glycosaminoglycans will not be considered, because they are discussed in detail in other chapters.

EXTRACELLULAR MATRIX OF NORMAL LIVER

The ECM of normal human liver is concentrated in the capsule, portal tracts, perisinusoidal space of Disse, and around central veins. The distribution, organization, and composition of the hepatic ECM in these anatomical structures is not homogeneous, reflecting different specialized functions. Many data on ECM metabolism *in vivo* and *in vitro* are derived from animal models, particularly rat and mouse. In adult rodent liver, however, ECM content is lower than in humans; therefore, information on ECM organization and metabolism obtained in these models may not necessarily reflect that of human liver.

Each liver cell type theoretically has the genetic potential to express ECM genes and secrete the corresponding proteins. However, it is generally accepted that *in vivo*, because of the influence of local regulatory signals and the development of a specialized phenotype, only a limited subset of liver cells is involved in matrix production. In this context, hepatic mesenchymal cells, namely portal and lobular (myo)fibroblasts[3-7], perisinusoidal fat-storing cells[8-23], and endothelial cells[16-18,24] have been indicated as main producers of hepatic ECM. In addition, some data suggest that bile duct epithelial cells may be involved in the synthesis of the ECM constituting their basement membranes[18,25-27].

Capsule

The liver capsule is a thin layer of connective tissue separated from the peritoneal space by a single line of mesothelial cells resting on a basement membrane. The interstitial matrix of the capsule contains interstitial collagen types I and III, associated with collagen types V and VI. Immunohistology also demonstrates variable amounts of collagen type IV and non-collagenous glycoproteins such as fibronectin, undulin, and laminin[28,29]. The basement membrane underlying mesothelial cells contains laminin, collagen type IV, and entactin[28]. *In-situ* hybridization to mRNAs shows that gene expression for interstitial collagen types I and III is low and limited to mesenchymal cells embedded in the interstitial matrix[27]. In these cells low levels of RNA transcripts for collagen type IV[27] and undulin[29] can also be appreciated,

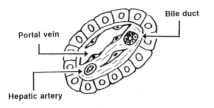

Basement membranes:

Collagen IV
Laminin

Portal stroma:

Collagen I, III, IV, V, VI
Laminin
Fibronectin
Undulin

Fig. 1 Scheme of portal tract of normal liver. Extracellular matrix is localized in basement membranes surrounding bile ducts and vessels and in portal stroma. Interstitial collagen types I, III, V, VI and fibronectin are distributed exclusively in the stroma. Laminin and collagen type IV are present in both basement membranes and stroma

but not laminin[25], possibly because of the low turnover of this latter protein in normal liver.

Portal tracts

The portal tracts contain bile ducts, the terminal branches of portal veins and hepatic arteries, and occasional nerve fibres surrounded by interstitial matrix containing smooth-muscle cells and (myo)fibroblasts (Fig. 1).

Bile ductular epithelial, endothelial, smooth-muscle cells and occasional Schwann cells of nerve fibres are separated from the interstitium by a thin basement membrane, showing, by electron microscopy, an electron-dense layer adjacent to the interstitium and an electron-lucent layer adjacent to the cell membrane[11]. In basement membranes, immunoelectron microscopy shows a preferential localization of collagen type IV in the lamina densa, and laminin in the lamina rara[28]. In human liver, the interstitial stroma contains collagen types I (Fig. 2A), III (Fig. 2B)[30,31], V[32], and VI[33], limited amounts of collagen type IV (Fig. 2C), as well as non-collagenous glycoproteins, as undulin[29], fibronectin[17], and laminin.

The rate of synthesis of these proteins in normal portal tracts is low, as suggested by the low levels of RNA expression demonstrated by *in-situ* hybridization. Basement membrane components are likely to be synthesized, at least in part, by the same cell types which have a basement membrane.

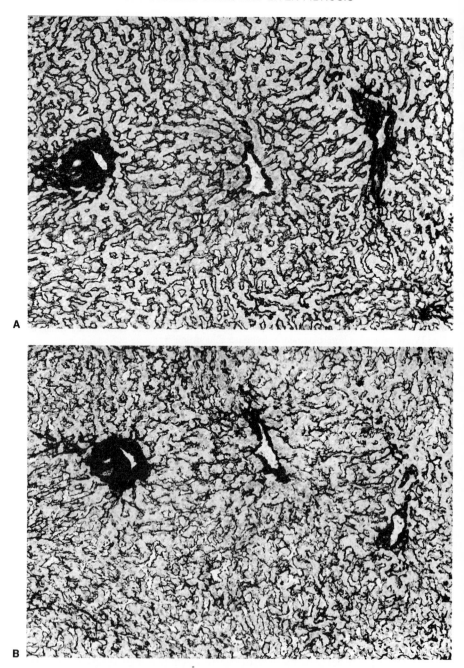

Fig. 2 Immunohistological patterns of collagen types I, III, IV, and tenascin distribution in normal human liver. Variable amounts of immunoreactive collagen types I (A), III (B), and IV (C) are distributed along sinusoids, central vein walls, and portal tract stroma. Collagen type

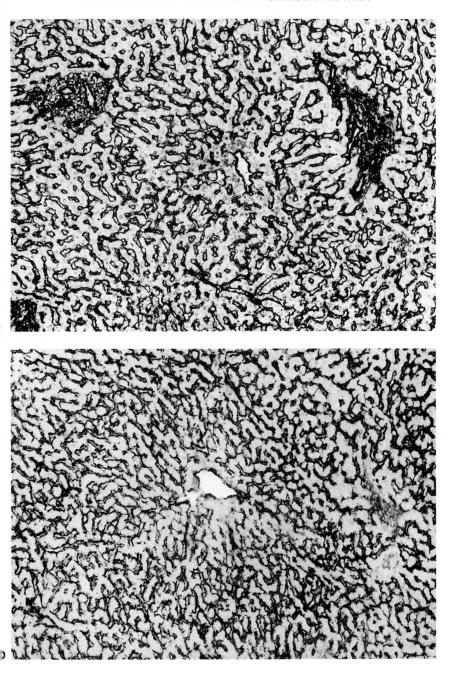

IV is also concentrated along the basal lamina of vessels and bile ducts. Tenascin (D) is distributed along sinusoids and, in limited amounts, subendothelial layers of central veins. (APAAP, original magnification ×80)

Laminin B1 RNA transcripts have indeed been found in epithelial bile duct cells and endothelial cells of normal and fibrotic human liver[25-27]. Low levels of laminin B1 and collagen α_1 (IV) gene transcripts have also been described in mesenchymal cells of the portal stroma in human liver, reflecting the limited amounts of immunoreactive laminin and collagen type IV present in that space[25-27]. However, the exact cell type responsible for their expression (fibroblast, myofibroblast, smooth-muscle cells?) is not yet characterized. In the portal stroma, the synthesis of interstitial collagen types I and III, as well as undulin, appears to be a function of mesenchymal cells localized in the matrix[27,29] (Fig. 3A), whereas the cellular sources of collagen types V, and VI, and fibronectin have not yet been elucidated.

Lobule

In the hepatic lobule, the ECM is concentrated in the thin space (perisinusoidal space or space of Disse) separating the laminae of hepatocytes from the sinusoidal endothelium (Fig. 4). As illustrated in another chapter of this book, within the perisinusoidal space are located liver-specific pericytes rich in lipid droplets (fat-storing cells, Ito cells). Electron microscopic studies show that the perisinusoidal space is almost devoid of ECM except for occasional fibres of collagen and a thin amorphous matrix[28]. Basement membranes are lacking either along the fenestrated endothelium or along the sinusoidal aspect of hepatocyte cell membranes. The absence of basement membrane along hepatic sinusoids and the endothelial fenestration facilitate the exchange of solutes between plasma and hepatocytes. However, basement membrane components as collagen type IV and laminin have been demonstrated by immunohistology in the perisinusoidal space of human liver[34], but not in rodent liver[11,28]. Whether this reflects different specificity of the antibodies or interspecies variation in the distribution of this protein it is not yet clear. By the same method, interstitial collagen type I shows a continuous pattern of fibres extending from portal tracts to central veins. Collagen type III is relatively less abundant, and it appears as sparse thin filaments mainly concentrated in periportal and centrilobular areas[30,31]. The perisinusoidal distribution of collagen type VI appears homogeneous[33], although, by electron microscopy, it can be resolved as thin filaments interconnecting groups of collagen fibres. Small amounts of undulin are present as regularly undulating fibres lining the perisinusoidal space[29]. Fibronectin shows a continuous deposition along the sinusoids[34]. The presence of tenascin (Fig. 2D), a glycoprotein typical of rapidly growing mesenchyme, has recently been reported along sinusoids of normal human liver[35], in the form of homogeneous deposition discontinued at the margin of portal tract stroma.

The cellular origin of ECM proteins in the perisinusoidal space has been long debated. Current concepts indicate fat-storing cells as the main source of ECM proteins at this site. Immunological, biochemical and gene expression analysis of ECM protein expression in fat-storing cells isolated from human and rat liver[8-10,13-15,20-23], together with the localization of immunoreactive

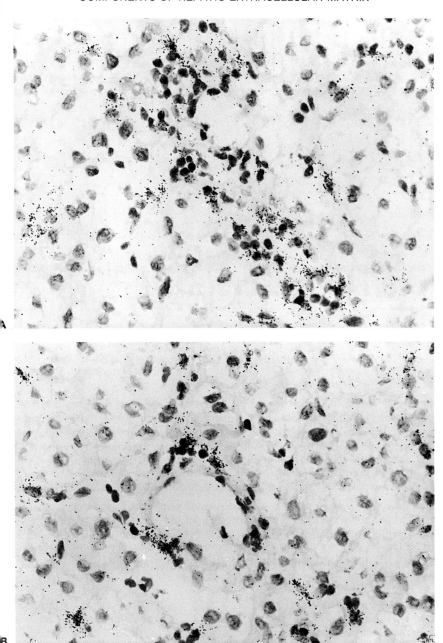

Fig. 3 *In situ* hybridization labelling patterns with [^{35}S]-labelled antisense RNA probe for procollagen α_1(I) RNA transcripts in normal human liver. In portal fields (**B**), mesenchymal cells of portal stroma are labelled. Periportal sinusoidal cells but not hepatocytes display procollagen α_1(I) expression. In central veins (**A**), transcripts are localized in mesenchymal cells of central vein walls and perisinusoidal cells. (Exposure: 10 days, original magnification: × 380)

43

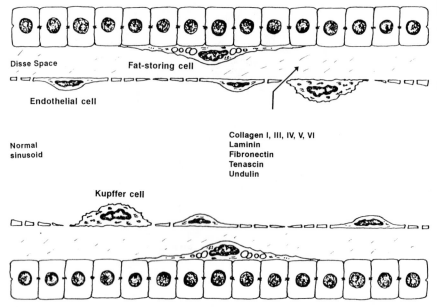

Fig. 4 Scheme of the perisinusoidal space of Disse in normal human liver. The perisinusoidal space contains small amounts of extracellular matrix components accumulated between the fenestrated endothelium and the laminae of hepatocytes. Fat-storing cells located in the space are likely to synthesize most of these ECM components. Basement membranes are absent, but basement membrane components as laminin and collagen type IV are deposited

material and RNA expression in fat-storing cells *in vivo* by electron microscopy[11,12,16,17] and *in-situ* hybridization (Fig. 2B)[7,19,29] suggest that these cells are a main source of interstitial collagen type I, III, IV, laminin, fibronectin, and undulin in the normal perisinusoidal space. Recent data suggest that they may also contribute to the synthesis of collagen type VI[33] and tenascin[36].

The role of sinusoidal endothelial cells in this context requires further elucidation; however, studies on endothelial cells freshly isolated from rat liver have shown that they may express collagen type I, III, IV, laminin B1, fibronectin, and undulin[14,15,18,36]. Hepatocytes, long considered as a source of collagens and other non-collagenous ECM proteins[37–40] do not appear to play a relevant role in normal adult liver, but they have been suggested to contribute to matrix synthesis in fetal liver[33,40].

Central veins

The veins of the central spaces consist of endothelial cells resting on a basement membrane. They are surrounded by smooth-muscle cells and myofibroblasts embedded in limited amounts of ECM containing collagen types I, III, V, VI, fibronectin, undulin[28–33]. Basement membranes contain collagen type IV, laminin.

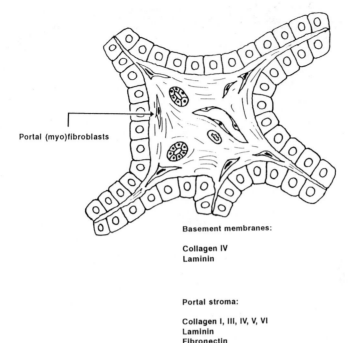

Portal (myo)fibroblasts

Basement membranes:

Collagen IV
Laminin

Portal stroma:

Collagen I, III, IV, V, VI
Laminin
Fibronectin
Undulin

Fig. 5   Scheme of fibrotic portal tract in human liver. The expansion of portal tracts is associated with increased deposition of ECM components in portal stroma and the formation of newly formed bile ducts and vessels. Portal (myo)fibroblasts, endothelial cells, and bile duct epithelial cells may contribute to the synthesis of fibrotic ECM

EXTRACELLULAR MATRIX OF FIBROTIC LIVER

The deposition of excessive connective tissue, i.e. hepatic fibrosis, is the response to chronic injury caused by a number of noxious agents (viral, toxic, immune, metabolic). The area at which ECM accumulation begins depends on the type of injury. In chronic hepatitis, portal and periportal areas are primarily involved, whereas in chronic alcoholic liver disease fibrosis may initially develop in centrilobular areas, around central veins and sinusoids. In severe chronic active hepatitis the deposition of connective tissue follows the development of necrosis and inflammation, with formation of septa extending from portal tracts to midlobular and centrilobular areas (Fig. 5). In cirrhotic liver most ECM is organized in fibrotic septa surrounding nodules of regenerating hepatocytes[41].

Although fibrosis in each liver disease may have its own morphological and pathophysiological distinctive characters, the ECM components deposited in excess are basically the same, regardless of aetiology, but their amount and relative ratio may dramatically change. In advanced cirrhosis, collagen type I predominates over type III, but even minor components such as collagen types IV and VI may have a 10-fold increase[2-42].

45

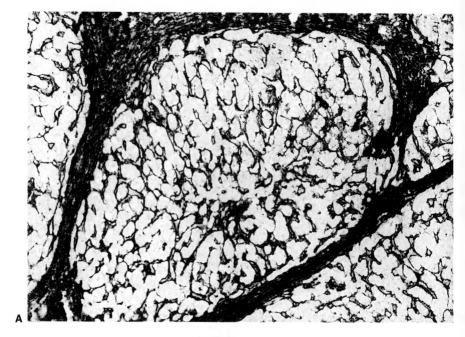

Fig. 6 Immunohistological patterns of collagen types I, III, and IV in cirrhotic human liver. Increased amounts of collagen types I (**A**), III (**B**), and IV (**C**) are deposited in fibrous septa and adjacent sinusoids of regenerative nodules. (APAAP, original magnification ×80)

In chronic active hepatitis and cirrhosis, immunohistology demonstrates increased amounts of collagen types I (Fig. 6A), III (Fig. 6B), V, and VI[30-33] distributed within expanding portal tracts and fibrous septa. Basement membrane components such as collagen type IV (Fig. 6C) and laminin are increased not only around newly formed vessels and bile ducts, but also, to a lesser extent, in the fibrous matrix[34]. Fibronectin[34] and undulin[29] increase in the fibrous stroma, whereas tenascin undergoes a selective increase in areas of piecemeal necrosis and fibrogenesis, but not in mature connective tissue[35]. In addition to increased amounts of ECM, fibrotic septa of cirrhotic liver contain a higher number of mesenchymal cells (myofibroblasts, fibroblasts, endothelial cells of newly formed vessels, smooth-muscle cells, inflammatory cells and epithelial cells of newly formed bile ducts[41-44]).

Conventional and immunoelectron microscopy show that the organization of sinusoidal ECM undergoes important modifications, as a morphologically distinct basement membrane-like structure containing collagen type IV and laminin appears along the perisinusoidal face of endothelial cells (Fig. 4). In addition, conventional immunohistology demonstrates increased amounts of collagen types I, III, IV, V, VI, fibronectin, tenascin and undulin along sinusoids[29-35]. These changes are associated with an alteration of the number and phenotype of sinusoidal cells. Endothelial cells reduce their fenestrations and form tight junctions[45]. Fat-storing cells increase in number and acquire

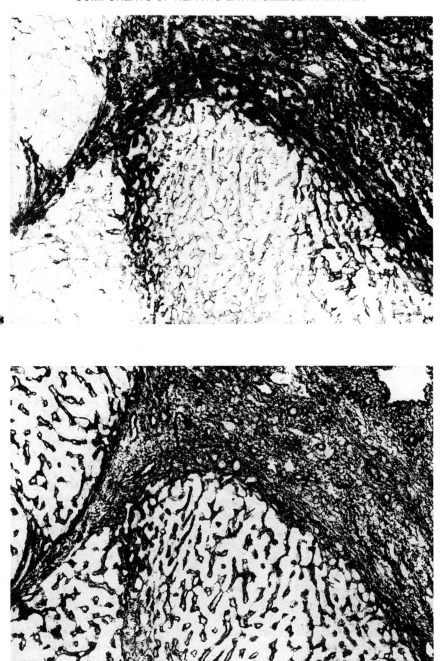

Fig. 6 *continued*

47

Myofibroblast

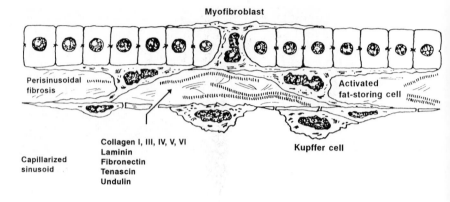

Perisinusoidal
fibrosis

Activated
fat-storing cell

Collagen I, III, IV, V, VI
Laminin
Capillarized   Fibronectin
sinusoid   Tenascin
                      Undulin

Kupffer cell

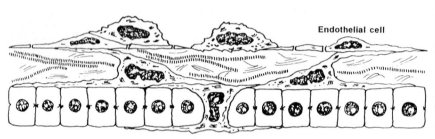

Endothelial cell

Fig. 7 Scheme of the perisinusoidal space of Disse in fibrotic human liver. Large amounts of ECM components are deposited within the space of Disse, leading to the so-called 'capillarization' of the sinusoid. Fat-storing cells become activated, acquiring a 'myofibroblast-like' phenotype, whereas endothelial cells lose their fenestration. A morphologically evident basement membrane appears in the space of Disse

an activated phenotype, with reduction of the number and size of vitamin A droplets and development of a prominent rough endoplasmic reticulum[45,46] (Fig. 7).

The increased deposition of these ECM molecules in human and rat fibrotic liver is generally associated with high levels of RNA expression of the corresponding genes[47-50], suggesting that increased synthesis is likely to be the main mechanism of accumulation. However, as described in another chapter of this book, decreased degradation collagens and non-collagenous proteins by specific proteolytic enzymes may also be involved in the excessive deposition of ECM[51].

In the past 15 years the search for a potential cellular target for antifibrotic therapies has prompted several studies aimed at the identification of the cell types which synthesize ECM molecules in fibrotic liver. Studies on human and rodent hepatic cells, either freshly isolated or cultured *in vitro*, have shown that mesenchymal cells, namely activated fat-storing cells, endothelial cells, and myofibroblasts, have a high potential for ECM synthesis and secretion which can be enhanced by stimulation with fibrogenic cytokines and growth factors[8-10,13-15,18,20-24,52-55]. *In vivo*, *in-situ* hybridization combined with immunohistology for desmin and/or immunoelectron

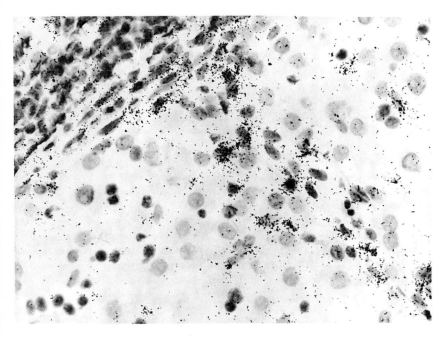

Fig. 8 *In situ* hybridization with [^{35}S]-labelled procollagen α_1(I) antisense RNA probe on cirrhotic human liver. Autoradiographic signal is localized mainly over mesenchymal cells of fibrotic septa and sinusoids; epithelial cells are not labelled. (Exposure time 6 days, original magnification × 380)

microscopy suggest that perisinusoidal fat-storing cells and their activated counterpart are principal sources of collagens and non-collagenous proteins (collagen types I, III, IV, VI, fibronectin, laminin, undulin) in fibrotic rat and human liver[7,19,29]. Indirect evidence suggests that hepatic myofibroblasts and fibroblasts[7,29] may also be involved in the synthesis of ECM in the septa of fibrotic liver (Fig. 8), but their role has to be conclusively demonstrated.

Gene expression for ECM components (collagen types I, III, IV, laminin B1) has also been shown *in vitro* in endothelial cells freshly isolated from fibrotic rat liver[16] and *in vivo*, in some sinusoidal endothelial cells of fibrotic human liver[7,29]. This suggests that they may be involved, together with fat-storing cells, in the so-called 'capillarization' of the hepatic sinusoids. Biliary epithelial cells of newly formed bile ducts express type IV collagen and laminin-B1 RNA transcripts in rat (Fig. 9) and human liver[18,23,26,27], suggesting that they may contribute to the formation of basement membranes surrounding bile ducts (Fig. 10). In human and rat fibrotic liver, hepatocytes have been shown by immunoelectron microscopy to contain immunoreactive collagens and laminin associated with the cisternae of rough endoplasmic reticulum[12,28,33]. However, the absence of detectable amounts of intracellular gene transcripts for the corresponding genes[25-27,29] raises doubts on their participation in the synthesis of these proteins.

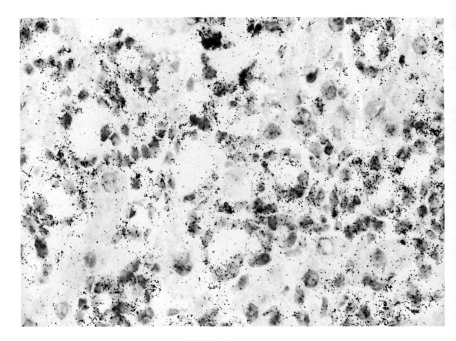

Fig. 9 *In situ* hybridization with [^{35}S]-labelled procollagen α_1(IV) antisense RNA probe on rat liver 3 weeks following bile duct obstruction. Autoradiographic signal is localized over mesenchymal and bile duct epithelial cells of newly formed bile ductules occupying expanding portal tracts. (Exposure time 6 days, original magnification × 380)

CONCLUSIONS

The analysis of the distribution and expression of ECM components in the liver has revealed that each molecule has a specific localization in the different districts of the organ. This has suggested the existence of specialized matrices containing different types and amounts of ECM components. ECM composition, which is normally regulated by homeostatic mechanisms in normal liver, undergoes important changes in response to chronic liver injury.

In the presence of severe chronic liver damage most ECM components accumulate in excess, forming fibrous septa dissecting the lobules and perisinusoidal basement membranes which interfere with the exchange of solutes between hepatocytes and plasma.

These changes have important consequences on the overall function of the organ, not only for their physical and mechanical implications, but also for the biological effects of the modified matrix on the function of adjacent cells.

In this sense immunohistological and molecular biological techniques analysing ECM distribution and gene expression in human and animal liver have offered the unique opportunity to correlate the presence of ECM molecules with peculiar aspects of tissue organization or injury. This, in

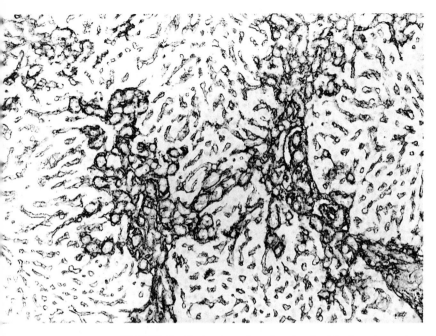

Fig. 10 Procollagen type IV (NC1) distribution in rat liver 3 weeks after bile duct obstruction. Large amounts of procollagen type IV are localized along basal laminae of bile ducts and in the stroma of expanding portal fields. (APAAP, original magnification × 80)

conjunction with the information derived from cell culture studies, has helped to shed a new light on the role of ECM in the function of the liver.

Despite some controversy, mesenchymal cells, and particularly fat-storing cells, have emerged as the main source of sinusoidal ECM. They have been implicated in the excessive deposition of fibrotic matrix taking place in the lobule, which may lead to the formation of fibrotic septa. As pointed out in other chapters, these cells may increase the synthesis of ECM molecules after stimulation *in vitro* by various soluble factors, most of which are released by inflammatory cells, platelets, and hepatocytes. Studies *in vivo* have confirmed this role, demonstrating that activated fat-storing cells are able to increase ECM gene expression in areas of inflammation and tissue damage, thus providing a potential target for antifibrotic therapies aimed at the selective inhibition of ECM synthesis and accumulation. However, data highlighting the role of activated fat-storing cells in hepatic fibrogenesis are mostly derived from animal models of hepatic fibrosis in the rat, or from human and baboon alcoholic liver disease. Thus, it is not clear whether fat-storing cells play a relevant role in the development of hepatic fibrosis caused by other agents such as viral infections or autoimmune liver disease, which primarily involve portal and periportal areas. In these diseases, portal fibroblasts and myofibroblasts might be at least equally important.

The complexity of hepatic ECM is still far from being completely elucidated.

ECM proteins may exist in multiple molecular forms, deriving from differential splicing of a common gene[56] or a different pattern of glycosylation. Well-known proteins such as laminin may reveal a heterogeneous composition, resulting from the assemblage of different constitutive chains[57]. Obviously, these differences must have implications on the biological function of these proteins. However, a characterization of distribution and regulation of these variant molecules *in vivo* has not yet been attempted in the liver. Thus, their possible role in the regulation of hepatic function and involvement in hepatic fibrogenesis is still to be investigated.

References

1. Schuppan D, Herbst H, Milani S. Matrix, matrix synthesis and molecular networks in hepatic fibrosis. In: Zern M, Reid L, editors. Extracellular matrix: its chemistry, biology and pathobiology. New York: Marcel Dekker. 1993:201–53.
2. Schuppan D. Structure of the extracellular matrix in normal and fibrotic liver. Semin Liver Dis. 1992;1:1–10.
3. Nakano M, Lieber CS. Ultrastructure of initial stages of perivenular fibrosis in alcohol-fed baboons. Am J Pathol. 1982;106:145–55.
4. Rudolph R, McClure WJ, Woodward M. Contractile fibroblasts in chronic alcoholic cirrhosis. Gastroenterology. 1979;76:704–9.
5. Savolainen ER, Leo MA, Timpl R et al. Acetaldehyde and lactate stimulate collagen synthesis of cultured baboon liver myofibroblasts. Gastroenterology. 1984;87:777–87.
6. Nakano M, Worner TM, Lieber CS. Perivenular fibrosis in alcoholic liver injury: ultrastructure and histologic progression. Gastroenterology. 1982;83:777–85.
7. Herbst H, Heinrichs O, Milani S et al. Immunophenotype of procollagen-expressing cells in rat and human liver. (Submitted.)
8. McGee J, Patric RS. The role of perisinusoidal cells in hepatic fibrogenesis. An electron microscopic study of acute carbon tetrachloride liver injury. Lab Invest. 1972;265:429–40.
9. Kent G, Gay S, Inouye T et al. Vitamin A-containing lipocytes and formation of type III collagen in liver injury. Proc Natl Acad Sci USA. 1976;73:3719–22.
10. Minato Y, Hasumura Y, Takeuchi J. The role of fat-storing cells in Disse space fibrogenesis in alcoholic liver disease. Hepatology. 1983;3:559–66.
11. Martinez-Hernandez A. The hepatic extracellular matrix. I. Electron immunohistochemical studies in normal rat liver. Lab Invest. 1984;51:57–74.
12. Martinez-Hernandez A. The hepatic extracellular matrix. II. Electron immunohistochemical studies in rats with CCl_4-induced cirrhosis. Lab Invest. 1985;53:166–86.
13. Friedmann SL, Roll FJ, Boyles J et al. Hepatic lipocytes: the principal collagen-producing cells of normal rat liver. Proc Natl Acad Sci USA. 1985;82:8681–5.
14. DeLeeuw AM, McCarthy SP, Geerts A et al. Purified rat liver fat-storing cells in culture divide and contain collagen. Hepatology. 1984;4:392–403.
15. Tsutsumi M, Takada A, Takase S et al. Connective tissue components in cultured parenchymal and nonparenchymal cells of rat liver. Immunohistochemical studies. Lab Invest. 1988;58:88–92.
16. Takahara T, Kojima T, Miyabayashi C et al. Collagen production in fat-storing cells after carbon tetrachloride intoxication in the rat. Immunoelectron microscopic observation of type I, type III collagens, and prolyl-hydroxylase. Lab Invest. 1988;59:509–21.
17. Clement B, Grimaud JA, Campion JP et al. Cell types involved in collagen and fibronectin production in normal and fibrotic human liver. Hepatology. 1986;6:225–34.
18. Maher JJ, McGuire RF. Extracellular matrix gene expression increases preferentially in rat lipocytes and sinusoidal endothelial cells during hepatic fibrosis *in vivo*. J Clin Invest. 1990;86:1641–8.
19. Nakatsukasa H, Nagy P, Evarts RP et al. Cellular distribution of transforming growth factor-$\beta1$ and procollagen types I, III, and IV transcripts in carbon tetrachloride-induced rat liver fibrosis. J Clin Invest. 1990;85:1833–43.

20. Weiner FR, Giambrone MA, Czaja MJ et al. Ito-cell gene expression and collagen regulation. Hepatology. 1990;11:111–17.
21. Moshage H, Casini A, Lieber CS. Acetaldehyde selectively increases collagen synthesis in cultured rat fat-storing cells but not in hepatocytes. Hepatology. 1990;12:511–18.
22. Knittel T, Schuppan D, Meyer zum Buschenfelde K-H et al. Differential expression of collagen types I, III and IV by fat-storing (Ito) cells in vitro. Gastroenterology. 1992;102: 1724–35.
23. Casini A, Pinzani M, Milani S et al. Regulation of extracellular matrix synthesis by transforming growth factor-β1 in human fat-storing cells. Gastroenterology. 1993;105: 245–53.
24. Irving MG, Roll FJ, Huang S et al. Characterization and culture of sinusoidal endothelium from normal rat liver: lipoprotein uptake and collagen phenotype. Gastroenterology. 1984;87:1233–47.
25. Milani S, Herbst H, Schuppan D et al. Laminin gene transcripts in normal and fibrotic human liver. Am J Pathol. 1989;134:1175–82.
26. Milani S, Herbst H, Schuppan D et al. Procollagen expression by non-parenchymal rat liver cells in experimental biliary fibrosis. Gastroenterology. 1990;98:175–84.
27. Milani S, Herbst H, Schuppan D et al. Cellular localization of procollagen type I, III, and IV gene transcripts in normal and fibrotic human liver. Am J Pathol. 1990;137:59–70.
28. Martinez-Hernandez A, Amenta PS. Morphology, localization, and origin of hepatic extracellular matrix. In: Zern M, Reid L, editors. Extracellular matrix: its chemistry, biology and pathobiology. New York: Marcell Dekker; 1993:255–327.
29. Vigano S, Milani S, Schuppan D et al. Distribution of a new extracellular matrix glycoprotein, undulin, in normal and pathologic human liver. Ital J Gastroenterol. 1990;22:269.
30. Konomi H, Sano J, Nagai Y. Immunohistochemical localization of type I, III and IV (basement membrane) collagens in the liver. Acta Pathol Jpn. 1981;31:973–8.
31. Voss B, Rauterberg J, Allam S et al. Distribution of collagen type I, type III and of two non-collagenous components of basement membrane in human liver. Pathol Res Pract. 1980;170:50–60.
32. Schuppan D, Becker J, Boehm J et al. Immunofluorescent localization of type V collagen as fibrillar component of interstitial connective tissue of human oral mucosa, artery and liver. Cell Tissue Res. 1986;243:535–43.
33. Loréal O, Clément B, Schuppan D et al. Distribution and cellular origin of collagen type VI during development and in cirrhosis. Gastroenterology. 1992;102:980–7.
34. Hahn EG, Wick G, Pencev D et al. Distribution of basement membrane proteins in normal and fibrotic human liver: collagen type IV, laminin, and fibronectin. Gut. 1980;21:63–71.
35. Van Eyken P, Sciot R, Desmet VJ. Expression of the novel extracellular matrix component tenascin in normal and diseased human liver. J Hepatol. 1990;11:43–52.
36. Knittel T, Armbrust T, Schwogler S et al. Distribution and cellular origin of undulin in rat liver. Lab Invest. 1992;67:779–87.
37. Diegelmann RF, Guzelian PS, Gay R et al. Collagen formation by the hepatocyte in primary monolayer culture and in vivo. Science. 1983;219:1343–5.
38. Chojkier M. Hepatocyte collagen production in vivo in normal rats. J Clin Invest. 1986;78:333–9.
39. Clement B, Laurent M, Guguen-Guillouzo C et al. Types I and IV procollagen gene expression in cultured rat hepatocytes. Collagen Rel Res. 1988;8:349–59.
40. Rescan PY, Clement B, Grimaud JA et al. Participation of hepatocytes in the production of basement membrane components in human and rat liver during perinatal period. Cell Diff Develop. 1989;26:131–44.
41. Popper H. General pathology of the liver: light microscopic aspects serving diagnosis and interpretation. Semin Liver Dis. 1986;6:175–84.
42. Rojkind M, Giambrone MA, Biempica L. Collagen types in normal and cirrhotic liver. Gastroenterology. 1979;76:710–19.
43. Bhunchet E, Wake K. Role of mesenchymal cell populations in porcine serum-induced rat liver fibrosis. Hepatology. 1992;16:1452–73.
44. Schmitt-Gräff A, Krüger S, Borchard F et al. Modulation of alpha smooth muscle actin and desmin expression in perisinusoidal cells of normal and diseased human livers. Am J

Pathol. 1991;138:1233–42.

45. Burt AD, LeBail B, Balabaud C et al. Morphologic investigation of sinusoidal cells. Semin Liver Dis. 1993;13:21–38.

46. Mak KM, Leo MA, Lieber CS. Alcoholic liver injury in baboons: transformation of lipocytes to transitional cells. Gastroenterology. 1984;87:188–200.

47. Ala-Kokko L, Pihlajaniemi T, Myers JC et al. Gene expression of type I, III and IV collagens in hepatic fibrosis induced by dimethylnitrosamine in the rat. Biochem J. 1987;244:75–9.

48. Pierce RA, Glaug MR, Greco RS et al. Increased procollagen mRNA levels in carbon tetrachloride-induced liver fibrosis in rats. J Biol Chem. 1987;262:1652–8.

49. Annoni G, Czaja MJ, Wiener FR et al. Increased transforming growth factor beta 1 gene expression in human liver disease. Hepatology. 1988;8:1227.

50. Castilla A, Prieto J, Fausto N. Transforming growth factors $\beta 1$ and α in chronic liver disease. Effects of interferon alpha therapy. N Engl J Med. 1991;324:933–40.

51. Arthur MPJ. Matrix degradation in the liver. Semin Liver Dis. 1990;10:47–55.

52. Matsuoka M, Pham NT, Tsukamoto H. Differential effects of interleukin-1a, tumor necrosis factor α, and transforming growth factor $\beta 1$ on cell proliferation and collagen formation by cultured fat-storing cells. Liver. 1989;9:71–8.

53. Matsuoka M, Tsukamoto H. Stimulation of hepatic lipocyte collagen production by Kupffer cell-derived transforming growth factor β: implication for a pathogenetic role in alcoholic liver fibrogenesis. Hepatology. 1990;11:599–605.

54. Geerts A, Vrijsen R, Rauteberg J et al. In vitro differentiation of fat-storing cells parallels marked increase of collagen synthesis and secretion. J Hepatol. 1989;9:59–68.

55. Friedman SL, Rockey DC, McGuire RF et al. Isolated hepatic lipocytes and Kupffer cells from normal human liver: morphological and functional characteristics in primary culture. Hepatology. 1992;15:234–43.

56. Kornblihtt AR, Umezawa K, Vibe-Pedersen K et al. Primary structure of human fibronectin: differential splicing may generate at least ten polypeptides from a single gene. EMBO J. 1985;4:1755–9.

57. Chung AE. Laminin. In: Zern M, Reid L, editors. Extracellular matrix: its chemistry, biology and pathobiology. New York: Marcell Dekker; 1993:25–48.

6
Liver fibrosis: ultrastructural aspects

A. M. JEZEQUEL, A. BENEDETTI, E. BRUNELLI, R. MANCINI,
C. BASSOTTI and F. ORLANDI

Fibrosis has long been considered an unattractive field of research, due largely to the image of 'fibrosis' as a result of tissue collapse, following a sequence of passive events. Recent years have seen an explosion of knowledge in this field following progress in the understanding of extracellular matrix composition, improved structural and functional characterization of the various cell types involved, advances in immunohistochemistry and molecular biology.

In the process of liver fibrosis the normal balance between the various components of the extracellular matrix is modified so that the relative amounts, not the nature of the components themselves, are altered. The development of fibrosis is part of an unspecific pattern response to injury, but peculiar features associated with tissue repair in the liver are worth considering. Progress in this area is largely due to the contribution of ultrastructural studies. Of particular interest are the changes affecting the architecture of the sinusoidal wall, the modulation of non-parenchymal cells involved in the deposition of extracellular matrix components and the formation of cirrhotic nodules which, together with the septa, are the main features in conventional definition of cirrhosis. Modifications of the parenchymal cells forming the nodules have been the subject of early studies[1], and have shown that in long-standing cirrhosis the ultrastructure of liver cells from the multilayered cells plates is well preserved. The main alteration consists in the presence of occasional intracytoplasmic 'glycogen bodies' and of numerous microvilli forming on the cell surface, projecting into the pericellular canals. These are thought to facilitate the access of substrates to hepatocytes in the widened cell plate. These are, however, late events associated with the remodelling of the liver architecture. In recent years attention has focused on early events leading to cirrhosis, especially on new relationships which develop between parenchymal and non-parenchymal cells, or between parenchymal cells and the hepatic microcirculation with a special interest in the sinusoidal and perisinusoidal compartments, an area of strategic importance for normal liver function.

The normal structure of the sinusoidal wall has already been extensively described, either in experimental animals or in human liver[2-5]. The barrier between circulating blood and parenchymal cells is made up of fenestrated endothelial cells and Kupffer cells, separated from hepatocytes by the space of Disse, which contains perisinusoidal cells (fat-storing cells, lipocytes) (Fig. 1). Occasional mast cells have been observed in human liver[6], as well as nerve endings[5]. The membrane of hepatocytes facing the space of Disse exhibits numerous microvilli which increase the surface of exchange between parenchymal cells and extracellular milieu. In normal conditions a well-defined basement membrane is lacking along the subendothelial aspect of the sinusoids.

'Capillarization' of sinusoids, as described by Schaffner and Popper[7], is a modification of the sinusoidal wall and of the extracellular matrix with alterations in size and decreased number of fenestrae of the endothelial cells, formation of a well-defined basement membrane, disappearance of microvilli with flattening of the hepatocyte plasma membrane[8-10]. While diffuse sinusoidal capillarization has been observed in an experimental model of nodular regenerative hyperplasia[11], the morphology of sinusoids in human cirrhotic liver appears heterogeneous: true capillaries are present in scar tissue but capillarization of sinusoids seems to occur in 'patchy' areas in the parenchyma[12]. Equally important for the circulatory abnormalities occurring in cirrhotic liver is probably the relative decrease of the sinusoidal area due to remodelling of liver architecture and thickening of liver cell plates[12]. Structural alterations of the sinusoidal exchange area are probably accompanied by alterations of the blood–lymph barrier, since the space of Disse is the first collecting area of lymph flowing towards the portal spaces[9]. This aspect has received little attention until now[13].

These modifications of the space of Disse are accompanied by structural changes of perisinusoidal cells (lipocytes) which tend to lose their characteristic lipid droplets and assume the appearance of fibroblasts with well-developed rough endoplasmic reticulum, or of myofibroblasts with fusiform indented nuclei, cytoplasmic bundles of filaments and hemidesmosomes (Figs 2 and 3). Proliferation *in situ* of lipocytes occurs during the development of fibrosis and formation of septa as shown by immunohistochemistry in an experimental model[14]; that this is indeed cell replication, and not only increased DNA synthesis, was shown in ultrastructural data with evidence of mitosis in characteristic lipocytes[15] (Fig. 4).

Criteria for identification of lipocytes on ultrastructural grounds are well defined in the normal animal or human liver, due to their roughly triangular shape, their perisinusoidal location, the presence of cytoplasmic droplets displacing a large, globular nucleus and the poorly developed endoplasmic reticulum. The presence of lipid droplets facilitates the quantitative analysis of lipocytes in normal liver at the light microscope level[16] but takes into consideration only part of the population of Ito cells: in fact, cells lacking lipid droplets may occasionally be observed in the perisinusoidal space in normal tissue, with location, shape, nuclear and cytoplasmic features similar to lipocytes. Such elements assume the appearance of undifferentiated mesenchymal cells or pericytes, and escape observation using the optical microscope.

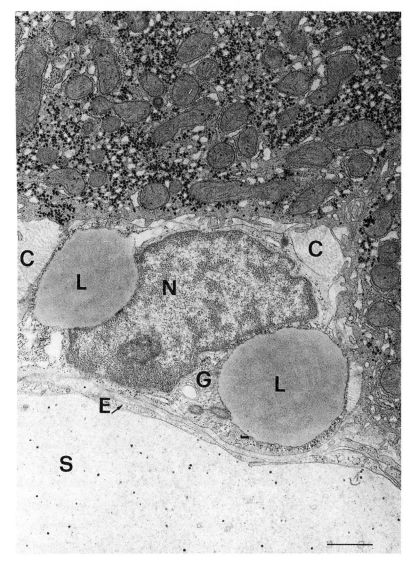

Fig. 1 Ultrastructural appearance of an Ito cell in normal human liver. The lipocyte is located in the subendothelial space, closely apposed to the endothelium (E) on one side and to the basolateral membrane of hepatocytes on the other side. Most of the cell body is occupied by two large cytoplasmic lipid droplets (L) pressing against the large nucleus (N). A few cisternae of rough endoplasmic reticulum are present, and a small Golgi apparatus (G) may be seen next to two centrioles. Bundles of collagen fibres (C) are located around the lipocyte, mainly along the juxtahepatocytic areas, while the juxta-endothelial area contains flocculent material but no evidence of basement membrane. S = sinusoid. (Bar = 1 μm). Reproduced from G Millward-Sadler and AM Jezequel, in Wright's liver and biliary disease, Vol. 1. London: WB Saunders, 1992:12, with permission of the publisher.

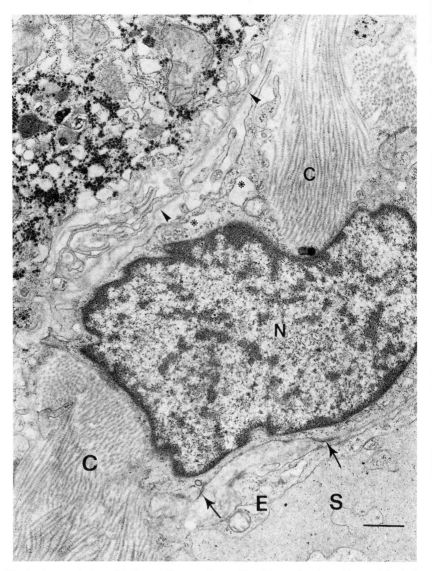

Fig. 2 Aspect of a Ito cell in human liver, as observed in a biopsy showing evidence of alcoholic hepatitis. The general architecture is preserved but the relationships between the Ito cell and the neighbouring hepatocyte are modified due to the presence of a basement membrane closely apposed to the liver cell microvilli (arrowheads). Large bundles of collagen fibrils (C) are seen in the subendothelial space. The cytoplasm of the Ito cell is scanty and contains dilated cisternae of rough endoplasmic reticulum (asterisks). Subplasmalemmal densities are evident along the cell membrane (arrows). No lipid droplets are seen in the plane of section. E = Endothelium, S = sinusoid. (Bar = 1 μm)

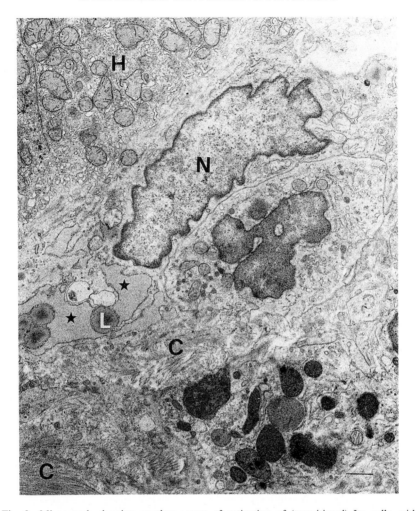

Fig. 3 Micrograph showing another aspect of activation of (transitional) Ito cells, with prominent dilated cisternae of the rough endoplasmic reticulum (stars) encircling small lipid droplets (L). The nucleus of the cell (N) appears modified, elongated in shape, with numerous indentations reminiscent of myofibroblast nuclear morphology. The intercellular relationships are deeply modified by the associated inflammatory reaction and deposition of collagen (C). H = Hepatocyte (Bar = 1 μm)

In some areas of the parenchyma, and especially around the terminal hepatic vein, the subendothelial space exhibits an organization more complex than in the rest of the lobule. The subendothelial space in this area is wider, and may contain two or three layers of cells. Some appear as typical myofibroblasts with fusiform cell body and elongated indented nucleus, and are probably part of the vascular wall. Others exhibit the morphology of fibroblasts and have been considered as interstitial fibroblasts or 'second-layer cells'[17]. In a particular model of experimental fibrosis without necrosis

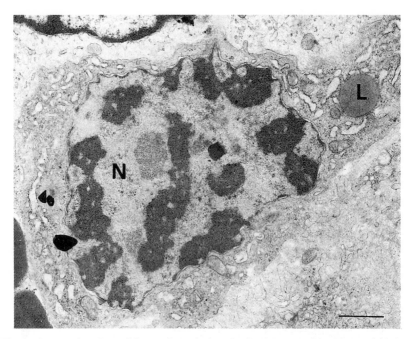

Fig. 4 Aspect of an Ito cell in prophase during the development of experimental cirrhosis induced by dimethylnitrosamine in the rat, giving evidence of active cell division *in situ*. Together with the configuration of chromatin, the activation of the Ito cell is shown by the development of rough endoplasmic reticulum assuming a fibroblast-like distribution. A small lipid droplet (L) is still present. (Bar = 1 μm.) (Reproduced from A.M. Jezequel *et al.* J Hepatol. 1989;8:42, with permission of the publisher)

or formation of nodules these cells appear able to proliferate and participate in the formation of septa[17]. However, in this particular model, modulation of the cell phenotype with development and dilatation of the cisternae of rough endoplasmic reticulum seems to occur at advanced stages of fibrosis[17], contrary to the early changes appearing in other models of experimental fibrosis (Figs 3, 5 and 6): these changes have been taken as an expression of activation of the Ito cells, and sometimes transition to myofibroblasts such as observed in alcoholic liver disease[18-20]. All transitional aspects may be observed in association with excess deposition of extracellular matrix in experimental model as well as in human pathology (Figs 7–10). Typical myofibroblasts share the ultrastructural features of fibroblasts and smooth muscle cells, with elongated cell body, well-developed endoplasmic reticulum, fusiform indented nuclei and cytoplasmic bundles of filaments about 7 nm. They are a widespread element of granulation tissue and their contractile properties[21] are supported by positive staining for alpha smooth muscle actin. The phenotypic plasticity of this cell type has been shown during experimental wound healing by the transient expression of alpha smooth muscle actin[22], an observation also made in experimental cirrhosis, in association with the development of septa[17].

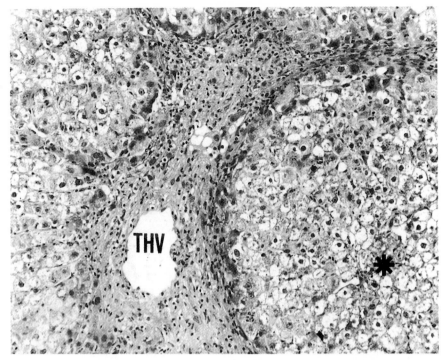

Fig. 5 General view of the hepatic parenchyma in a rat given dimethylnitrosamine for 3 weeks. Micronodular cirrhosis is evident with formation of centro-central septa. A modified terminal hepatic vein is seen lying deep in the midst of the fibrous septa (THV), while a small portal space (asterisk) is present in the centre of the parenchymal nodule. The corresponding ultrastructural appearance is shown in Fig. 6

Activation of Ito cells in response to injury is part of the more general phenomenon of activation of mesenchymal cells associated with repair mechanisms. As already pointed out, pathological matrix deposition occurs earliest in those regions of the acinus where cell injury and inflammation is greatest[23]. The site of initial injury is thus a determinant for the pattern of developing fibrosis. The absence of typical fibroblasts in the acinus is only apparent since Ito cells can modulate their phenotype and participate in the repair mechanism if needed. When the initial injury affects the intralobular biliary epithelium, as for instance in primary biliary cirrhosis, proliferation of interstitial fibroblasts of the portal space occurs with increased production of extracellular matrix components, accounting for the periductular fibrosis characteristic of the disease (Fig. 11). Dutular proliferation associated with stimulation of mesenchymal cells, increase of extracellular matrix components, and progressive periportal fibrosis may be observed in a variety of pathological or experimental situations characterized by long-standing cholestasis with changes of periportal parenchyma.[24].

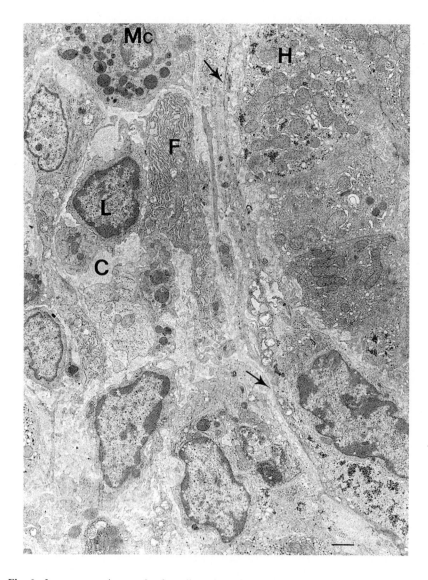

Fig. 6 Low-power micrograph of rat liver tissue from the same animal as in Fig. 5. The periphery of a nodule is shown, with evidence of the deposition of basement membrane-like material along the hepatocytes and along cellular remnants of an altered sinusoidal wall (arrows). Closely apposed to the edge of the nodule, fibroblasts (F), lymphocytes (L) and macrophages (Mc) are dispersed in the abundant extracellular matrix. H = Hepatocytes. (Bar = 1 μm.) (Reproduced from A.M. Jezequel *et al.* J Hepatol. 1990;11:206, with permission of the publisher)

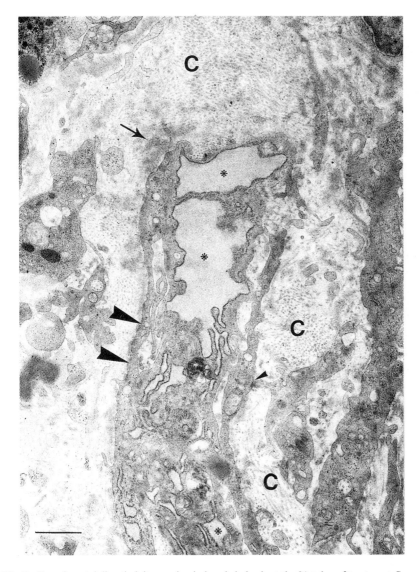

Fig. 7 Experimental dimethylnitrosamine-induced cirrhosis at the 21st day of treatment. Some cellular elements present in the midst of fibrous septa exhibit the features of fibroblasts actively engaged in protein synthesis, as shown by the abundant cytoplasm and prominent cisternae of the rough endoplasmic reticulum (asterisks). They are surrounded by well-defined collagen fibrils (C) or amorphous dense material (arrows) along the cell membrane. Subplasmalemmal densities are seen (large arrowheads) as well as junctional complexes between fibroblasts (small arrowhead). (Bar = 1 μm)

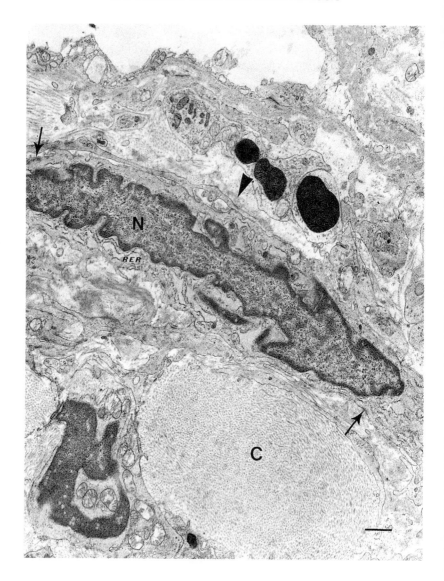

Fig. 8 Experimental dimethylnitrosamine-induced cirrhosis at the 28th day of treatment. Typical myofibroblasts are also present in the fibrous septa and exhibit elongated cell body with a fusiform, indented nucleus (N), abundant rough endoplasmic reticulum (RER) and subplasmalemmal densities (arrow). A discontinuous, basement membrane-like material may be seen along the cell membrane (arrowhead). (Bar = 1 μm.) (Reproduced from AM Jezequel *et al.* J Hepatol. 1987;5:174, with permission of the publisher)

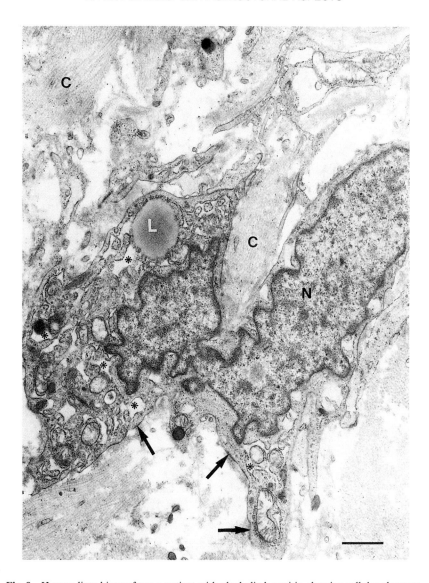

Fig. 9 Human liver biopsy from a patient with alcoholic hepatitis, showing cellular elements, exhibiting the structural features of myofibroblasts, possibly in late telophase. The general appearance is similar to that of the myofibroblasts observed in cirrhotic rat liver with subplasmalemmal densities (arrows), rich cisternae of rough endoplasmic reticulum (asterisks), and indented nucleus (N). A lipid droplet (L) is also present. Bundles of collagen fibres (C) are dispersed in the extracellular matrix which also contains thin cytoplasmic extensions, probably from other fibroblasts, and clumps of dense basement membrane-like material along the cell body. (Bar = 1 μm)

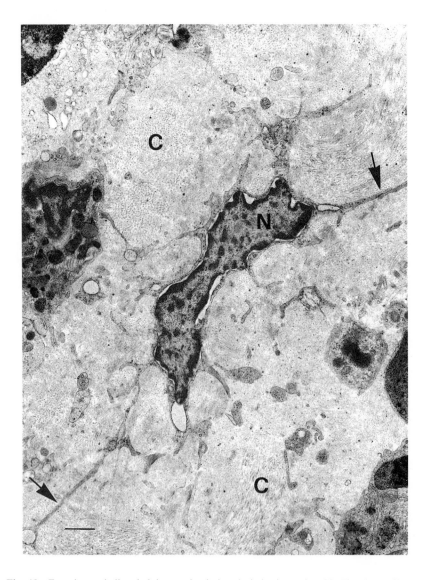

Fig. 10 Experimental dimethylnitrosamine-induced cirrhosis at day 35. The dense fibrous septa contain typical fibroblasts apparently in a resting state. The slender spider-like cell body exhibits long thin cytoplasmic extensions (arrows) with rare organelles, inconspicuous rough endoplasmic reticulum limited to the perinuclear compartment and a nucleus (N) rich in heterochromatin. The extracellular matrix is packed with bundles of collagen fibres (C) of variable diameter. (Bar = 1 μm.) (Reproduced from AM Jezequel *et al.* J Hepatol. 1987;5:174, with permission of the publisher)

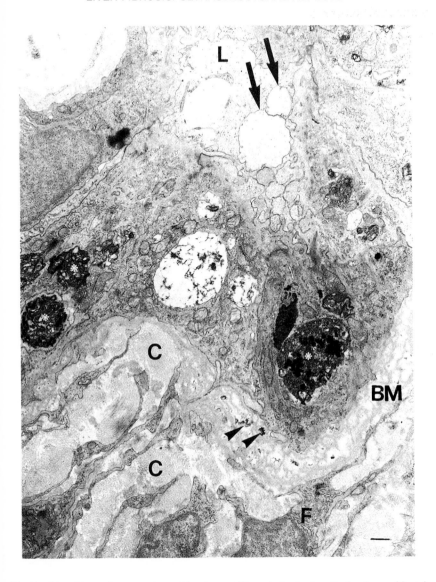

Fig. 11 Liver biopsy from a patient with primary biliary cirrhosis, stage 2, showing periductal fibrosis developing around damaged bile ductules. The lumen of a ductule (L) is surrounded by biliary epithelial cells showing various structural alterations, from retention of dense residual lamellar bodies (asterisks), to the fragmentation of the luminal membrane and formation of blebs eliminated in the lumen (arrows). Eventually the rupture of the luminal membrane is followed by leakage of the cell content in the lumen and the periductular spaces. Such leaked material (arrowheads) may be seen along the basal aspect of biliary epithelial cells, entrapped in the network of a multilayered basement membrane (BM). The periductular area is occupied by dense connective tissue containing collagen fibrils (C) and numerous fibroblasts (F). (Bar = 1 μm)

Acknowledgements

Thanks are due to A. Fava and L. Trozzi for excellent technical assistance. The work was realized in part with research grants from MURST and the National Research Council (CNR): targeted project 'Prevention and control of disease factors'.

References

1. Steiner JW, Jezequel AM, Phillips MJ et al. Some aspects of the ultrastructural pathology of the liver. In: Popper H, Schaffner F, editors. Progress in liver diseases, vol. 2. New York: Grune & Stratton; 1965:303–72.
2. Fahimi HD. Sinusoidal endothelial cells and perisinusoidal fat-storing cells. Structure and function. In: Arias I, Popper H, Shafritz DA, editors. The liver: biology and pathobiology. New York: Raven Press; 1982:495–506.
3. Jones EA, Summerfield JA. Functional aspects of hepatic sinusoidal cells. Semin Liver Dis. 1985;5:157–74.
4. Millward-Sadler GH, Jezequel AM. Normal histology and ultrastructure. In: Millward-Sadler GH, Wright R, Arthur MJP, editors. Wright's liver and biliary disease, vol. 1. London: WB Saunders; 1992:12–42.
5. Balabaud C, Boulard A, Quinton A et al. Light and transmission electron microscopy of sinusoids in human liver. In: Bioulac-Sage P, Balabaud C, editors. Sinusoids in human liver: health and disease. Rijswijk: Kupffer Cell Foundation; 1988:87–110.
6. Jezequel AM, Macarri G, Brunelli E et al. A hitherto undescribed component of the perisinusoidal space in normal human liver: the mast cell. In: Rozen P, editor. Frontiers of gastrointestinal research, vol. 9. Basel: Karger; 1986:126–31.
7. Schaffner F, Popper H. Capillarization of hepatic sinusoids in man. Gastroenterology. 1963;44:239–42.
8. Bioulac-Sage P, Lafon ME, Le Bail B et al. Ultrastructure of sinusoids in liver disease. In: Bioulac-Sage P, Balabaud C, editors. Sinusoids in human liver: health and disease. Rijswijk: Kupffer Cell Foundation; 1988:233–78.
9. Henriksen JH, Horn T, Christoffersen P. The blood–lymph barrier in the liver. A review based on morphological and functional concepts of normal and cirrhotic liver. Liver. 1984;4:221–32.
10. Sherman IA, Pappas SC, Fisher MM. Hepatic microvasculature changes associated with development of liver fibrosis and cirrhosis. Am J Physiol. 1990;258(Heart Circ Physiol 27):H460–5.
11. Dubuisson L, Bedin C, Gonzalez P et al. Sinusoidal capillarization in a model of regenerative hyperplasia induced by selenium intoxication in the rat. In: Wisse E et al., editors. Cells of the hepatic sinusoid, Vol. 3. Leiden: Kupffer Cell Foundation; 1991:222–5.
12. Le Bail B, Janvier G, Boulard A et al. Morphologic heterogeneity of sinusoids in human cirrhotic nodules. In: Wisse E et al., editors. Cells of the hepatic sinusoid, Vol. 3. Leiden: Kupffer Cell Foundation; 1991:211–14.
13. Witte MH, Borgs P, Way DL et al. Alcohol, hepatic sinusoidal microcirculation and chronic liver disease. Alcohol. 1992;9:473–80.
14. Mancini R, Jezequel AM, Benedetti A et al. Quantitative analysis of proliferating sinusoidal cells in dimethylnitrosamine-induced cirrhosis. J Hepatol. 1992;15:361–6.
15. Jezequel AM, Mancini R, Rinaldesi ML et al. Dimethylnitrosamine-induced cirrhosis. Evidence for an immunological mechanism. J Hepatol. 1989;8:42–52.
16. Giampieri MP, Jezequel AM, Orlandi F. The lipocytes in normal human liver. A quantitative study. Digestion. 1981;22:165–9.
17. Bhunchet E, Wake K. Role of mesenchymal cell populations in porcine serum-induced liver fibrosis. Hepatology. 1992;16:1452–73.
18. French SW, Miyamoto K, Wong K et al. Role of the Ito cell in the liver parenchymal fibrosis in rat fed alcohol and a high fat–low protein diet. Am J Pathol. 1988;132:73–85.
19. Mak KM, Leo AM, Lieber CS. Alcoholic liver injury in baboons: transformation of lipocytes

to transitional cells. Gastroenterology. 1984;87:188–200.
20. Mak KM, Lieber CS. Lipocytes and transitional cells in alcoholic liver disease. A morphometric study. Hepatology. 1988;8:1027–33.
21. Rudolph R, McClure WJ, Woodward M. Contractile fibroblasts in chronic alcoholic cirrhosis. Gastroenterology. 1979;76:705–9.
22. Darby I, Skalli O, Gabbiani G. Alpha smooth muscle actin is transiently expressed by myofibroblasts during experimental wound healing. Lab Invest. 1990;63:21–9.
23. Friedman SL, Millward-Sadler GH, Arthur MJP. Liver fibrosis and cirrhosis. In: Millward-Sadler GH, Wright R, Arthur MJP, editors. Wright's liver and biliary disease, Vol. 2. London: Saunders; 1992:821–81.
24. Desmet VJ. Cirrhosis: aetiology and pathogenesis: cholestasis. In Boyer JL, Bianchi L, editors. Liver cirrhosis. Lancaster: MTP Press; 1987:101–18.

Section II
Fat-storing cells

7
Fat-storing cells and vitamin A metabolism: modulation of collagen synthesis

B. H. DAVIS

INTRODUCTION

The hepatic Ito cell (or stellate cell or fat-storing cell) undergoes marked morphological and phenotypic changes during hepatic injury and subsequent fibrogenesis. The cellular transformation which occurs *in vivo* in humans and experimental animals is simulated *in vitro* during short-term culture[1]. Unlike the *in vivo* process, which develops gradually over months and years, *in vitro* transformation occurs within $\approx 1-2$ weeks following isolation. The relatively rapid *in vitro* changes have provided a model to begin to examine some of the intracellular and extracellular forces which may combine to regulate the transformation/activation cascade. The functional hallmarks of activation *in vivo*, as well as *in vitro*, include excessive cellular proliferation and abundant extracellular matrix protein production. The matrix proteins which are produced by the activated Ito cell *in vitro* include the interstitial collagens, basement membrane collagens and glycoproteins, and proteoglycans[1,2]. Previous studies of matrix accumulation *in vivo* during cirrhosis have demonstrated a similar array of proteins[1,3]. Activated, proliferating Ito cells have been demonstrated *in vivo* adjacent to matrix deposition in the abnormal space of Disse and circumferentially at the periphery of fibrotic nodules. These observations, as well as *in situ* hybridization studies which have detected abundant collagen mRNA within Ito cells, suggest that the activated Ito cell may be largely *responsible* for the deposition of these proteins[1,3,4]. During the activation/transformation process *in vitro*, the quiescent non-proliferating Ito cell changes to a cytokine-responsive proliferating cell[1,5-8]. This shift has been noted by several laboratories, and is also associated with a change in collagen phenotype – from low levels of type III collagen synthesis to high levels of type I collagen production (e.g. in activated cells, the type I/type III collagen ratio is generally $> 3:1$)[1,6,9]. Another major feature of the activation process is the Ito cell's cytokine responsiveness.

73

Previous studies have demonstrated responsiveness to insulin, corticosteroids, epidermal growth factor, transforming growth factor (TGF) α and β, platelet-derived growth factor (PDGF), as well as colony-stimulating factor[4]. Receptor expression studies suggest that the acquired cytokine responsiveness is related to the activated cell's expression of the appropriate surface receptor (e.g. the PDGF receptor and the family of TGF-β receptors)[5,10,11].

The regulatory factors which maintain the Ito cell's quiescent state are unknown. During activation these factors are either suppressed or bypassed. Agents which suppress activation may partially simulate the quiescent state. Studies of these suppressive agents have begun to provide insight into the key steps in the activation cascade.

BACKGROUND

Morphological studies *in vivo* and *in vitro* initially suggested that retinoids might function in a suppressive capacity[4,8,12,13]. During fibrogenesis *in vivo* or during the initial days of *in vitro* culture, the Ito cell's prominent cytoplasmic lipid droplets diminish in size and number[14]. These droplets contain stored vitamin A, predominantly as retinyl palmitate[14]. This loss of vitamin A was found to coincide with a gradual shift in the proliferative capacity of the cultured cells as well as the *de novo* expression of the PDGF-β surface receptor[5,15]. The initial studies utilized rat cells exclusively, but recent work with human cells suggests a similar pattern (see Results)[16]. When vitamin A in the form of retinol was then reintroduced into the cell cultures, suppression of activation was observed[15]. Retinol reduced both cell proliferation and collagen synthesis, the major components of activation.

The Ito cell response was examined with regard to other retinoids with higher potency. In addition, recent studies imply that retinoic acid may be the active metabolite which mediates the retinol effect[14]. Retinoic acid (RAc) profoundly suppressed serum-induced [^{3}H]-thymidine incorporation during Ito cell culture and was 1000 times more potent on a molar basis versus retinol[17]. RAc was similarly found to suppress the production of Ito cell type I and type III collagen, as well as the endogenous production of TGF-β, as measured by ELISA. This suppression was dose-dependent, and when normal rats and mice were administered RAc there were profound reductions in the abundance of total liver type I collagen mRNA transcripts with no change in simultaneously examined fibronectin or apolipoprotein E mRNA transcript abundance. Similar findings were then confirmed in purified fresh Ito cell RNA extracts from rats treated with RAc. This work then confirmed that retinoids have the capacity to alter Ito cell behaviour *in vivo*. RAc effectively suppresses major components of both the proliferation and collagen synthesis components of activation.

Further mitogenesis studies were pursued using the PDGF-specific agonist as it is likely to play a significant role *in vivo* when the activated Ito cell expresses the PDGF receptor[18]. Ito cells were found to be sensitive to PDGF (either AB or BB isoforms)-induced mitogenesis in the dose range described for most cell types (5–15 ng/ml). When Ito cells were *pretreated* with RAc the PDGF mitogenic response was depressed to levels comparable to unstimulated cells[19]. If RAc and PDGF were given simultaneously there was no RAc suppression. This suggested that the RAc effect required a series of preceding intracellular events (consistent with the known RAc-generated nuclear sites of action).

The RAc-sensitive steps would be predicted to be central, pharmacologically modulatable features of mitogenesis. The detailed steps associated with RAc suppression in rat cells are unknown, but a post-receptor mechanism is likely to be involved, as RAc caused no effect on the abundance of the rat Ito cell's PDGF-β receptor.

The present study further explored the mechanism of action of RAc in human-derived cells. The RAc mechanism has been pursued as a tool to further dissect the Ito cell activation cascade. The emphasis has been on the proliferation component of activation, but future studies are needed to examine the regulators of the collagen component of activation as well.

MATERIAL AND METHODS

Cell isolation and culture

Segments of normal human liver obtained at the time of organ preparation prior to transplantation were used for cell preparations. Liver cell isolation was performed as previously described for baboon liver[16]. Following collagenase perfusion the cells were sedimented twice at $50g$ for 5 min, adjusted to approximately 1×10^6 cells/ml in Williams' medium E supplemented with 10 mmol/l HEPES-KOH + 10% FCS and plated on flasks coated with Primaria (Falcon). After 48 h of culture the medium was changed (depending on the desire to maintain either hepatocytes or mesenchymal cells) to a serum-free formulation previously described for hepatocyte culture or the medium was changed to Dulbecco's MEM containing 10% calf serum/10% fetal calf serum (Ito medium)[16]. The latter Ito medium was changed daily and during the subsequent 5–10 days of culture there was a gradual loss of hepatocytes coincident with the prominent appearance of stellate-like cells. To enrich for stellate cells, and to reduce the percentage of remaining viable hepatocytes, the mixed cell cultures were trypsinized (0.5% trypsin/0.02% EDTA) when the stellate cells (which had lost most of their lipid droplets) appeared to occupy > 50–60% of the available surface area. The released cells were centrifuged ($50g$ for 2 min) and the pellet and the supernatant were cultured separately. The pellet contained a mixture of non-viable cells as well as predominantly hepatocytes and rare stellate cells (< 20%). The supernatant fraction yielded a homogeneous stellate cell population which was subsequently passaged and maintained on type I collagen flasks as previously described for rat Ito cells[6]. As this method was primarily an outgrowth technique, precise yields cannot be quantitated. The cells were split at a 1 : 3 ratio and were characterized at passages 1–3. Some cells were also studied at later passage (passages 5 and 6) as noted separately. The current report includes passaged cells from three separate human donors.

Morphologic and phenotypic characterization

The passaged cells (subcultured on 24-well type I collagen coated plates) were characterized immunohistochemically with regard to collagen synthetic phenotype and Ito cell-like features (desmin and α-smooth muscle actin staining). Staining was performed as described below using either rabbit polyclonal calf procollagen I or III, rabbit polyclonal chicken desmin (courtesy of Dr J. Madri, Yale University), or mouse monoclonal α-smooth muscle actin (Sigma) antisera. Cells were initially fixed in 10% formalin/0.2% Triton X-100. Control wells either excluded the primary antibody or contained equal amounts of normal rabbit serum or mouse IgG.

Cell proliferation

Cells (groups of four parallel wells) were cultured on 24-well plates under sub-confluent conditions in 0.4% fetal calf serum (FCS) $\pm$ RAc for 18 h. The medium was then replaced with fresh medium containing PDGF (10 ng/ml) $\pm$ RAc. Eight hours later the cultures were pulsed with [^{3}H]-thymidine and incubated for an additional 16 h. The degree of labelling was previously found to correlate with changes in cell number as well as *in situ* bromodeoxyuridine nuclear labelling in the analogous rat cell culture system[19].

PDGF receptor abundance

Cell cultures initially maintained in media containing 10% fetal calf serum (FCS) were changed to media with 0.4% FCS $\pm$ RAc (10^{-6} mol/l) for 18–24 h. When the acute effects of PDGF were assessed, PDGF was added directly to the tissue culture medium for the last 15 min at a final concentration of 30 ng/ml. The medium was then removed, the cells were washed twice in iced phosphate buffered saline (PBS) and then scraped directly into RIPA (50 mmol/l Tris/HCl, pH 7.5; 150 mmol/l NaCl, 1% Triton X-100, 0.5% deoxycholate, 0.1% SDS, 1 mmol/l Na orthovanadate, 2 mmol/l EDTA, 10 mmol/l Na fluoride, 10 μg/ml leupeptin, 10 μg/ml aprotonin, 300 μg/ml PMSF) buffer, and centrifuged at 12000g for 15 min to remove insoluble cell material. Aliquots of equivalent protein concentrations were run on a 7.5% SDS-polyacrylamide gel and then electroblotted and probed (4°C for 18 h or room temperature for 1 h) with either rabbit polyclonal PDGF human α- or β-receptor (courtesy of Dr J. Escobedo and L. Williams, UCSF) or rabbit polyclonal phosphotyrosine antiserum (East Acres and courtesy of Dr J. Avruch, MGH). Similar blots were probed with a monoclonal human α-smooth muscle actin antiserum (Sigma) as previously described[19]. The blots were then probed with peroxidase conjugated anti-rabbit or anti-mouse secondary antibodies (Amersham) followed by the ECL Amersham method.

Assessment of PDGF-induced cascade

To consider some of the distal events which follow PDGF receptor activation, two potential signal 'transducers' were examined: (a) activation and translocation of the cytoplasmic proto-oncogene c-Raf, and (b) nuclear expression of the fos, jun, and egr-1 proteins. Based on previous studies, these 'transducers' are sequentially linked and critically involved in the cascade at progressively more distal or nuclear levels[20].

Raf activation

The cRaf serine/threonine kinase activation which occurs upon exposure to PDGF is due to tyrosine, serine and threonine phosphorylation, and may be detected as a change in the electrophoretic migration pattern seen on a 7.5% SDS gel[20]. Cell lysates were processed in RIPA as described above, and were then immunoprecipitated overnight at 4°C using monoclonal human PBB1 Raf antibody purified from mouse ascites with a protein G column[20]. The characteristic 72 kDa Raf protein identified by the monospecific antibody is completely blocked by preincubation with the Raf protein[20]. Immunoprecipitation was performed with protein A agarose beads prebound with a horse anti-mouse IgG (Vector) linker. The Raf antigen–antibody complexes were loaded directly onto a 7.5% SDS gel. The gel was electroblotted as described above and the transferred proteins probed with either the PBB1 raf monoclonal or a rabbit polyclonal raf antibody[20]. Following activation, the Raf kinase then phosphorylates a series of proteins ranging from 55 to 170 kDa. Raf kinase function was assessed using the Raf-bound protein A agarose immunoprecipiates obtained after a 3-h incubation as previously described after incubation for 10 min at room temperature in kinase buffer with [^{32}P]-ATP (10 μCi/reaction) and histone 1 protein (24 μg/reaction; Worthington) as an exogenous substrate for phosphorylation[20]. Eluates were loaded on a 12.5% SDS gel and the gel containing the resolved proteins was subsequently fixed, stained, dried, and exposed to Kodak XAR-5 film and intensifying screens at -70°C.

The activated Raf protein has been strongly implicated as a cytoplasmic transmitter leading to nuclear transcriptional events, and is required for serum-induced initiation of mitogenesis in some cell culture systems[20,21]. The cytoplasm to nucleus signal transmission may in part relate to the physical translocation of the Raf protein which has been observed in some cell lines[20]. The Raf cytoplasm to perinuclear translocation was assessed during cell culture in response to PDGF stimulation $\pm$ RAc pretreatment. This enabled an assessment of the capacity of the activated Raf kinase (as demonstrated above) to physically shift its localization, which might be important in the further downstream transmission of the PDGF cascade. Cells were cultured in 24-well plates and made quiescent with overnight culture in 0.4% FCS as described above, and then exposed to PDGF (30 ng/ml) for 15 min. After fixation and blocking, the wells were then incubated with PBB1 (5 μg/well) diluted in PBS/BSA for 1 h. Control wells either excluded the primary antibody or used equal amounts of purified mouse IgG. Following three washes with PBS/BSA the wells were incubated with a biotinylated horse anti-mouse secondary antibody (Vector) followed by the avidin–biotin peroxidase complex and the final brown/black reaction product was produced using diaminobenzidine as previously described[16].

Nuclear proto-oncogene expression

To determine whether the PDGF-initiated cascade ultimately produced nuclear events generally associated with the initiation of mitogenesis and the G_0 to G_1 shift, the enhanced expression of the nuclear fos, jun, and egr-1 protein was determined immunocytochemically following FCS or PDGF stimulation $\pm$ RAc. The nuclear expression of these transcriptional inducers is generally associated with the rapid and transient transcription of their respective genes, and would imply that the PDGF cascade has reached the nuclear level[22]. Immunocytochemical staining was performed using the same technique described above, with minor modifications. Primary antibody staining utilized a rabbit polyclonal fos or c-jun anti-serum (3 and $2 \mu g$/well respectively, Oncogene Science) for 1 h at room temperature or a rabbit polyclonal egr-1 antiserum (R5232) (1 : 500, courtesy of V. Sukhatme, University of Chicago) for 1 h at 37°C. Control staining included comparable amounts of rabbit IgG.

Statistical analysis

Differences between the means of various subgroups were assessed by Student's t-test by using the Statworks statistical package.

RESULTS AND DISCUSSION

Morphologic/phenotypic characterization

Non-parenchymal cells were found adjacent to hepatocytes in liver cell cultures maintained in serum containing media. The spherical hepatocytes with contracted cytoplasm appear brighter under phase microscopy and are readily distinguished from the flatter, stellate-shaped cells with their greater cytoplasm/nucleus ratio. These latter cells resemble primary cultures of human and rat hepatic Ito cells or lipocytes as well as passaged cultures of the rat Ito cell/myofibroblast[1-9,23]. Stellate cell growth in these mixed cultures may relate to a hepatocyte paracrine factor. The passaged stellate cell number/confluent T75 was similar to rat Ito cells: $675 \pm 130 \times 10^3$ cells ($n = 8$). Immunostaining of the passaged human cells revealed that the majority ($> 80\%$) displayed desmin and α-smooth muscle actin cytoplasmic filaments as well as procollagen I protein cytoplasmic granules. Procollagen III reactivity was much less than procollagen I reactivity, which is consistent with quantitative data from passaged rat Ito cell/myofibroblasts showing type I collagen dominance[4,6]. Since these early passaged cells shared many of the commonly described features of the rat Ito cell/myofibroblast, it was important to determine whether similar factors regulate mitogenesis in both the human and rat systems.

Table 1 PDGF-induced DNA synthesis ($[^3H]$-thymidine incorporation) (cpm/well)

PDGF	Retinoid acid (mol/l)	
−	−	4670 ± 1360*
+	−	9271 ± 1740*
+	10^{-7}	3560 ± 670*
+	10^{-8}	5140 ± 1190
+	10^{-9}	7000 ± 2500*
		(mean ± SD, $n = 4$)

Subconfluent passaged human myofibroblasts were made quiescent in media containing 0.4% fetal calf serum and then exposed to PDGF-BB (10 ng/ml) for 24 h. Proliferation was assessed via $[^3H]$-thymidine uptake during the final 16 h. Retinoic acid (or ethanol vehicle) was added as indicated during the initial 24 h pretreatment culture in 0.4% serum containing media and during the addition of PDGF.
*$p < 0.002$; $F = 10.3$

Regulation of cell proliferation

As shown in Table 1, the early passaged human myofibroblasts are responsive to PDGF-BB as previously reported for rat Ito cells as well as numerous other mesenchymal cell types. It has previously been demonstrated that retinol or retinoic acid can suppress serum and PDGF-induced mitogenesis in the rat-derived Ito cell[15-17,24]. While the precise mechanism of the retinoid suppressive effect is not clear, this responsiveness was felt to be a central feature in Ito cell mitogenesis and relevant to the overall fibrogenic process. The human cells were found to be similarly sensitive to RAc suppression. Pretreatment with RAc produced a concentration-dependent inhibition of the PDGF stimulus (Table 1) using the 10^{-7}–10^{-9} mol/l RAc dose range used in numerous other studies. This experiment performed in quadruplicate culture was representative of the retinoid inhibition seen in cells obtained from each of the three human liver donors. The RAc doses did not cause any apparent change in cell morphology or viability.

The proliferation data demonstrate marked similarities to the reported studies involving primary and passaged rat Ito cells. The rat studies demonstrated that retinoid inhibition of $[^3H]$-thymidine incorporation directly mirrored *in situ* nuclear thymidine incorporation as well as reversible changes in cell number. In addition, when later passaged human cells were used in the current study (> passage 5), the retinoid sensitivity was lost. Similar loss of retinoid responsiveness was noted in later passage rat cells, suggesting the likely requirement of persistent expression of retinoid receptors and/or response elements which may wane with increasing length of culture[15]. It also implies that a non-specific toxic retinoid effect is less likely. These studies collectively suggest that the passaged human cell type corresponds well to the predicted behaviour of an activated Ito cell/myofibroblast. Since an understanding of the mechanism(s) of activation or repression of activation should also have ultimate clinical significance, we chose to explore several levels of the PDGF activation cascade in the presence of the RAc repressor.

PDGF receptor abundance and activation

The PDGF receptor phenotype was initially examined in human cells and contrasted to the passaged rat Ito cell previously described[5,19]. As shown in Figs 1A and 1B, the human cell type differs from the rat Ito cell in that it contains abundant quantities of both the PDGF-α receptor and the PDGF-β receptor, while the rat cell contains predominantly the PDGF-β receptor. The slight difference in electrophoretic mobility between the human and rat PDGF-β receptors may relate to previously described differences in glycosylation patterns which occur during receptor processing[22]. When the human cells were exposed to 10^{-6} mol/l RAc, there was no significant change in the abundance of either receptor type. This is consistent with previous studies involving the rat PDGF-β receptor[19]. To assess the receptor's functional capacity for activation following ligand binding $\pm$ RAc, *in vivo* tyrosine phosphorylation of the receptor was assessed via phosphotyrosine immunoblotting (Fig. 2C). A single band corresponding to the PDGF receptor was found following a 15-min exposure to PDGF and the relative intensity of this band was similar $\pm$ RAc, suggesting that receptor activation and tyrosine kinase activity were not the alterations responsible for RAc repression of mitogenesis. Since a smooth muscle actin was demonstrated immunohistochemically in these cells, and has been suggested as a marker of an activated myofibroblast, similar blots were probed with a monoclonal α-smooth muscle actin antibody (Fig. 2D). There was no change in the abundance of this marker in the presence of RAc as previously reported for rat cells[19]. Furthermore, despite equal loading of human and rat cell lysates the human cells appear to contain significantly greater amounts of this actin isoform. These differences do not appear to be secondary to unequal antigen–antibody affinities, as other studies suggest this antibody stains intracellular human and rat actin equally well. The significance of these inter-species differences is unclear, but may relate to differences in contractile function as recent data demonstrate both rat and human Ito cells have the capacity to contract in response to agonist stimulation[4,7].

Raf activation

The cytoplasmic raf proto-oncogene plays a key role in transmitting surface receptor (i.e. PDGF receptor) and cytoplasmic activation signals to the nucleus during the initiation of cellular proliferation[20]. Through the use of transfections involving constitutively activated Raf constructs, it has been demonstrated in numerous cell types that Raf activation alone is sufficient to activate the large repertoire of nuclear transcription activators and initiate DNA synthesis and cell proliferation[20]. The capacity of PDGF to activate raf in Ito cells $\pm$ RAc was therefore examined. This activation was studied at the three levels associated with raf activation, as it is likely that all three components are necessary for signal transmission. These levels include phosphorylation of the raf protein, raf's kinase capacity, and raf's ability to translocate. Figure 2 demonstrates that PDGF induced the characteristic shift

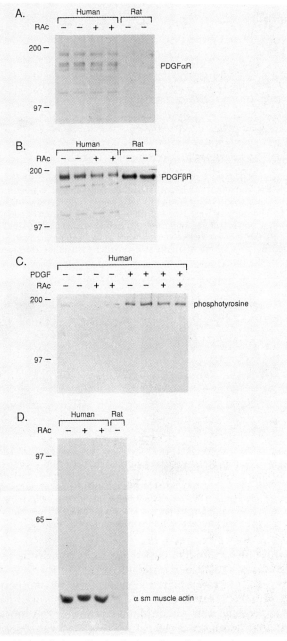

Fig. 1 Retinoic acid modulation of 'activation' markers. Quiescent human myofibroblasts or passaged rat Ito cells ± PDGF-BB (30 ng/ml for 15 min) were extracted in RIPA buffer. Lysates were normalized for comparable amounts of cell protein, further solubilized into Laemmli loading buffer and separated on a 7.5% SDS-polyacrylamide gel, transblotted and subsequently probed with either (**A**) polyclonal PDGFα receptor antisera (PDGFαR), (**B**) polyclonal PDGFβ receptor antisera (PDGFβR), (**C**) polyclonal phosphotyrosine antisera, or (**D**) monoclonal α-smooth muscle actin antisera. Molecular weight markers are indicated on the left of each gel

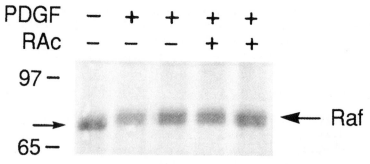

Fig. 2 Raf activation. Human myofibroblasts were exposed to PDGF-BB (30 ng/ml for 15 min), solubilized in RIPA, and after protein normalization the lysates were immunoprecipitated with monoclonal PBB1 raf antiserum prebound to horse anti-mouse linked protein A agarose beads for 18 h at 4°C. The samples were resolved on a 7.5% SDS polyacrylamide gel, transblotted and probed with a polyclonal raf antiserum. Molecular weight markers indicated on the left side of the gel. PDGF induces a characteristic shift in electrophoretic mobility ± retinoic acid (RAc) (indicated by large arrow at right) as compared to baseline raf protein (indicated by smaller arrow at left)

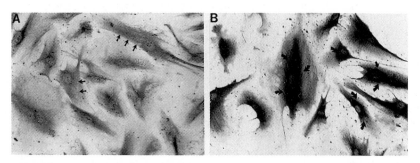

Fig. 3 Raf perinuclear translocation. The raf protein was immunolocalized using the PBB1 raf antisera (5 μg/well) after initial methanol (10 min) fixation. Antibody localization was via biotinylated secondary antibody, avidin–biotin peroxidase complex and diaminobenzidine. (Final magnification: 200 ×, phase). **A:** Baseline raf distribution in quiescent sub-confluent myofibroblasts maintained in 0.4% serum containing media. Note diffuse cytoplasmic localization (arrows). **B:** Perinuclear raf redistribution following PDGF-BB for 15 min (arrows). Similar redistribution was observed in cultures pretreated with retinoic acid

in raf's electrophoretic mobility (attributed to its transient phosphorylation) following 15 min of PDGF exposure ± RAc.

Immunoprecipitated raf displayed kinase activity by phosphorylating three endogenous proteins (MW ≈ 120, 55, and 33 kDa) as well as exogenously added histone 1 equally well ± RAc (data not shown). The diffuse cytoplasmic distribution of raf in quiescent cell culture (Fig. 3A) was observed to change acutely secondary to its perinuclear relocalization following 15 min of PDGF exposure (Fig. 3B). Background staining was minimal. This similar translocation occurred in RAc-pretreated cells exposed to PDGF (data not shown), further reinforcing the findings that RAc's repressive effect appears independent of raf function. Since raf activation alone can initiate proliferation in the absence of other upstream stimulants, the data collectively suggest that RAc is functioning at either a distal/nuclear level or via a parallel pathway required for the complete mitogenic response. There have been no other studies to date which have shown RAc alterations in raf function.

Nuclear proto-oncogene expression

PDGF or serum induction of nuclear fos, jun, and egr proteins was examined in cells $\pm$ RAc. Previous work suggests these proteins are critical for the mitogenic process and the shift to the G_1 phase of mitosis[22,25]. In addition, transfection experiments demonstrate that raf activation alone can induce their expression, as well as initiating proliferation. As shown in Fig. 4, RAc did not cause any apparent reduction in the expression of these transcriptional mediators. In other cell types the induction of the proto-oncogenes within their nuclear site of action correlated highly with radiolabelling studies as well as RNA transcription data, collectively implying that new mRNA transcription and *de novo* protein synthesis were initiated following raf activation[22,25]. Subtle changes in nuclear protein levels may have escaped detection. In addition, alterations in the nuclear protein's differential phosphorylations and dephosphorylations associated with the activated state were not examined. However, the simultaneous demonstration of all three major proteins in > 95% of the cells suggests that the cytoplasm-originated signal had at least reached a nuclear level. This further corroborates that raf activation, as well as other pre-nuclear cascade steps required for the stimulation of these nuclear proteins, were unlikely to have been altered by RAc exposure. While it is possible that RAc's effect is mediated by a more proximal parallel pathway required for mitogenesis, the majority of RAc studies to date imply that its mode of action is at a nuclear level[14].

In summary, the current work has characterized a potential human hepatic fibrogenic effector cell and considered one system of mitogenic stimulation and repression which has been suggested by numerous studies to be relevant during *in vivo* injury and fibrosis. Though the human cells are PDGF-responsive, they differ from their rat counterparts in the expression of abundant amounts of both the α and β receptors, which could have potential relevance *in vivo* as it relates to the regulation of Ito cell activation.

The human cells herein were shown to be sensitive to retinoid suppression, which again emphasizes their similarity to the rat cell and further implies that retinoids in general may be relevant in the regulation of this cell and the activation process which occurs during fibrogenesis. The RAc suppressive effect was shown either to occur via a parallel pathway unrelated to raf activation and the induction of fos, jun, and egr, or to involve a more distal mechanism.

Acknowledgements

The author especially acknowledges Dr David Beno's major contributions to the human retinoid studies as well as Drs U. Rapp (NCI), J. Escobedo

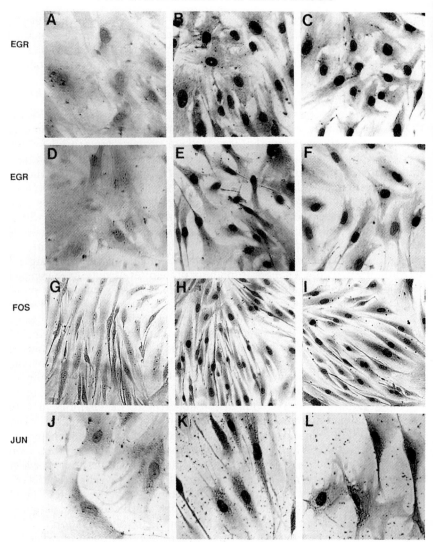

Fig. 4 Proto-oncogene nuclear localization. The EGR, FOS, and JUN proteins were immuno-localized to the nucleus as indicated 90 min following either fetal calf serum (10%) (**B**), fetal calf serum + retinoic acid (**C**), PDGF-BB (**E, H, K**) or PDGF-BB + retinoic acid (**F, I, L**) stimulation. In **A**, quiescent cells were stained with normal rabbit serum. In **D, G**, and **J**, quiescent cells were stained with the corresponding antibodies as indicated on the left side of the figure. Antibody localization was via biotinylated secondary antibody, avidin–biotin peroxidase complex and diaminobenzidine. (Relative cell density was high in FOS-stained groups.) (Final magnification: 300 ×, phase)

and L. Williams (UCSF), J. Avruch (MGH) and V. Sukhatme (University of Chicago) for advice and supply of antisera as well as S. Skarosi and N. Davidson for allowing access to human-derived primary cell cultures. This work was supported in part by the Liver Research Fund, University of

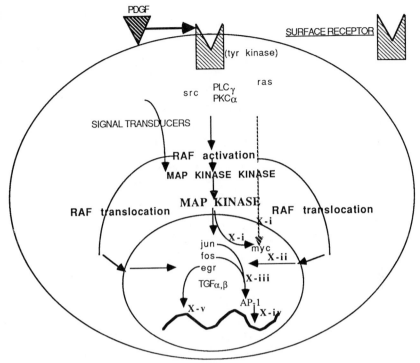

FAT-STORING CELLS AND VITAMIN A METABOLISM

Fig. 5 Putative Ito cell activation cascade. The × marks indicate potential major areas of regulation by retinoids and other suppressive agents

Chicago, and National Institute of Health grants DK40223, DK 42086, and DK 07074-18.

References

1. Laskin DL. Nonparenchymal cells and hepatoxicity. Semin Liver Dis. 1990;10:293–304.
2. Meyer DH, Krull N, Dreher KL *et al.* Biglycan and decorin gene expression in normal and fibrotic rat liver: Cellular localization and regulatory factors. Hepatology. 1992;16:204–16.
3. Clement B, Grimaud J-A, Campion J-P *et al.* Cell types involved in collagen and fibronectin production in normal and fibrotic human liver. Hepatology. 1986;6:225–34.
4. Mak KM, Leo MA, Lieber CS. Alcoholic liver injury in baboons: transformation of lipocytes to transitional cells. Gastroenterology. 1984;87:188–200.
5. Friedman SL, Arthur MJP. Activation of cultured rat hepatic lipocytes by Kupffer cell conditioned medium. J Clin Invest. 1989;84:1780–5.
6. Davis BH. Transforming growth factor beta responsiveness is modulated by the extracellular collagen matrix during hepatic ito cell culture. J Cell Physiol. 1988;136:547–53.
7. Pinzani M, Failli P, Ruocco C *et al.* Fat storing cells as liver-specific pericytes: spatial dynamics of agonist-stimulated intracellular calcium transients. J Clin Invest. 1992;90:642–6.
8. Shiratori Y, Takafumi I, Geerts A *et al.* Modulation of collagen synthesis by fat-storing cells, isolated from CCl4- or vitamin A-treated rats. Dig Dis Sci. 1987;32:1281–9.
9. Friedman SL, Roll FJ, Boyles J. Hepatic lipocytes: the principal collagen-producing cells of normal rat liver. Proc Natl Acad Sci USA. 1985;82:8681–5.

10. Davis BH, Beno DWA. PGE inhibits hepatic and Ito cell collagen gene expression independent of TGFβ and PDGFβ receptor modulation. Hepatology. 1991;14:115A.
11. Friedman SL, Yamasaki G. Characterization of TGFβ receptors in cultured rat lipocytes: Enhanced receptor expression accompanies cellular activation. Hepatology. 1991;14:113A.
12. Ballardini G, Esposti SD, Bianchi FB et al. Correlation between Ito cells and fibrogenesis in an experimental model of hepatic fibrosis: a sequential stereological study. Liver. 1983;3:58–63.
13. Kent G, Gay S, Inouye T et al. Vitamin A-containing lipocytes and formation of type III collagen in liver injury. Proc Natl Acad Sci USA. 1976;73:3719–22.
14. Blomhoff R, Wake K. Perisinusoidal stellate cells of the liver: important roles in retinol metabolism and fibrosis. FASEB J. 1991;5:272–7.
15. Davis BH, Vucic A. The effect of retinol on ito cell proliferation in vitro. Hepatology. 1988;8:788–93.
16. Davis BH, Coll D, Beno DWA. Retinoic acid suppresses the PDGF response in human hepatic Ito cell-like myofibroblasts: a post-receptor mechanism independent of RAF/FOS/-JUN/EGR activation. Biochem J. 1993 (In press).
17. Davis BH, Kramer RT, Davidson NO. Retinoic acid modulates rat ito cell proliferation, collagen and transforming growth factor β production. J Clin Invest. 1990;86:2062–70.
18. Friedman SL, Yamasaki G, Wong L et al. 14-Hydroxy 4,14-retro-retinol (14-HRR): A novel metabolite of retinol produced by activated rat lipocytes in vivo and in culture. Hepatology. 1992;16:143A.
19. Davis BH, Rapp UR, Davidson NO. Retinoic acid and transforming growth factor β differentially inhibit platelet-derived growth-factor-induced Ito-cell activation. Biochem J. 1991;278:43–7.
20. Rapp U. Role of Raf-1 serine/threonine protein kinase in growth factor signal transduction. Oncogene. 1991;6:495–500.
21. Kolch W, Heidecker G, Lloyd P et al. Raf-1 protein kinase is required for growth of induced NIH/3T3 cells. Nature. 1991;349:426–8.
22. Williams LT. Signal transduction by the platelet-derived growth factor receptor. Science. 1989;243:1564–70.
23. Friedman SL, Rockey DC, McGuire RF et al. Isolated hepatic lipocytes and Kupffer cells from normal human liver: Morphological and functional characteristics in primary culture. Hepatology. 1992;15:234–43.
24. Pinzani M, Gentilini P, Abboud HE. Phenotypical modulation of liver fat-storing cells by retinoids: influence on unstimulated and growth factor-induced cell proliferation. J Hepatol. 1992;14:211–20.
25. Cao X, Koski RA, Gashler A et al. Identification and characterization of the egr-1 gene product, a DNA-binding zinc finger protein induced by differentiation and growth signals. Mol Cell Biol. 1990;10:1931–9.

8
Proteoglycan expression during fat-storing cell activation

A. M. GRESSNER, N. KRULL and M. G. BACHEM

INTRODUCTION

Glycoconjugates in liver extracellular matrix (ECM) are present as structural glycoproteins[1] and as a large group of proteoglycans[2-4]. The latter comprise a heterogeneous class of protein-polysaccharide complexes consisting of a protein backbone (core protein) which is N- or O-glycosidically substituted with highly polyanionic, sulphated and linear (unbranched) carbohydrate polymers (glycosaminoglycans)[5]. In healthy liver three main types of sulphated glycosaminoglycans are known: in order of decreasing concentrations they are heparan sulphate (ca. 60% of total glycosaminoglycans), dermatan sulphate and chondroitin sulphate[2,4,6,7]. Keratan sulphate could not be detected to date[8,9] and only trace amounts of its de novo synthesis have been reported several years ago[10]. Under pathological conditions such as liver fibrosis the entire amount of proteoglycans increases several-fold, paralleled by a redistribution of the pattern of the glycosaminoglycan types and their histological rearrangement. Dermatan sulphate and chondroitin sulphate isomers display a dramatic, absolute and relative increase, forming the preponderant body of glycosaminoglycans in the diseased liver, whereas heparan sulphate follows only a slight increase, which counts thus for its relative (fractional) decrease[2,11] (Fig. 1). Hyaluronan, an unsulphated, glucuronic acid–glucosamine polymer of high molecular weight not covalently linked with a core protein, is present only in trace amounts in normal liver (about 4% of all glycosaminoglycans) but increases 6–10-fold in the cirrhotic extracellular matrix (ECM).

In the past, proteoglycans have been classified almost exclusively by the composition of the repeating disaccharide unit polymerized in the glycosaminoglycan side-chain[12,13]. However, sequencing and molecular cloning of the core proteins have established a great heterogeneity of extracellular, intracellular and membrane-intercalated proteoglycans independent of the composition of the glycosaminoglycans[5]. Based on molecular characterization of the respective core proteins the classification and nomen-

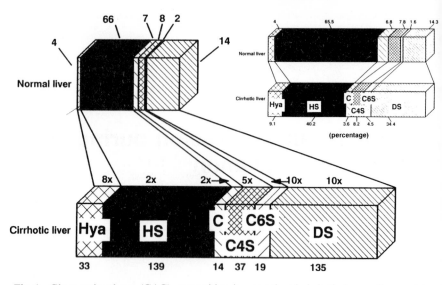

Fig. 1 Glycosaminoglycan (GAG) composition in normal and cirrhotic human liver matrix (μmol hexosamine per 100 g dry weight). Hya: hyaluronan; HS: heparan sulphate; C: chondroitin; C4S: chondroitin-4-sulphate; C6S: chondroitin-6-sulphate; DS: dermatan sulphate. The x-fold increases in cirrhotic liver are given. Inset: Percentage of GAG in normal and cirrhotic human liver

clature of proteoglycans has been redefined (Table 1). Very recently the presence of some of these newly identified proteoglycans in normal and fibrotic ECM of liver was established[14,15].

In previous studies, using experimental approaches of acute (D-galactosamine, thioacetamide) and chronic (thioacetamide) rat liver injury *in situ*, we established a biphasic modulation of overall proteoglycan synthesis in response to injury[10,16–18]: A rapid decline, preferentially of heparan sulphate, was followed by a strong elevation of chondroitin sulphate and dermatan sulphate formation ('overshoot'). This overshoot phenomenon was reversible after a single application of the injurious agent, but remained constant during chronic application of thioacetamide[18]. It expresses the activation of sulphated proteoglycan synthesis in diseased liver, which ultimately leads to the typical distribution profile of these components in liver fibrotic ECM (Fig. 1). Based on these initial findings consequent studies were concentrated on the following points:

1. What is (are) the principal cellular source(s) of sulphated proteoglycans (and of hyaluronan) in the healthy and diseased liver?
2. Do the patterns of the proteoglycans secreted by a defined cell type change in the process of liver fibrosis?
3. Do cytokines such as TGF-α and TGF-β influence the expression of the proteoglycans, and, if yes, in what terms and by what potential pathways?
4. What is the source of the above-mentioned traces of keratan sulphate in the liver?

Table 1 Proteoglycans (PG) characterized by sequencing and cloning of the core protein

Proteoglycan	Alternate name(s)	Glycosamino-glycan(s)
Secreted/extracellular matrix proteoglycans		
Aggrecan	Large aggregating cartilage PG	CS/KS
Versican	PG 350	CS/DS
Decorin	PGII, PG40	CS/DS
Biglycan	PGI	CS/DS
Periecan	Basement membrane PG	HS
Type IX collagen	—	CS
Betaglycan	Type III TGFβ receptor	HS/CS
Fibromodulin	Collagen-binding 59 kDa	KS
Intracellular granule proteoglycans		
Serglycin	PG 19	CS/DS
Membrane-intercalated proteoglycans		
Syndecan	—	HS/CS
MHC Invariant chain*	—	CS
Betaglycan	Type III TGFβ receptor	HS/CS
Transferrin receptor*	—	HS
Thrombomodulin*	—	HS
Lymphocyte homing receptor*	—	CS

*part-time PG
CS = chondroitin sulphate
DS = dermatan sulphate
HS = heparan sulphate
KS = keratan sulphate

MATERIALS AND METHODS

Experimental rat liver fibrosis

For the purpose of *in situ* hybridization, female Uje-Wist rats, body weight approx. 150 g, were used. Thioacetamide was administered at a concentration of 0.03% (w/v) in drinking water, to which the animals had unlimited access. The treatment was performed over a period of 3 months, without withdrawal of thioacetamide prior to sacrifice[14,19]. Fibrosis was induced also by prolonged bile duct ligation[14]. For all other purposes, male Sprague-Dawley rats aged 3–5 months and 1 year (FSC isolation), respectively, were used.

Cell isolation and culture

Non-parenchymal cells (fat-storing cells and Kupffer cells) were isolated by the pronase-collagenase method of de Leeuw et al.[20] with slight modifications described elsewhere[21,22].

Fat-storing cells were purified from the cell suspension by a single-step density gradient centrifugation with Nycodenz[21]. The purity of the cell fraction was estimated by light microscopy, transmission electron microscopy, positive indirect immunofluorescence staining for desmin, vimentin and iso-α-smooth muscle actin, and vitamin A-specific autofluorescence. Cells were kept in culture in DMEM containing glutamine (4 mmol/l), FCS (10%), penicillin/streptomycin (1%), in a humid atmosphere containing 5% CO_2; the medium was changed at 2-day intervals. For subcultivation, primary cultures were split at a 1 : 5 ratio after trypsinization.

Kupffer cells were extracted from the non-parenchymal fraction by centrifugal elutriation, with subsequent dish-adherence purification[23]. Assessment of the purity of the prepared cells was performed by light and electron microscopy, peroxidase staining, positive immunofluorescence staining for vimentin and negative for desmin, and by phagocytosis of latex beads.

Parenchymal cells were isolated by a slight modification[24] of the collagenase perfusion method of Seglen[25]. The cells were cultured in Hank's F12 medium containing 0.2% BSA, 20 mU/ml insulin, penicillin/streptomycin (1%). The viability of isolated parenchymal cells was verified by trypan blue exclusion. Contamination with non-parenchymal cells was checked by vimentin/desmin staining.

In situ hybridization

Liver tissue was snap-frozen in liquid nitrogen. Serial cryostat sections of a uniform thickness of 8 μm were lyophilized at $-70°C$ for 2 h prior to the fixation in 4% paraformaldehyde/PBS, pH 7.4 for 10 min at 4°C. To reduce the background due to the 'stickiness' of the probes, slides were acetylated in a 0.5% solution of acetic anhydride in 0.1 mol/l triethanolamine, pH 8.0, for 10 min at room temperature. Probes for biglycan, decorin and aggrecan were constructed after a computer-aided comparison of the sequences; fragments displaying the lowest homology were further subcloned in pBSK-KS II (Stratagene). Single stranded, $[\alpha\text{-}^{35}S]$-radioactively labelled probes complementary (anti-sense) or complementary (sense probe; control) were synthesized using T3 and T7 RNA polymerases. The hybridization procedure was performed according to Tecott *et al.*[26], hybridization taking place for 16 h at 25°C below the T_m (melting point temperature) calculated for each probe separately. Unspecifically bound probe was digested with RNAase A (0.02 mg/ml) and RNAase T1 (2500 Kunitz U/ml), and washed off in a series of washes with increasing stringency up to 0.1 × SSC at 25°C below the calculated T_m, for 15 min.

Autoradiography was performed by use of the liquid NTB2 nuclear tracking emulsion (Kodak). After exposure for 11 days at 4°C, autoradiographs were developed in D19 developer (Kodak) for 2 min, rinsed with 1% acetic acid and fixed in ADEFO fixer (ADEFO Nuremberg). For better orientation, cellular structures were counterstained with cresyl violet.

Immunocytochemistry

Cultured cells were fixed in 4% paraformaldehyde in 0.1 mol/l sodium cacodylate, pH 7.4. Prior to the immunocytochemical staining by a three-step immunoperoxidase procedure, a digestion with 0.1 U/ml chondroitin ABC-lyase (Sigma) for 90 min at 37°C in the presence of proteinase inhibitors was introduced. Monoclonal antibodies against chondroitin (C)-0,4,6-sulphate isomers (ICN Chemicals), all recognizing as epitopes an unsaturated hexuronic acid at the non-reducing end of a chondroitin sulphate 'stub' generated by the action of chondroitin ABC-lyase. The primary antibodies were applied for 30 min at room temperature, followed by incubation with rabbit anti-mouse and finally with swine anti-rabbit immunoglobulins conjugated to horseradish peroxidase. The reaction product was visualized by a colour development subsequent to a chemical reaction between the peroxidase and 3-amino-9-ethylcarbazole/H_2O_2 for 10 min at room temperature. For better histological orientation the cell nuclei were stained with Mayer's hemalum.

Northern blotting and hybridization

Total RNA extraction was performed according to the method of Chirgwin et al.[27]. After electrophoretic separation onto 1.3% agarose/formaldehyde gels the RNA was blotted onto nitrocellulose membranes (Hybond N, Amersham-Buchler). Northern blots were hybridized with the decorin cDNA probe comprising the entire sequence, and with the biglycan cDNA comprising the 3'-terminal part of the gene (bp 483-2446). Both probes were a generous gift of Dr K. L. Dreher, Research Triangle Park, USA. As fibromodulin probe a PCR generated 660 bp long fragment spanning two-thirds of the coding region, was used. Lumican probe originated from the chicken (entire sequence) and was a kind donation of T. Blochberger, Pennsylvania University, USA.

Determination of proteoglycan (PG) synthesis

The synthesis of sulphated PGs was determined by the incorporation of [^{35}S]sulphate into the GAGs during a labelling period of 24 h. Labelled PGs were determined in the medium, because fat-storing cells were shown to secrete nearly 80% of newly synthesized PGs into the cultured medium[21]. The medium was removed, centrifuged and mixed with 3 ml buffer A (7 mol/l urea, 0.13 mol/l Tris.Cl, 1 mmol/l EDTA, 1 mmol/l PMSF, 10 mmol/l NEM, 0.1% CHAPS, pH 7.5) and unlabelled GAGs were added as carrier. Then the PGs were bound to DEAE-Sephacel equilibrated with the same buffer. After washing the resin with buffer B (= buffer A + 0.1 mol/l NaCl + 10 mmol/l thymidine, pH 7.5) total PGs were eluted with buffer C (= buffer A + 0.8 mmol/l NaCl, pH 7.5). An aliquot of the supernatant was counted for radioactivity.

Determination of specific types of proteoglycans

PGs were subjected to consecutive degradations with nitrous acid to yield the incorporation of [^{35}S]sulphate into heparan sulphate (HS) and to enzymatic digestions with chondroitin AC- and ABC-lyases, to obtain the fractions of chrondroitin-4,6-sulphate (CS) and dermatan sulphate (DS), respectively. Details of these methods have been reported previously[21,28].

Stimulation of cells by cytokines

The cytokines were added in the presence of 0.5% fetal calf serum to primary cultured fat-storing cells or secondary cultured myofibroblasts 48 h after seeding. Twenty-four hours later the cytokines were again added for another medium change and cultures were labelled with radionuclides ([^{35}S]sulphate or [^{3}H]leucin).

SDS-PAGE and fluorography of labelled proteoglycans

The synthesis of proteoglycans and proteoglycan-core proteins was visualized by fluorography using [^{3}H]leucin incorporation. Cells were labelled for 24 h with 200 μCi [^{3}H]leucin/ml medium. Proteoglycans were isolated after solubilization in 7 mmol/l urea by binding to DEAE-Sephacel (Pharmacia Fine Chemicals, Uppsala, Sweden), equilibrated with 0.3 mol/l sodium acetate buffer (pH 6.6), extensively washed with the same buffer, and thereafter eluted using 2.2 mol/l NaCl. To get the core proteins an aliquot of the eluate was treated with chondroitin-ABC-lyase. The small proteoglycans and proteoglycan core proteins of decorin and biglycan were fractionated in 4–12% gradient- or 10% slab-gel (SDS-PAGE), the gels were dried, and proteins visualized by fluorography using Hyperfilm MP.

Determination of soluble fibronectin

Fibronectin was determined by time-resolved immunofluorometric assay using europium chelate[29,30]. Fibronectin was captured from medium by solid-phase coated gelatin. Rabbit anti-fibronectin antiserum used as first antibody was detected by a biotinylated anti-rabbit IgG antibody. Time-resolved fluorescence (Delfia, LKB Wallace) was measured after incubation with streptavidin-BCPDA [4,7-bis(chlorosulphophenyl)-1,10-phenanthroline-2,9-dicarboxylic acid] and europium[30].

RESULTS AND DISCUSSION

Expression of genes encoding mRNAs of biglycan and decorin core proteins in liver and isolated liver cells

The investigation of the proteoglycan as well as glycosaminoglycan synthesis was performed both *in vivo* and *in vitro*, by use of immunocytochemical staining and the technique of *in situ* hybridization in order to reveal potential discrepancies of the results obtained by both methods, and thus delineate the applicability of the *in vitro* obtained results to the *in vivo* processes.

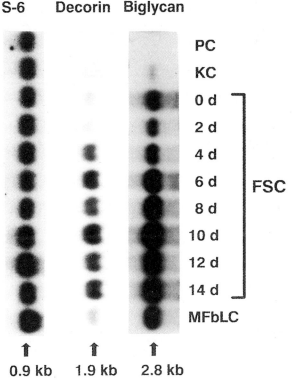

S-6   Decorin Biglycan

PC

KC

0 d ⌉

2 d

4 d

6 d   FSC

8 d

10 d

12 d

14 d ⌋

MFbLC

↑   ↑   ↑

0.9 kb   1.9 kb   2.8 kb

Fig. 2 Northern blot hybridization of biglycan and decorin core protein mRNAs in freshly isolated hepatocytes (PC), Kupffer cells (KC) and fat-storing cells (FSC) at various time-points (days, d) of culture and in myofibroblasts (MFbLC). Each lane contains 15 µg of RNA. Autoradiographic signals were developed after 13 h (biglycan) and 24 h (decorin), respectively

Data accumulated in cell cultures have shown that hepatocytes from normal[24] but also from fibrotic liver[31] do synthesize neither chondroitin nor dermatan sulphate glycosaminoglycans. No transcripts of *biglycan* and *decorin* mRNA, respectively, could be detected by Northern blot hybridization[14]. RNA from freshly isolated Kupffer cells hybridized weakly both with biglycan and decorin cDNAs, these signals probably originating from contaminating fat-storing cells. Fat-storing cells were the only population studied which consistently and clearly expressed both biglycan and decorin transcripts. The steady-state levels of the respective mRNAs increased dramatically (biglycan: threefold, decorin: fourfold) during primary culture. With the phenotypic transition of the fat-storing cells to fully developed myofibroblasts in tertiary culture, however, the levels of biglycan transcripts dropped slightly, those of decorin significantly, compared to the primary culture (Fig. 2). These data combined with those obtained with [35S]sulphate labelling studies of glycosaminoglycans during phenotypic transition of fat-storing cells to myofibroblasts in primary and secondary culture[32] indicate that the modulation of the steady-state levels of decorin and biglycan mRNAs

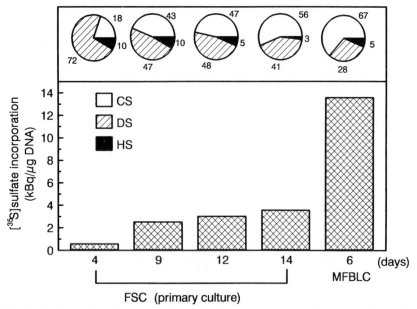

Fig. 3 Synthesis of medium proteoglycans during spontaneous transformation of fat-storing cells (FSC) in primary (4th–14th culture day) and in secondary culture (6th day) when myofibroblasts (MFBLC) have been developed. The fractional distribution (percentages) of chondroitin sulphate (CS), dermatan sulphate (DS), and heparan sulphate (HS) are given in the upper row of the figure. Proteoglycan synthesis was studied by incorporation of [^{35}S]sulphate into the glycosaminoglycan side-chains of the respective molecules

in fat-storing cells and myofibroblasts is not reflected by changes of the synthesis rates of sulphated medium glycosaminoglycans, in particular of chondroitin sulphate (Fig. 3). The latter increases strongly in myofibroblasts. Potential causes of this disparity are: (1) enhanced translational efficiency of core protein mRNAs in myofibroblasts, (2) increased sulphation and/or chain length, (3) increased number of sulphated carbohydrate polymers attached to a core protein, (4) reduced degradation of proteoglycans and/or reduced endocytosis, and (5) additional presence of specific chondroitin sulphate proteoglycans in the medium not identical with decorin and biglycan. The latter aspect has already found experimental support[33]. The results of the *in situ* hybridization show that in the thioacetamide-induced fibrosis model, solely cells identified histologically and immunocytochemically as fat-storing cells and myofibroblasts, respectively, exhibit positive hybridization signals with the biglycan and decorin probes, the intensity of the decorin signals being albeit about one-third of those of biglycan. The signals were accumulated in periportal fields and along the forming septa, and coincided in the early stages with the intensity and extent of the fibrotic process. The temporal and spatial co-distribution with the TGF-β_1 mRNA, which was studied in parallel, pointed to a possible, yet not elucidated, correlation among these genes (Fig. 4).

In the fully developed cirrhosis characterized by distortion of the parenchy-

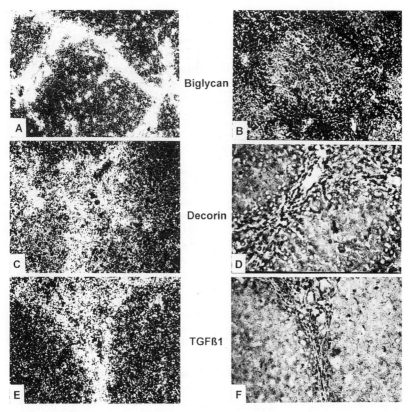

Fig. 4 *In situ* hybridization depicting the coordinated expression of biglycan (**A, B**), decorin (**C, D**) and TGF-β_1 (**E, F**) at 2 months after the onset of the thioacetamide treatment. The signals (left: dark field, signals appear bright; right: bright field, signals appear black) are distributed in the periportal fields. Biglycan and TGF-β_1 follow the entire length of the forming septa, whereas decorin signals can be traced only partially, centrifugally to the periphery ($\times$ 58)

mal architecture, a segregation of the signals between biglycan and decorin occurred. For biglycan the signal intensity per cell decreased slightly, but the distribution along the fibrotic septa remained unaltered. For decorin, on the contrary, the signal disappeared almost entirely and remained detectable only in those periportal fields in which a massive proliferation of bile ducts was appreciated. It coincided inversely with the extent of luminalization of the bile ducts: the large, already luminalized bile ducts were surrounded by cells expressing high levels of decorin, whereas cells surrounding small bile ducts delivered only weak hybridization signals.

The study was accomplished by immunocytochemical detection of the distribution patterns of chondroitin (C)-0,-4, and -6-sulphate isomers by use of monoclonal antibodies onto cultured primary and transformed fat-storing cells[34]. In early primary culture (up to 6 days), immunoreactivity for C-0-S dominated over that of C-4- and C-6-S. In myofibroblast cultures, on the

Primary culture (5 days)   Secondary culture (4 days)

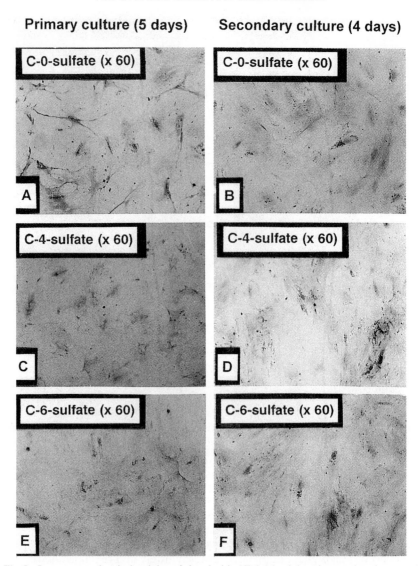

Fig. 5 Immunocytochemical staining of chondroitin (C)-0,4,6-sulphate isomers in primary and secondary cultures of rat liver fat-storing cells. Original magnification is given in parentheses

contrary, staining for C-4-S prevailed, followed by C-6-S and finally C-0-S (Fig. 5).

Thus, summarizing the data obtained, the principal cellular sources of sulphated glycosaminoglycans in the liver, as deduced both from the *in vitro*[28] and *in vivo* experiments[14,15,35], are the fat-storing cells and their phenotypically transformed counterpart, the myofibroblasts. Similar results were obtained for hyaluronan, which also is synthesized exclusively in fat-storing cells[36,37].

Further on, response to mitogenic stimuli at different stages of the phenotypic transformation of the fat-storing cell was investigated[14]. Untransformed fat-storing cells and myofibroblasts showed a different response to mitogenic stimuli with respect to the expression of the core proteins of biglycan and decorin. TGF-β_1, as well as transiently acidified conditioned media from Kupffer cells and myofibroblasts, enhanced the relative abundance of biglycan and decorin mRNAs up to five times in the primary cultures of fat-storing cells, but remained ineffective in myofibroblasts. On the contrary, TGF-α and native conditioned media, both ineffective in primary cultures of fat-storing cells, were most effective in increasing the steady-state levels of both proteoglycan mRNA transcripts in fully transformed myofibroblasts. These data provide evidence for a differential expression (signalling?) for both proteoglycans in dependence of the degree of phenotypic transformation of the fat-storing cell.

Gene expression of keratan sulphate bearing core proteins (fibromodulin, lumican, aggrecan) in liver

Subsequent to the proteoglycans biglycan and decorin, both belonging to the family of small proteoglycans consisting of leucin-rich, repeating motifs, we have investigated two further members of this family, *fibromodulin* and *lumican*. The proteoglycans mentioned are supposed to have arisen from a common ancestral gene[38]. They are shown to be capable of binding TGF-β_1[39], fibronectin[40] and collagen[41] via their core proteins and of influencing (with the exception of biglycan) the synthesis rate and properties of the collagen fibrils as well as the cell adhesion. In contrast to biglycan and decorin, the core proteins of fibromodulin[42] and lumican[43] have been demonstrated to possess keratan sulphate glycosaminoglycan side-chains in the tissues studied, i.e. in the tendon, cartilage and cornea. Because genes of common ancestral origin do often display co-ordinated expression patterns with respect to the cell type, it seemed not illogical to investigate the expression of fibromodulin and lumican in the liver. If this could prove true the proteoglycans mentioned could account, at least partially, for the spurious trace amounts of keratan sulphate synthesis reported in the liver[10]. For completion, aggrecan, another representative of the keratan sulphate bearing proteoglycans, was included in our investigation. It is, however, not definitely elucidated whether this proteoglycan in rat does possess keratan sulphate chains because of its lack of the so-called HABR (*h*yaluronic *a*cid-*b*inding *r*egion) where in other species the majority of keratan sulphate glycosaminoglycan chains is attached.

At the beginning of our studies only the aggrecan homologue of the rat gene was sufficiently characterized; thus, it was the only suitable candidate for *in situ* hybridization. The technique revealed expression of the core protein gene of this proteoglycan during the acute inflammatory response of the liver parenchyma subsequent to thioacetamide poisoning (time point of

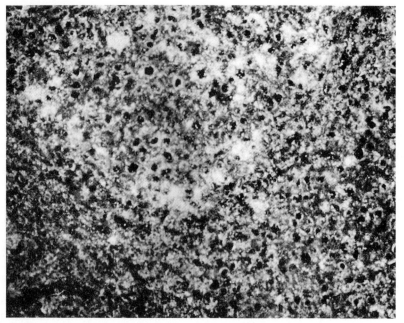

Fig. 6 Dark field micrograph of an *in situ* hybridization of aggrecan in a regeneration node of a cirrhotic rat liver. Signals (bright spots) appear predominantly in cells localized at the limiting plate adjacent to the septum

2 weeks since the onset of thioacetamide administration). Thereafter, the expression levels dropped substantially, scattered cells localized at the limiting plate of proliferating nodes remained but signal positive even in the fully developed cirrhotic stage (Fig. 6). The expressing cells showed good correlation up to the cirrhotic stage with the immunocytochemical staining using the BMA 0370 antibody which is directed against an epitope present on (human) sessile tissue macrophages and Kupffer cells. From now on, discrepancies in terms of positive *in situ* signal but negative immunocytochemistry occurred. To clarify this we have performed an RNAase A protection assay (RPA) using the mRNA extracted from entire acute inflamed liver, hepatocytes and Kupffer cells. This method has confirmed the Kupffer cells as the most potent source of aggrecan. A protected fragment of the predicted 228 bp length was, anyway, present also in the hepatocyte mRNA, though at extremely low intensity. The reason for this observation was most probably the presence of impurities in the hepatocyte cell preparation caused by Kupffer cells[15].

The fibromodulin and lumican rat homologues had to be characterized prior to their application for *in situ* hybridization purposes. A computer-aided inter-species comparison between bovine fibromodulin and chicken lumican revealed a homology of more than 50%; the homology of the chicken lumican to its rat pendant was estimated to approximately the same extent based on the results obtained by genomic blots so that a clear-cut

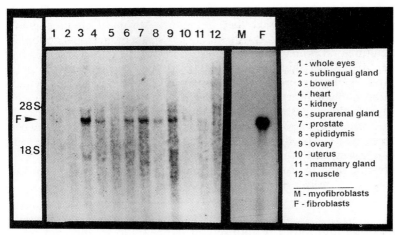

Fig. 7 Northern blot hybridization of rat fibromodulin (F). Total RNA extracted from whole organs and cultured cells was applied at 30 μg per lane, autoradiographs were exposed for 24 h at −70°C. Myofibroblasts are devoid of fibromodulin mRNA

interpretation of the eventually obtained results could prove difficult. The blots containing rat genomic DNA revealed a homology to the bovine fibromodulin of approximately 80–90%, thus focusing our search primarily on this gene. By use of PCR with degenerated oligonucleotides a fragment of the rat homologue was identified, cloned and sequenced. It shared a 97% homology at the amino acid level, the amino acid exchanges being preponderantly of conservative type. Subsequent Northern hybridization with various rat tissues, in order to define the most suitable RNA for the construction of a cDNA bank, revealed strong signals in the skin and tendon fibroblasts (Fig. 7), moderate signals in the sternal cartilage, the bowel and stomach and signals of low intensity but predicted length of about 3.5 kb in other parts of the gastrointestinal tract, RNA extracted from whole eyes, various parts of the male and female genitourinary tract, from the brain and from the muscle. Cultured myofibroblasts did not allow detection of a hybridization signal with the fibromodulin cDNA. Although *in situ* hybridization results are lacking at present, it may, based on the data obtained, be expected that fibromodulin is expressed in the liver in fibroblasts, mainly those accompanying the major branches of the portal vein, but not in transformed fat-storing cells (myofibroblasts).

Rat lumican has not been extensively studied yet. It represents a single-copy gene on the rat genome with a homology between the rat and chicken genes estimated to about 65%. As in the chicken, Northern blot hybridization of rat tissues reveals a closely spaced doublet of 1.8 kb length, the probe hybridizing selectively but tissue-specifically either to the upper, to the lower or to both parts of this doublet. This finding suggests a tissue-specific splicing by either a cassette splicing or, more probably, by alternate polyadenylation. In the liver, the cDNA hybridizes solely to the upper part of this doublet[15]. The intensity of the signal does not change substantially during the process of liver fibrosis, thus suggesting a relatively constant population of liver cells.

It remains to be added that immunocytochemical staining delivered consistently negative results with keratan sulphate monoclonal antibodies in the cultured rat primary and transformed fat-storing cells. This could be due either to the fact that fat-storing cells do not contribute to the putative keratan sulphate expression or, alternatively, the proteoglycans defined as keratan sulphate bearing in other tissues do possess in the liver side-chains, if any, of other kinds than keratan sulphate.

In conclusion, we could prove that the genes of the core proteins of certain proteoglycans defined as keratan sulphate glycosaminoglycan bearing in other tissues are expressed in the liver tissue. In case of aggrecan its expression shows a distinct temporal and spatial pattern during the process of development of liver fibrosis.

Cytokines mediating proteoglycan expression in cultured fat-storing cells

Previously obtained results have shown that supernatants from cultured Kupffer cells, myofibroblasts and platelet lysate promote proliferation[23,44-48] and proteoglycan synthesis[22,47] of fat-storing cells in monolayer culture. Interestingly, transient acidification of the conditioned media whereby latent TGF-β_1 is activated, increased proteoglycan synthesis and reduced proliferation of fat-storing cells[45,47]. To demonstrate that TGF-β_1 represented the fibrogenic activity in Kupffer cell- and myofibroblast-conditioned media these fluids were incubated for 1 h with the neutralizing antibodies to TGF-β_1 before they were added to fat-storing cells. As shown in Fig. 8, increasing doses of anti-TGF-β_1 depressed proteoglycan synthesis and converted the growth-inhibiting activity to a growth stimulation. These results demonstrate that TGFβ_1 is responsible for at least a part of the effects obtained with media conditioned by Kupffer cells and myofibroblasts (Fig. 8). TGF-α is suggested to represent the responsible mitogen in these media[47]. The mRNAs of both TGFs could be detected in Kupffer cells, preferentially in activated Kupffer cells[47] and in myofibroblasts[45].

Studies evaluating the dose response to TGF-α and TGF-β_1 stimuli have shown that TGF-α (5 ng/ml) stimulated glycosaminoglycan synthesis of fat-storing cells to a maximum of 1.2–1.4-fold, TGF-β_1 (2.0 ng/ml) to a maximum of 2.2-fold[49]. However, since TGF-α stimulated proliferation of early cultured fat-storing cells too, glycosaminoglycan synthesis was stimulated to a maximum of 1.9-fold per culture well by 5 ng/ml TGF-α. Northern blot hybridization (data not shown) and slot–blot hybridization experiments have shown that TGF-β_1 enhanced the steady-state levels of the decorin mRNA in fat-storing cells 2.7-fold and that of biglycan 2.4-fold of controls (Fig. 9). TGF-α was ineffective to elevate decorin or biglycan mRNA in fat-storing cells. In contrast to primary cultures TGF-α (but not TGF-β) in myofibroblasts (tertiary cultures) enhanced the steady-state levels of decorin (1.35-fold) and biglycan (1.75-fold) mRNA (Fig. 9). These results have been confirmed at the glycosaminoglycan- and core-protein level[49]. As shown in

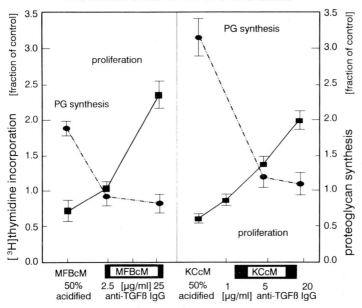

Fig. 8 Effect of neutralizing anti-TGF-β_1 IgG on myofibroblast and Kupffer cell-induced stimulation of proteoglycan synthesis and inhibition of fat-storing cell proliferation. Anti-TGF-β IgG (2.5, 12.5 and 25 μg/ml) was added to MFB- and KC-conditioned media and incubated for 1 h at 21°C on a rotating platform. Thereafter these media were added to FSC monolayers in the appropriate concentrations at the 3rd and 4th day after seeding. Proteoglycan synthesis was quantified by β-counting after [^{35}S]sulphate incorporation and binding of the proteoglycans to DEAE-Sephacel. Proliferation was determined by [^{3}H]thymidine incorporation into DNA

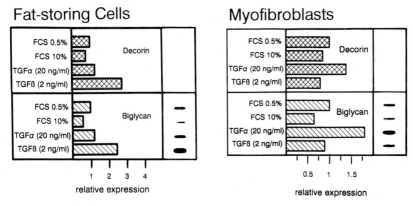

Fig. 9 Effects of TGFs on the expression of the decorin and biclycan mRNAs in fat-storing cells and myofibroblasts. Cultured fat-storing cells and myofibroblasts were exposed for 48 h to 20 ng/ml TGF-α and 2 ng/ml TGF-β_1, respectively. Total cellular RNA (each slot 15 μg) was analysed by slot–blot hybridization under high-stringency conditions. The intensity of the autoradiographic signals was quantitated by laser densitometry and expressed as relative densitometric units compared to the signal intensity of fat-storing cells and myofibroblasts grown in 0.5% fetal calf serum after correction for ribosomal S6 expression

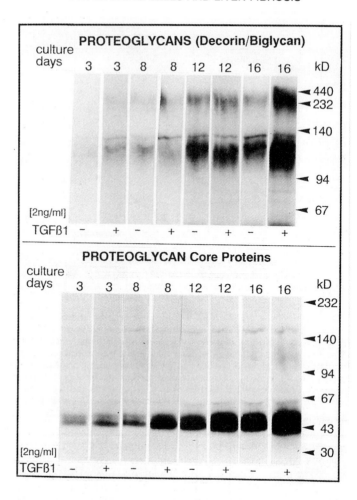

Fig. 10 Spontaneous and TGF-β_1-induced increase in proteoglycan- and core-protein synthesis during primary culture of fat-storing cells. TGF-β_1 (2 ng/ml) was added at the 2nd, 7th, 11th and 15th day, respectively. Cells were labelled during 24 h with 200 μCi [^{3}H]leucin/ml medium. Medium proteoglycans were isolated by binding to DEAE-Sephacel. An aliquot of the isolated proteoglycans was subjected to chondroitin-ABC-lyase. Proteoglycans were fractionated using a 4–12% gradient gel, for proteoglycan core proteins a 7% gel was used. Fluorography was performed during 48 h using Hyperfilm MP with an intensifying screen. Molecular weight standards are indicated

Fig. 10 by fluorography after SDS electrophoresis the synthesis of the small proteoglycans and proteoglycan–core proteins which are suggested to represent decorin and biglycan increasing during primary culture from the 3rd to the 16th day. Addition of TGF-β_1 (2 ng/ml) significantly increased [^{3}H]leucin incorporation into these core proteins (Fig. 10).

Since Kupffer cells, platelets and myofibroblasts release additional cyto-

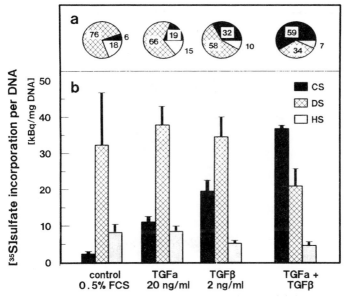

Fig. 11 Effects of TGF-α, TGF-β_1 and a combination of both TGFs on the synthesis of specific types of glycosaminoglycans secreted by fat-storing cells. TGFs were added at the 2nd and 3rd day after seeding alone and in combination to cultured fat-storing cells. Glycosaminoglycan side-chains were determined after enzymatic and chemical degradation of total proteoglycans as described in Methods. (**a**) Relative amount; (**b**) absolute amount

kines including platelet-derived growth factor, interleukin-1 and -6, basic fibroblast growth factor, tumour necrosis factor α and insulin-like growth factor, of which a variable combination will challenge fat-storing cells and myofibroblasts *in vivo* simultaneously, the effects of these cytokines alone and in various combinations on proteoglycan synthesis of fat-storing cells were determined. Platelet-derived growth factor, insulin-like growth factor I and II, interleukins 1 and 6, and basic fibroblast growth factor displayed no significant effect on proteoglycan synthesis of fat-storing cells. However, as shown in Figs 11 and 12, proteoglycan synthesis of fat-storing cells might be potentiated by combining different growth factors. While addition of 20 ng/ml TGF-α to cultured fat-storing cells resulted in a 3-fold increase of chondroitin sulphate synthesis and TGF-β_1 (2 ng/ml) caused an 8-fold increase of chondroitin sulphate synthesis, the combination of both TGFs enhanced chondroitin sulphate synthesis 15-fold, whereas the synthesis of dermatan sulphate and heparan sulphate slightly decreased (Fig. 11). In fat-storing cells predominantly chondroitin sulphate synthesis was stimulated by TGFs, in myofibroblasts the synthesis of all types of glycosaminoglycans was stimulated by TGFs (data not shown). Furthermore, as shown by Fig. 12, the synthesis of the core proteins of decorin and biglycan is stimulated to a higher extent by a combination of TGF-β_1 with TNF-α compared to the sum of the effects of the single growth factors (2 ng/ml TGF-β_1 2.2-fold of control, 8 ng/ml TNF-α 1.6-fold and the combination of TGF-β_1 and

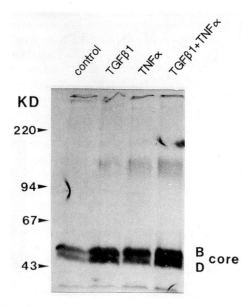

Fig. 12 Effects of TGF-β_1, TNF-α and a combination of both on the synthesis of the decorin and biglycan core proteins. Cultured fat-storing cells were stimulated with 2 ng/ml TGF-β_1 and 8 ng/ml TNF-α on the 3rd and 4th day after seeding. Cells were labelled with 200 μCi [^{3}H]leucine/ml medium. Medium proteoglycans were isolated by binding to DEAE-Sephacel and glycosaminoglycan side-chains were cleaved using chondroitin-ABC-lyase. Decorin and biglycan core proteins were fractionated in 10% gel (SDS-PAGE) and visualized by fluorography. Molecular weight standards are indicated

TNF-α 4.6-fold). Maximum stimulation of proteoglycan synthesis was obtained by a synthetic medium consisting of Dulbecco's modification of Eagle's medium with 4 ng/ml TGF-β_1, 50 ng/ml TGF-α, 20 ng/ml IGF-1, 20 ng/ml PDGF (BB), 20 ng/ml TNF-α and 2.5 U/ml thrombin (Fig. 13). The stimulatory effect of this medium was even higher than the effect obtained by 10% fetal calf serum.

Furthermore, since (1) myofibroblasts expressed the type I and II TGF-β receptors as well as the EGF/TGF-α receptor[49], (2) myofibroblasts respond to added TGFs by enhanced proteoglycan[50] and fibronectin synthesis[51] and (3) myofibroblasts synthesize TGFs[49], autocrine stimulatory mechanisms are suggested. To prove this hypothesis neutralizing anti-TGF-α and anti-TGF-β_1 immunoglobulins were added to highly active myofibroblasts. Hereby proteoglycan (Fig. 14) and fibronectin synthesis (data not shown) were reduced significantly. The modest effects of only 20–30% reduction of proteoglycan synthesis obtained by the use of neutralizing antibodies might be explained by the facts that (1) TGFs probably represent not the only fibrogenic mediators produced by myofibroblasts, (2) TGF-β, which is secreted in the latent form, might not bind to anti-TGF-β, and (3) the factors might bind even intracellularly to their receptors as shown in v-sis-transformed cells for PDGF[52]. To overcome some of these difficulties we used

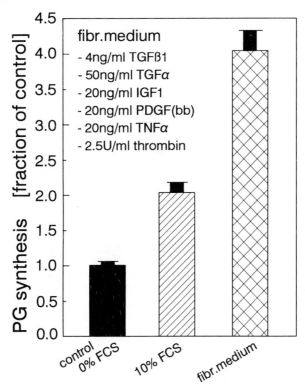

Fig. 13 Effect of a combination of several growth mediators and thrombin on proteoglycan synthesis fat-storing cells. Cultured fat-storing cells were stimulated with 50 ng/ml TGF-α, 4 ng/ml TGF-β_1, 20 ng/ml IGF-1, 20 ng/ml PDGF(BB), 20 ng/ml TNF–α and 2.5 U/ml thrombin (in the absence of fetal calf serum) or alternatively with 10% fetal calf serum on the 3rd and 4th day after seeding. Cells were labelled for 24 h with 30 μCi [^{35}S]sulphate/ml medium. Medium proteoglycans were quantified by β-counting after isolation using binding to DEAE-Sephacel. Control represents unstimulated cells (without fetal calf serum)

a TGF-β_1-antisense oligonucleotide to block TGF-β_1 synthesis. Addition of 1, 5 and 10 μmol/l TGF-β_1 antisense thiophosphonate-oligonucleotide to highly active myofibroblasts in culture reduced fibronectin synthesis significantly by 25%, 42% and 48% respectively (Fig. 15) and proteoglycan synthesis by 12–23%. These results provide strong evidence that in particular TGF-β_1 represents a positive autocrine regulator of matrix synthesis in myofibroblasts.

Acknowledgements

The financial support of the Deutsche Forschungsgemeinschaft by grant Gr 463/10-1, technical assistance by Birgit Lahme, Brigitte Heitmann, Markus Fischer and Lothar Scheckel, and the excellent secretarial help of Inge Schmidt are gratefully acknowledged.

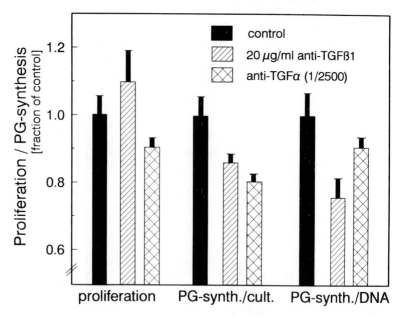

Fig. 14 Effects of neutralizing anti-TGF-β_1 IgG and anti-TGF-α IgG on autocrine stimulated proteoglycan synthesis in myofibroblasts. Anti-TGF-β and anti-TGF-α were added to cultured myofibroblasts. Proteoglycan synthesis was quantified by β-counting after [^{35}S]sulphate incorporation and binding of the proteoglycans to DEAE-Sephacel

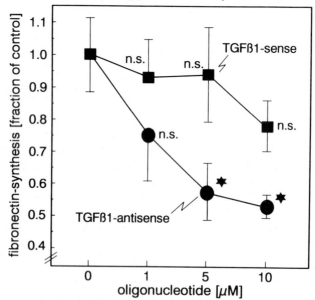

Fig. 15 Effects of an TGF-β_1-antisense oligonucleotide on autocrine-stimulated fibronectin synthesis in myofibroblasts. Thiophosphonate-oligonucleotides (1, 5 and 10 μmol/l TGF-β_1 antisense and TGF-β_1-sense) were added to cultured myofibroblasts (in the absence of fetal calf serum). Medium was harvested 48 h later and fibronectin was determined by time-resolved fluorescence

References

1. Schuppan D. Structure of the extracellular matrix in normal and fibrotic liver: collagens and glycoproteins. Semin Liver Dis. 1990;10:1–10.
2. Gressner AM. Liver fibrosis: perspectives in pathobiochemical research and clinical outlook. Eur J Clin Chem Clin Biochem. 1991;29:293–311.
3. Gressner AM. Hepatic fibrogenesis: the puzzle of interacting cells, fibrogenic cytokines, regulatory loops, and extracellular matrix molecules. Z Gastroenterol. 1992 (Suppl. 1):30: 5–16.
4. Gressner AM. Hepatic proteoglycans – a brief survey of their pathobiochemical implications. Hepato-Gastroenterol. 1983;30:225–9.
5. Ruoslahti E. Structure and biology of proteoglycans. Annu Rev Cell Biol. 1988;4:229–55.
6. Murata K, Akashio K, Ochiai Y. Changes in acidic glycosaminoglycan components at different. Hepato-Gastroenterol. 1984;31:261–5.
7. Murata K, Ochiai Y, Akashio K. Polydispersity of acidic glycosaminoglycan components in human liver and the changes at different stages in liver cirrhosis. Gastroenterology. 1985;89:1248–57.
8. Galambos JT, Shapira R. Natural history of alcoholic hepatitis. Glycosaminoglycuronans and collagen in the hepatic connective tissue. J Clin Invest. 1973;52:2952–62.
9. Stuhlsatz HW, Vierhaus S, Gressner AM et al. The distribution pattern of structural differences of the glycosaminoglycans in normal and cirrhotic human liver. In: Popper H, Reutter W, Gudat F, Köttgen E, editors. Structural carbohydrates in the liver. Lancaster: MTP Press; 1983:650–1.
10. Gressner AM, Pazen H, Greiling H. The biosynthesis of glycosaminoglycans in normal rat liver and in response to experimental hepatic injury. Hoppe Seyler's Z Physiol Chem. 1977;358:825–33.
11. Olds RG, Finegan C, Kresina TF. Dynamic of hepatic glycosaminoglycan accumulation in murine *Schistosoma japonicum* infection. Gastroenterology. 1986;91:1335–42.
12. Poole AR. Proteoglycans in health and disease: structures and functions. Biochem J. 1986;236:1–14.
13. Kjellen L, Lindahl U. Proteoglycans – structures and interactions. Annu Rev Biochem. 1991;60:443–76.
14. Meyer DH, Krull N, Dreher KL et al. Biglycan and decorin gene expression in normal and fibrotic rat liver: cellular localization and regulatory factors. Hepatology. 1992;16:204–16.
15. Krull N, Gressner AM. Differential expression of keratan sulfate proteoglycans fibromodulin, lumican and aggrecan in normal and fibrotic rat liver. FEBS Lett. 1992;312:47–52.
16. Gressner AM, Heinrigs S, Grouls P. The sequence of changes in the biosynthesis of sulfated glycosaminoglycans in acute, experimental liver disease. J Clin Chem Clin Biochem. 1982;20:15–24.
17. Gressner AM, Köster-Eiserfunke W. Synthesis of hepatic glycosaminoglycans in the early stages of galactosamine hepatitis: a rapid decline of heparan sulfate is followed by elevation of chondroitin sulfate and dermatan sulfate. J Clin Chem Clin Biochem. 1981;19:363–70.
18. Gressner AM, Pazen H, Greiling H. The synthesis of total and specific glycosaminoglycans during development of experimental liver cirrhosis. Experientia. 1977;33:1290–2.
19. Krull N, Zimmermann T, Gressner AM. Spatial and temporal patterns of gene expression for the proteoglycans biglycan and decorin and for transforming growth factor-beta 1 revealed by in situ hybridization during experimentally induced liver fibrosis in the rat. Hepatology. 1993;18:581–9.
20. DeLeeuw AM, McCarthy SP, Geerts A et al. Purified rat liver fat-storing cells in culture divide and contain collagen. Hepatology. 1984;4:392–403.
21. Schäfer S, Zerbe O, Gressner AM. The synthesis of proteoglycans in fat-storing cells of rat liver. Hepatology. 1987;7:680–7.
22. Gressner AM, Zerbe O. Kupffer cell-mediated induction of synthesis and secretion of proteoglycans by rat liver fat-storing cells in culture. J Hepatol. 1987;5:299–310.
23. Zerbe O, Gressner AM. Proliferation of fat storing cells is stimulated by secretions of Kupffer cells from normal and injured liver. Exp Mol Pathol. 1988;49:87–101.
24. Gressner AM, Pfeiffer T. Preventive effects of acute inflammation on liver cell necrosis and inhibition of heparan sulfate synthesis in hepatocytes. J Clin Chem Clin Biochem.

1986;24:821–9.
25. Seglen PO. Preparation of isolated rat liver cells. In: Prescott DM, editor. Methods in cell biology, Vol. 8. New York: Academic Press; 1987:29–83.
26. Tecott LH, Eberwine JH, Barchas JD *et al.* Methodological considerations in the utilization of in situ hybridization. In: Valentino KL, Eberwine JH, Barchas JD, editors. In situ hybridization. Oxford: Oxford University Press; 1987:3–24.
27. Chirgwin JM, Przybyla AE, MacDonald RJ *et al.* Isolation of biologically active ribonucleic acid from sources enriched in ribonuclease. Biochemistry. 1979;18:5294–9.
28. Gressner AM, Schäfer S. Comparison of sulphated glycosaminoglycan and hyaluronate synthesis and secretion in cultured hepatocytes, fat storing cells, and Kupffer cells. J Clin Chem Clin Biochem. 1989;27:141–9.
29. Kropf J, Bötel T, Gressner AM. Time-resolved immunoassay for cell-bound antigens in the solid phase status using cultured cells. Fresenius Z Anal Chem. 1992;334:54–5.
30. Kropf J, Quitte E, Gressner AM. Time-resolved immunofluorometric assays with measurement of a europium chelate in solution. Anal Biochem. 1991;197:258–65.
31. Meyer DH, Zimmermann T, Müller D *et al.* The synthesis of glycosaminoglycans in isolated hepatocytes during experimental liver fibrogenesis. Liver. 1990;10:94–105.
32. Gressner AM. Time-related distribution profiles of sulfated glycosaminoglycans in cells, cell surfaces and media of cultured rat liver fat-storing cells. Proc Soc Exp Biol Med. 1991;196:307–15.
33. Witsch P, Kresse H, Gressner AM. Biosynthesis of small proteoglycans by hepatic lipocytes in primary culture. FEBS Lett. 1989;258:233–5.
34. Ross RS, Eyken Van P, Desmet VJ *et al.* Immunocytochemical monitoring of different glycosaminoglycans in cultures of rat liver fat storing cells. In: Gressner AM, Ramadori G, editors. Molecular and cell biology of liver fibrogenesis [Proceedings of International Falk Symposium, Marburg]. Dordrecht: Kluwer; 1992:155–8.
35. Krull N, Zimmermann T, Lehnhardt A *et al.* Detection of expression of the proteoglycans biglycan and decorin and of TGFb1 by means of in-situ hybridization during experimentally induced liver fibrosis in rat. In: Gressner AM, Ramadori G, editors. Molecular and cell biology of liver fibrogenesis [Proceedings of the International Falk Symposium, Marburg]. Dordrecht: Kluwer; 1992:137–44.
36. Gressner AM, Haarmann R. Hyaluronic acid synthesis and secretion by rat liver fat storing cells (perisinusoidal lipocytes) in culture. Biochem Biophys Res Commun. 1988;151:222–9.
37. Gressner AM, Haarmann R. Regulation of hyaluronate synthesis in rat liver fat-storing cell cultures by Kupffer cells. J Hepatol. 1988;7:310–18.
38. Fisher LW, Heegaard AM, Vetter U *et al.* Human biglycan gene. J Biol Chem. 1991;266:14371–7.
39. Yamaguchi Y, Ruoslahti E. Expression of human proteoglycan in Chinese hamster ovary cells inhibits cell proliferation. Nature. 1988;336:244–6.
40. Winnemöller M, Schmidt G, Kresse H. Influence of decorin on fibroblast adhesion to fibronectin. Eur J Cell Biol. 1991;54:10–17.
41. Pringle GA, Dodd CM. Immunoelectron microscopic localization of the core protein of decorin near the d and e bands of tendon collagen fibrils by use of monoclonal antibodies. J Histochem Cytochem. 1990;38:1405–11.
42. Oldberg A, Antonsson P, Lindblom K *et al.* A collagen-binding 59-kd protein (fibromodulin) is structurally related to the small interstitial proteoglycans PG-S1 and PG-S2 (decorin). EMBO J. 1989;8:2601–4.
43. Blochberger TC, Vergnes JP, Hempel J *et al.* cDNA to chick lumican (corneal keratan sulfate proteoglycan) reveals homology to the small interstitial proteoglycan gene family and expression in muscle and intestine. J Biol Chem. 1992;267:347–52.
44. Bachem MG, Melchior R, Gressner AM. The role of thrombocytes in liver fibrogenesis: Effects of platelet lysate and thrombocyte-derived growth factors on the mitogenic activity and glycosaminoglycan synthesis of cultured rat liver fat storing cells. J Clin Chem Clin Biochem. 1989;27:555–65.
45. Bachem MG, Meyer DM, Melchior R *et al.* Activation of rat liver perisinusoidal lipocytes by transforming growth factors derived from myofibroblast-like cells – a potential mechanism of self perpetuation in liver fibrogenesis. J Clin Invest. 1992;89:19–27.
46. Friedman ASL, Arthur JP. Activation of cultured rat hepatic lipocytes by Kupffer cell

conditioned medium. J Clin Invest. 1989;84:1780–5.
47. Meyer DH, Bachem MG, Gressner AM. Modulation of hepatic lipocyte proteoglycan synthesis and proliferation by Kupffer cell-derived transforming growth factors type beta1 and type alpha. Biochem Biophys Res Commun. 1990;171:1122–9.
48. Shiratori Y, Geerts A, Ichida T et al. Kupffer cells from CCl4-induced fibrotic livers stimulate proliferation of fat-storing cells. J Hepatol. 1986;3:294–303.
49. Bachem MG, Meyer DH, Schäfer W et al. The response of rat liver perisinusoidal lipocytes to polypeptide growth regulator changes with their transdifferentiation into myofibroblast-like cells in culture. J Hepatol. 1993;18:40–52.
50. Bachem MG, Riess U, Melchior R et al. Transforming growth factors (TGF alpha and TGF beta 1) stimulate chondroitin sulfate and hyaluronate synthesis in cultured rat liver fat storing cells. FEBS Lett. 1989;257:134–7.
51. Bachem MG, Sell KM, Melchior R et al. Tumor necrosis factor alpha (TNFalpha) and transforming growth factor beta1 (TGFbeta1) stimulate fibronectin synthesis and the transdifferentiation of fat-storing cells in the rat liver into myofibroblasts. Virchows Arch B Cell Pathol. 1993;63:123–30.
52. Keating MT, Williams LT. Autocrine stimulation of intracellular PDGF receptors in v-sis-transformed cells. Science. 1988;239:914–16.

9
Matrix degradation in the liver

M. J. P. ARTHUR

INTRODUCTION

Liver fibrosis is characterized by excess deposition of matrix proteins (particularly collagen types I and III) in liver. These are largely synthesized and secreted by hepatic lipocytes (fat-storing or Ito cells) which have been activated to a myofibroblast-like phenotype. In addition to matrix synthesis, recent evidence indicates that altered matrix degradation plays an important pathogenic role in liver injury and fibrosis.

Degradation of extracellular matrix proteins is regulated by a family of enzymes called the matrix metalloproteinases. These are subdivided into three groups according to substrate profile: *collagenases* which degrade interstitial collagens (types I, II and III), *gelatinases* which degrade basement membrane (type IV) collagen and gelatins, and *stromelysins* which degrade a broad range of substrates including proteoglycans, laminin, gelatins and fibronectin. The extracellular activity of these enzymes is regulated by several mechanisms which include alterations in gene transcription and proenzyme synthesis, cleavage of secreted proenzymes to active forms, inhibition of proenzyme activation and specific inhibition of activated forms by tissue inhibitor(s) of metalloproteinases (TIMPs).

Studies have now demonstrated that activated hepatic lipocytes and other non-parenchymal liver cells secrete many of the matrix metalloproteinases (Table 1), as well as factors involved in both activation of these proenzymes and specific inhibition of active enzymes. These cells therefore have the ability both to degrade and regulate degradation of matrix proteins in liver. The role of this carefully regulated matrix-degrading system in normal and diseased liver is not yet clearly defined, but there is increasing evidence, to be reviewed in this chapter, for altered matrix turnover in liver injury, liver regeneration and liver fibrosis.

THE MATRIX METALLOPROTEINASES

The matrix metalloproteinases are a family of enzymes with many common biochemical properties that exhibit degradative activity against a variety of

Table 1 Nomenclature, substrate specificity and hepatic origin of metalloproteinases

New nomenclature	Synonyms	Substrate profile	Cellular origin in liver
Collagenases			
Interstitial collagenase	MMP-1	III > I, II, VII, X	Lipocytes
Neutrophil collagenase	MMP-5	I > III, II	—
Gelatinases			
Gelatinase A	MMP-2 72 kDa type IV collagenase/gelatinase	IV, ?V, VII, X, gelatin	Lipocytes
Gelatinase B	MMP-9 92 kDa type IV collagenase/gelatinase	IV, V, gelatin, ?III	Kupffer cells
Stromelysins			
Stromelysin-1	MMP-3, Transin (in rat), Proteoglycanase	III, IV, V, IX, laminin, proteoglycans, fibronectin, casein	Lipocytes?
Stromelysin-2	MMP-10, Transin-2 (in rat)	As for stromelysin-1	Not known
Matrilysin	MMP-7, PUMP-1	IV, proteoglycans, fibronectin, gelatins, elastin	Not known
Stromelysin-3	—	Not known	Not known
Others			
Metalloelastase	—	Elastin, fibronectin	Not known

111

extracellular matrix proteins. There are currently nine identifiable members of this gene family, each of which encodes for an enzyme with a specific matrix protein substrate profile. The modern nomenclature for these enzymes, synonyms, and substrate profile, together with current knowledge of their cellular origin in liver, is summarized in Table 1.

All metalloproteinases possess several common structural domains with conserved sequences that confer important properties on these enzymes (for detailed review, see *Matrisian Bioessays* 1992;14:455–63). These include the pre- and propeptide domains which contain the highly conserved PRCGVPDV amino acid sequence (which is involved in enzyme latency), an N-terminal domain and a catalytic zinc-binding domain (amino acid sequence HELGH). All except matrilysin contain a vitronectin-like domain, but an additional fibronectin-like domain is present in both gelatinase A and gelatinase B, with the latter also possessing a type V collagen-like domain[1,2]. These additional domains provide metalloproteinases with the ability to bind to and degrade different substrates, giving the family a wide profile of matrix degradative activity (Table 1). Individual metalloproteinases and their properties will be described, with information provided in the context of their specific or potential role in normal or diseased liver. In addition there is increasing evidence for changes in the activity of these enzymes in liver to be mediated not only by changes in biosynthesis but also by alterations in proenzyme activation and specific inhibition of active enzymes. The pathways involved in regulating metalloproteinase activity will therefore be described further.

METALLOPROTEINASE REGULATION

The biosynthesis and activity of matrix metalloproteinases are closely regulated, presumably to exert ordered control over degradation of all types of extracellular matrix. This may be important in regulating physiological processes such as organogenesis, morphogenesis, tissue regeneration and wound healing or repair. In contrast, disordered regulation of extracellular metalloproteinase activity may contribute to pathological processes such as neoplasia/metastasis, connective tissue destruction and progressive fibrosis.

Matrix metalloproteinases are regulated at several different levels, facilitating a fine level of control over their extracellular degradative activity. Mechanisms of regulation are complex and include: regulation of prometalloproteinase biosynthesis at the level of gene transcription, differing (and often regulated) pathways of extracellular prometalloproteinase activation, and specific inhibition of active metalloproteinases by TIMPs. More recent data indicate that TIMPs may also be involved in an additional level of regulatory control by binding to prometalloproteinases (at the carboxyl terminus) and preventing their autocleavage to active enzymes, i.e. prometalloproteinase stabilization.

Metalloproteinase gene expression

This is regulated in most cell types by a combination of growth factors, cytokines and retinoids. Many of these co-regulate expression of several members of the metalloproteinase family, but others specifically regulate expression of individual genes. Many of the effects of these factors are mediated via stimulation (or inhibition) of the proto-oncogenes c-fos and c-jun[3]. Products of the latter genes are transactivating factors which bind to the activator protein-1 (AP-1) promoter site of the metalloproteinase genes (particularly procollagenase and prostromelysin) and increase their transcription. The well-characterized effects of individual cytokines, growth factors and retinoids on metalloproteinase gene expression are summarized in Table 2.

The effects of two of these factors on metalloproteinase expression, TGF-β_1 and retinoids, are directly relevant to liver because of their known overall importance to the pathogenesis of liver fibrosis. TGF-β_1 is of major interest because it inversely co-regulates expression of different members of the metalloproteinase family; gelatinase A expression is increased, but expression of stromelysin-1 and interstitial collagenase is decreased[4,5]. Retinoic acid also inhibits expression of interstitial collagenase[6]. TGF-β_1 and retinoids also have marked stimulatory effects on the expression of metalloproteinase inhibitors (see below), thus their likely overall effect in liver would be to inhibit degradation of fibrillar interstitial matrix and promote the progression of liver fibrosis (see below).

Activation of prometalloproteinases

This is an important regulatory step in determining the extracellular activity of these enzymes. Metalloproteinases are secreted predominantly as latent proenzymes which must undergo activation before they exhibit degradative activity against extracellular matrix proteins. Activation is effected by disruption of the interaction between a cysteine residue in the propeptide domain and the zinc molecule at the catalytic site of the metalloproteinase. This leads to cleavage of the propeptide (~ 80 amino acids) and conversion to an activated metalloproteinase[7,8]. This is achieved by a variety of mechanisms, which can differ for individual metalloproteinases. *In vivo*, the best-characterized mechanism of metalloproteinase activation involves urokinase–plasminogen activator (uPA) or tissue plasminogen activator (tPA) which both initiate a proteolytic cascade converting plasminogen to plasmin (Fig. 1). This in turn partially activates both procollagenase and prostromelysin[9]. The active form of stromelysin then leads to full activation of interstitial collagenase[9,10]. The promoter region of uPA is known to contain an AP-1 binding site[11], implying that uPA expression may be coregulated with premetalloproteinase expression, enabling the cascade mechanism of activation to proceed. Plasminogen activator inhibitor-1 (PAI-1) may also be produced by cells that synthesize metalloproteinases[9], and this may play an important regulatory role by inhibiting this cascade

Table 2 Factors involved in regulating metalloproteinases and TIMPs

	Metalloproteinase expression		Inhibitor expression	
	Increased	*Decreased*	*Increased*	*Decreased*
TGF-β_1	Gelatinase A	Interstitial collagenase, stromelysin-1	TIMP-1	TIMP-2
Retinoic acid	—	Interstitial collagenase	TIMP-1	—
EGF or b-FGF	Interstitial collagenase	—	TIMP-1	—
IL-1 or TNF-α or PDGF	Interstitial collagenase	—	—	—

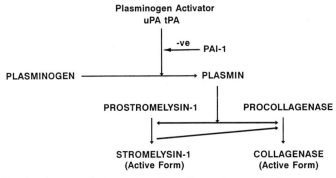

Fig. 1 The plasminogen activator system of metalloproteinase activation

mechanism. Other proteolytic enzymes are also involved in promoting metalloproteinase activation, including mast cell tryptase[12], neutrophil elastase, and cathepsin G[13]. In contrast, the plasminogen activator cascade and other proteolytic enzymes have no effect on progelatinase A, but this enzyme is activated by interaction with a cell membrane-associated protein[14,15]. Progelatinase A binds to an as yet unidentified protein in the cell membrane, and undergoes conformational change that promotes self-cleavage to active gelatinase A. This membrane-associated mechanism of activation is unique to progelatinase A and does not activate the proenzyme forms of other metalloproteinases[14].

Inhibition of active metalloproteinases

This is an important mechanism of regulating their extracellular degradative activity. Active metalloproteinases may be inhibited by entrapment within proteinase scavengers, such as α_2-macroglobulin[16,17] or by interaction with the specific TIMPs, which bind to the active site of metalloproteinases and inhibit their degradative activity[18]. Three members of the TIMP family have been described (TIMP-1, TIMP-2 and CHIMP or TIMP-3). Of these TIMP-1 and TIMP-2 have been characterized in detail, whereas TIMP-3 is recently described and less well characterized[19]. Each TIMP is the product of a separate gene, and although there is some sequence homology (40% homology between TIMP-1 and TIMP-2), TIMP-1 and TIMP-2 exhibit distinct properties and differ in their regulatory pathways (Table 2). Current evidence suggests that, for certain metalloproteinases, TIMP-1 and TIMP-2 can interact in a complex manner, binding either to the catalytic site of enzymes or at other sites on the proenzyme that can prevent cleavage of the propeptide and enzyme activation (see below). This notwithstanding, a broad overview indicates that TIMP-2 is particularly important in the inhibition of gelatinase A[20,21], whereas TIMP-1 is most relevant to the inhibition of interstitial collagenase, stromelysin and gelatinase B.

It is important to note that TIMP-1 and TIMP-2 gene expression can be regulated by the same growth factors and cytokines involved in regulating expression of metalloproteinase genes (see Table 2). Expression can be co-regulated, e.g. EGF and b-FGF increase both interstitial collagenase and TIMP-1 gene expression, or inversely co-regulated, e.g. TGF-β_1 decreases interstitial collagenase, stromelysin and TIMP-2 gene expression, but increases expression of TIMP-1 and gelatinase A[4,5,22,23]. Retinoids also inhibit expression of interstitial collagenase but increase expression of TIMP-1[6]. Several factors which are known to influence these regulatory pathways, e.g. cytokines, growth factors and retinoids are likely to be highly relevant in liver fibrosis.

Prometalloproteinase stabilization

This is a further, more recently recognized, mechanism involved in regulating extracellular activity of this class of enzymes. This occurs when either TIMP-1 or TIMP-2 binds to a prometalloproteinase, at a site other than the catalytic site, and inhibits proenzyme activation. This phenomenon was firstly clearly recognized for TIMP-2 which binds to the carboxyl terminus of progelatinase A and is often secreted from cells as a proenzyme–inhibitor complex[24-26]. When bound in this manner TIMP-2 can inhibit progelatinase A activation by the cell membrane-associated and other mechanisms[14,24,25]. Recent evidence suggests that this mechanism of regulating activation occurs for other members of the metalloproteinase family, as TIMP-2 has also been shown to bind to interstitial procollagenase and inhibit its proteolytic activation[27]. For progelatinase B, interaction occurs with TIMP-1 which binds to the carboxyl terminus, and this complex cannot be activated (unlike progelatinase B alone) by stromelysin or plasmin[28]. The described variety of molecular interactions between progelatinase B and TIMP-1 is the most complicated to date[28]; for example progelatinase B may form either a homodimer or a complex with interstitial collagenase, but formation of both is inhibited in the presence of TIMP-1. Once formed, however, the homodimer of progelatinase B does not bind TIMP-1 and may be activated by plasmin or stromelysin. In contrast, TIMP-1 can interact with the interstitial collagenase/progelatinase B complex, displacing active interstitial collagenase and binding preferentially to progelatinase B.

These data indicate that regulation of the extracellular activity of metallo-proteinases is much more complex than originally recognized, involving a wide variety of different and interactive mechanisms. Current concepts of the role of TIMPs include the selective inhibition of either proenzyme activation or inhibition of the catalytic site, with the intriguing possibility that different TIMPs may bind and affect individual members of the metalloproteinase family in differing ways.

MATRIX DEGRADATION IN THE LIVER

In comparison with other systems relatively little is known about matrix degradation in liver. This presumably reflects the relative inaccessibility of liver, and the inherent difficulties of studying a system as complex as the metalloproteinases and their inhibitors with earlier methodologies. The more recent application of improved liver cell culture methods (particularly sinusoidal liver cells) and molecular techniques has contributed to significant progress in our understanding of matrix degradation in the liver. Three principal areas of interest will be considered: matrix degradation in normal liver, matrix degradation in liver injury, and matrix degradation in liver fibrosis.

The role of matrix degradation in normal liver

This is undoubtedly the area about which there is the least knowledge. Metalloproteinases are generally produced in response to specific stimuli, but it is not clear whether there is a background of synthesis and release in normal tissues. There is presumably a need for matrix remodelling during organogenesis, but the author has no knowledge of studies of metalloproteinase expression in fetal liver. Similarly, there must be a requirement for a low level of matrix turnover in normal adult liver, e.g. remodelling of the basement membrane-like matrix in the space of Disse and turnover of the small quantities of pericellular and portal tract fibrillar collagens. Our own (unpublished) immunohistochemical studies have failed to detect metalloproteinases or their inhibitors at the protein level in normal human liver (even if monensin is used to enhance intracellular accumulation in biopsy material). Similarly we have not detected mRNA for metalloproteinases or their inhibitors by Northern analysis of total RNA prepared from normal human liver. If, however, we apply extremely sensitive RNAase protection assays, we have (to date) been able to detect extremely low levels of expression of mRNA for progelatinase A, interstitial collagenase and TIMP-1. The importance of being able to switch on an ordered matrix remodelling response is perhaps exemplified by the major changes required during liver regeneration. Recent preliminary data indicate that expression of transin (the rat equivalent of stromelysin) is indeed up-regulated rapidly after partial hepatectomy in the rat[29].

The role of matrix degradation in liver injury

The space of Disse contains a basement membrane-like matrix composed of type IV collagen, laminin and proteoglycans[3,30–33]. This normal liver matrix provides a critical functional role: by cell–matrix interaction(s) it maintains the specific differentiated gene functions of hepatocytes, e.g. albumin and cytochrome P450 expression[34,35] and also maintains hepatic lipocytes in a quiescent non-proliferative, non-fibrogenic phenotype[36]. Degradation of the normal liver matrix, as may occur in hepatic injury, therefore leads to major alterations in hepatocyte function and to conditions that promote the proliferation of fibrogenic hepatic lipocytes. This may in turn be an important event in the early stages of liver fibrosis. Three metalloproteinases with degradative activity against components of the normal liver matrix have been identified in liver: gelatinase A, gelatinase B and stromelysin-1.

Gelatinase A

Gelatinase A was originally described both as a type IV collagenase from studies of a murine tumour and as a gelatinase from rabbit bone cultures[37,38]. The nucleotide sequence was subsequently determined[39] and these studies confirmed that type IV collagenase and gelatinase were identical products of the same human gene. In addition to degrading native type IV collagen, gelatinase A also degrades collagen type VII, X and possibly V. In both rat and human liver our studies indicate that hepatic lipocytes are the main cellular source of gelatinase A, although Kupffer cells may also release small quantities[40-42]. These studies demonstrated that cultured hepatic lipocytes contain mRNA for gelatinase A, that immunoreactive gelatinase A could be detected in their cytoplasm and that both progelatinase and active gelatinase were present in cell culture media. Of particular interest was the observation that expression of progelatinase A was minimal or barely detectable in freshly isolated human hepatic lipocytes, with increased expression occurring in parallel with lipocyte activation in culture[42]. Lipocyte proliferation and activation is a well-recognized feature of liver injury[43,44], suggesting that gelatinase A expression occurs in, and contributes to, liver injury. Experimental evidence for this has been obtained in a rat model of macrophage-induced liver injury, in which we have demonstrated that gelatinase A expression occurs within 24–48 h of injury and that this enzyme was immunolocalized predominantly to proliferating lipocytes[45]. In diseased human liver we have demonstrated that expression of gelatinase A (as determined by immunohistochemical studies and RNAase protection analysis) is increased in comparison with normal human liver[46,47].

Gelatinase B

Gelatinase B (92–95 kDa) is the product of a metalloproteinase gene distinct from that for gelatinase A (72 kDa)[48], but the substrate profiles of the two enzymes have many similarities (see Table 1). It is released as a proenzyme predominantly from neutrophils and macrophages[49] which, when activated, exhibits degradative activity against gelatin and collagen types IV and V. In liver, Kupffer cells are the primary cellular source of this enzyme. From Kupffer cell media we have partially purified and characterized a 95 kDa enzyme which exhibited degradative activity against gelatin and native collagen types III, IV and V[50-52] and could be inhibited by EDTA, TIMP-1 or α_2-macroglobulin. In cell preparations from human liver we have demonstrated that Kupffer cells contain mRNA for gelatinase B, that the enzyme can be immunolocalized to these cells, and that they release progelatinase B and active lower molecular weight forms of the enzyme into culture medium[53,54]. For both rat and human Kupffer cells, release of enzyme activity is stimulated by factors known to promote Kupffer cell activation such as phorbol ester, zymosan or endotoxin. By immunohistochemical analysis we have also demonstrated that gelatinase B expression is increased in a proportion of diseased compared to normal human livers[53], indicating a possible role in liver injury, but sequential studies of the role of this enzyme in rat models (or other species) of liver injury are currently hampered by the lack of specific antibodies and cDNA probes.

Stromelysin-1

Stromelysin-1 is synthesized as two proenzyme species of 57 kDa (unmodified) and 60 kDa (glycosylated) respectively[55], which, when activated, exhibit degradative activity against a wide range of matrix protein and other substrates (see Table 1). Experimentally, degradative activity against casein (of appropriate molecular size at zymography) is used to detect and study stromelysin activity. In liver, this enzyme is of particular interest because of its ability to degrade all of the components of normal liver matrix: laminin, proteoglycans and type IV collagen. The cellular origin of stromelysin-1 in liver is currently under investigation. In preliminary studies we have demonstrated that activated and proliferating rat lipocytes release casein-degrading activity of appropriate molecular size, which is identified as transin (the rat equivalent of stromelysin-1) by immunoblotting. Other groups have demonstrated expression of mRNA for transin in rat liver injury induced by CCl_4 using in situ hybridization (ISH) of liver sections or Northern analysis of mRNA preparations[29,56]. By both techniques transin expression was minimal or absent in normal rat liver, but increased after CCl_4-induced liver injury, becoming detectable after 4–6 h, with peak expression occurring at 24 h. By ISH, mRNA transcripts were initially detectable over hepatocytes, but at 24–48 h were observed mainly over sinusoidal liver cells (which are probably lipocytes). To date there have been no studies of stromelysin-2 or matrilysin in liver.

In summary, several metalloproteinases with the ability to degrade normal liver matrix are synthesized by cultured sinusoidal liver cells and expressed in liver. Current evidence indicates that their expression is associated with lipocyte (or Kupffer cell) activation and liver injury. Because of the nature of their degradative activity and the functional importance of normal liver matrix, it is suggested these enzymes play a significant role in the pathogenesis of liver injury.

The role of matrix degradation in liver fibrosis

To separate the pathogenic events of liver injury from those of liver fibrosis is artificial, and many of the events described for liver injury may also be relevant to the early stages of liver fibrosis (see above). This section will concentrate on the role of metalloproteinases and their inhibitors in the more advanced or progressive stages of liver fibrosis. One principal concept that emerges is that this may occur, at least in part, due to a 'failure' of matrix degradation.

In progressive liver fibrosis there is net deposition of interstitial fibrillar collagens, which presumably occurs because the rate at which fibrillar collagens are synthesized and laid down in the extracellular space exceeds the rate of degradation by the relevant metalloproteinase, interstitial collagenase. Although the rate of collagen synthesis is clearly important, decreased collagen degradation could theoretically make a major contribution to the progression of liver fibrosis. Evidence from previous studies does indeed suggest that interstitial collagenase *activity*, and thus collagen degradation, are decreased as liver fibrosis progresses. There are several possible explanations for this observation, including: decreased procollagenase biosynthesis, decreased procollagenase activation, or specific inhibition of activated collagenase. These will be discussed with reference to the current state of knowledge in liver.

Interstitial collagenase

This has been cloned and sequenced in human fibroblasts[57] and the biochemical properties of the enzyme defined[58,59]. Interstitial collagenase is fundamentally important to the degradation of the fibrillar interstitial collagens that characterize fibrosis, because when activated it has the ability to cleave native collagens types I and III (Table 1), thus initiating degradation of these macromolecules. Cleavage occurs at a specific Gly–Ile bond forming characteristic TC^A and TC^B fragments of 1/4 and 3/4 of the original collagen molecule, respectively. These cleavage products partially denature and become susceptible to further degradation by other proteinases including the gelatinases.

In liver, earlier studies suggested that cultured Kupffer cells were the cellular source of interstitial collagenase *activity*[60,61], but these studies antedated the recognition of lipocyte contamination within Kupffer cell cultures, and are also difficult to interpret because of methodological difficulties in measuring this enzyme activity in the presence of other metalloproteinases, e.g. gelatinases. With the development of specific antibodies and cDNA probes for interstitial collagenase, and improved techniques for the purification and identification of individual sinusoidal liver cell populations, the cellular source of this enzyme in liver has been redefined. Recent data indicate that hepatic lipocytes, and not Kupffer cells, are the most important source of this enzyme. Initial evidence was obtained from studies of fibroblast-like cells prepared by outgrowth from a single human liver sample. When exposed to IL-1 or TNF-α passaged cells (of possible lipocyte origin) were demonstrated to express mRNA for interstitial collagenase and to release interstitial collagenase activity[62]. In subsequent studies we have immunolocalized interstitial collagenase to the cytoplasm of human lipocytes in primary culture[63], whilst others have detected mRNA for interstitial collagenase in total RNA prepared from human lipocytes by Northern analysis[64]. In our own studies we have found that relatively early primary human lipocyte cultures (4 days) express mRNA for interstitial collagenase, but that passaged cells prepared from these same cultures only express interstitial collagenase mRNA when exposed to cytokines such as TNF-α (unpublished observations). Milani and colleagues have reported that TGF-β_1 down-regulates interstitial collagenase expression by lipocytes[64], which is consistent with our data in passaged cells (as there is autologous expression of TGF-β_1 by such cells). In rat we have confirmed that rat hepatic lipocytes are the cellular source of interstitial collagenase (using a specific anti-rat collagenase antibody with dual immunostaining for desmin), but were unable to detect this enzyme in rat Kupffer (ED1-positive) cells. Release of interstitial collagenase activity into the culture medium of passaged rat hepatic lipocytes has also been demonstrated[65], and was recently reported to be stimulated by addition of polyunsaturated lecithin to acetaldehyde-treated lipocytes[66].

Following the original observation that liver explants obtained from CCl_4-treated rats degrade a type I collagen substratum more readily than explants from normal liver[67], there have been many attempts to study interstitial collagenase activity in progressive liver fibrosis. These studies have largely investigated interstitial collagenase activity in whole liver homogenates. Results have been widely discrepant, but a broad overview indicates that interstitial collagenase activity decreases as liver fibrosis progresses. This has been demonstrated in CCl_4-induced liver fibrosis in rat[68] and in advanced alcoholic cirrhosis in baboons and humans[69,70].

At present the biochemical basis for reduced collagenase activity is unclear, but one obvious explanation would be reduced *gene expression or biosynthesis of interstitial collagenase*. Using *in-situ* hybridization one preliminary study has reported that interstitial collagenase expression is either extremely low or absent in both normal and cirrhotic human liver, with the signal apparently located over the biliary epithelium[64]. We have recently studied interstitial collagenase expression in normal and diseased human liver by RNAase protection analysis. Using this sensitive technique we find a low level of interstitial collagenase mRNA expression in normal liver with no significant change in expression in either primary biliary cirrhosis or primary sclerosing cholangitis (liver explant material obtained from Birmingham liver transplant unit, UK). In contrast, expression of mRNA for interstitial collagenase was significantly increased in the liver of patients with autoimmune chronic active hepatitis (data presented at conference, see also TIMP-1 data below).

Decreased procollagenase activation

This is another possible explanation for the decreased interstitial collagenase activity observed in liver fibrosis. Although information about procollagenase activation in either normal or fibrotic liver is limited, there are some data for the plasminogen activating system (tPA, uPA and PAI-1). Hepatoma cell lines (HTC and Hep G2) express mRNA for, and synthesize the components of, this system including uPA[71], tPA and PAI-1[72-75]. In normal liver the pattern of expression is more restricted; tPA is expressed in normal rat liver, but uPA and PAI-1 expression are not found[76]. After systemic treatment with endotoxin there was a dramatic increase in liver PAI-1 mRNA levels, which was largely derived from sinusoidal endothelial cells[76]. The relevance of these observations to metalloproteinase activation in liver and to either liver injury or fibrosis has yet to be determined. An indication of the potential importance of this system is provided by the observation that plasminogen activator activity increases dramatically, in association with an increase in collagenase activity, as liver fibrosis resolves during treatment (with praziquantel) for murine hepatic schistomiasis[77,78]. Further studies of the mechanisms of metalloproteinase activation in liver are currently required.

Inhibition of activated collagenase

This is the final mechanism by which collagenase activity may be decreased in progressive liver fibrosis. Evidence for inhibition of collagenase activity was first obtained from studies of murine schistosomiasis[79–81]; interstitial collagenase synthesis (determined by immunoassay) and degradative activity in liver was maximal 8 weeks after experimental infection, but beyond this stage interstitial collagenase activity fell, in part due to decreased collagenase synthesis, but also due to increased synthesis of α_2-macroglobulin, which scavenges and inhibits interstitial collagenase[82]. α_2-Macroglobulin is synthesized predominantly by hepatocytes in liver, but both rat and human lipocytes have also been demonstrated to synthesize this proteinase scavenger[83,84]. It remains to be determined if local release of α_2-macroglobulin by lipocytes is important in regulating local activity of metalloproteinases in liver.

The specific metalloproteinase inhibitor, TIMP-1

This could also, by inhibition of interstitial collagenase and other metalloproteinases, play a critical role in the pathogenesis of progressive liver fibrosis. Because of the major role of hepatic lipocytes in both matrix synthesis and degradation, we have investigated whether these cells also synthesize metalloproteinase inhibitors. These studies have demonstrated TIMP-1 mRNA expression by cultured human lipocytes, have immunolocalized TIMP-1 to these cells and have confirmed release of immunoreactive TIMP-1 and TIMP-1 inhibitory activity into lipocyte culture medium[85]. The quantitative importance of TIMP-1 secretion into lipocyte medium was demonstrated by separating this inhibitor from metalloproteinases by gelatin-sepharose chromatography, which resulted in a 20-fold increase in detectable metalloproteinase activity. Furthermore by ELISA we have demonstrated that culture-activated human hepatic lipocytes release a 5–6-fold molar excess of TIMP-1 over interstitial collagenase. From these studies an important observation was that TIMP-1 mRNA expression was low or absent in freshly isolated hepatic lipocytes, but increased dramatically with lipocyte activation to a myofibroblast-like phenotype in cell culture[85]. This has led to the suggestion that in diseased human liver TIMP-1 secretion by activated hepatic lipocytes may, by preventing degradation of excess fibrillar collagens, promote progression of liver fibrosis. Supportive evidence for this hypothesis is provided by RNAase protection analysis of total RNA prepared from fibrotic liver explants (obtained from the Birmingham liver transplant centre, UK; data presented at conference). In these studies TIMP-1 mRNA expression was markedly increased in primary biliary cirrhosis, primary sclerosing cholangitis, and autoimmune chronic active hepatitis, compared with normal human liver. Thus in advanced human liver disease TIMP-1 expression is high, but the relative degree of importance of inhibition of collagenase activity to the overall pathogenesis of liver fibrosis requires further investigation. There is currently no information on TIMP-2 expression in liver.

CONCLUSIONS

Current evidence indicates that sinusoidal liver cells, particularly lipocytes which have become activated to a myofibroblast-like phenotype, synthesize many of the metalloproteinases and their inhibitors, TIMP-1 and α_2-macroglobulin. The role of these enzymes and their inhibitors in normal liver is not known, but they presumably regulate matrix remodelling and turnover. The principal areas of interest are: (1) degradation of the normal liver matrix by the gelatinases (A, B) and stromelysin and the role this has in the pathogenesis of liver injury, and (2) the respective roles of interstitial collagenase and TIMP-1 in the observed failure of degradation of excess fibrillar liver matrix and the relative importance of this to the progression of liver fibrosis. The past decade has witnessed a dramatic improvement in our general understanding of matrix degradation. Application of this knowledge to clinically important disease processes, such as liver fibrosis, is imperative if we are to develop new therapeutic strategies for their treatment.

Acknowledgements

My gratitude is extended to the Wellcome Trust, the Medical Research Council (UK), Action Research, and the Wessex Medical Trust for their generous support, and to Mrs Barbara Thomas for preparation of this manuscript.

References

1. Matrisian LM. Metalloproteinases and their inhibitors in matrix remodelling. Trend Genet. 1990;6:121–5.
2. Murphy G, Hembry RM, Hughes CE et al. Role and regulation of metalloproteinases in connective tissue turnover. Biochem Soc Trans. 1990;18:812–15.
3. Abrahamson DR, Caulfield JP. Distribution of laminin within rat and mouse renal, splenic, intestinal, and hepatic basement membranes identified after the intravenous injection of heterologous antilaminin IgG. Lab Invest. 1985;52:169.
4. Edwards DR, Murphy G, Reynolds JJ et al. Transforming growth factor beta modulates the expression of collagenase and metalloproteinase inhibitor. EMBO J. 1987;6:1899–904.
5. Overall CM, Wrana JL, Sudek J. Independent regulation of collagenase, 72 kDa progelatin-ase, and metalloendoproteinase inhibitor expression in human fibroblasts by transforming growth factor-beta. J Biol Chem. 1989;264:1860–9.
6. Clark SD, Kobayashi DK, Welgus HG. Regulation of the expression of tissue inhibitor of metalloproteinases and collagenase by retinoids and glucocorticoids in human fibroblasts. J Clin Invest. 1987;80:1280–8.
7. Springman EB, Angleton EL, Birkedal-Hansen H et al. Multiple modes of activation of latent human fibroblast collagenase: Evidence for the role of a Cys73 active-site zinc complex in latency and a 'cysteine switch' mechanism for activation. Proc Natl Acad Sci USA. 1990;87:364–8.

8. Van Wart HE, Birkedal-Hansen H. The cysteine switch: A principle of regulation of metalloproteinase activity with potential applicability to the entire matrix metalloproteinase gene family. Proc Natl Acad Sci USA. 1990;87:5578–82.
9. He C, Wilhelm SM, Pentland AP et al. Tissue cooperation in a proteolytic cascade activating human interstitial collagenase. Proc Natl Acad Sci USA. 1989;86:2632–6.
10. Suzuki K, Enghild JJ, Morodomi T et al. Mechanisms of activation of tissue procollagenase by matrix metalloproteinase 3 (stromelysin). Biochemistry. 1990;29:10261–70.
11. Nerlov C, Rorth P, Blasi F et al. Essential AP-1 and PEA3 binding elements in the human urokinase enhancer display cell type-specific activity. Oncogene. 1991;6:1583–92.
12. Gruber BL, Marchee MJ, Suzuki K et al. Synovial procollagenase activation by human mast cell tryptase dependence upon matrix metalloproteinase 3 activation. J Clin Invest. 1989;84:1657–62.
13. Okada Y, Nakanishi I. Activation of matrix metalloproteinase 3 (stromelysin) and matrix metalloproteinase 2 ('gelatinase') by human neutrophil elastase and cathepsin G. FEBS Lett. 1989;249:353–6.
14. Ward RV, Atkinson SJ, Slocombe PM et al. Tissue inhibitor of metalloproteinases-2 inhibits the activation of 72 kDa progelatinase by fibroblast membranes. Biochim Biophys Acta. 1991;1079 242–6.
15. Brown PD, Kleiner DE, Unsworth EJ et al. Cellular activation of the 72 kDa type-IV procollagenase/TIMP-2 complex. Kidney Int. 1993;43:163–70.
16. Enghild JJ, Salvesen G, Brew K et al. Interaction of human rheumatoid synovial collagenase (matrix metalloproteinase 1) and stromelysin (matrix metalloproteinase 3) with human alpha-2-macroglobulin and chicken ovostatin. J Biol Chem. 1989;264:8779–85.
17. Werb Z, Burleigh MC, Barrett AJ et al. The interaction of alpha-2-macroglobulin with proteinases. Binding and inhibition of mammalian collagenases and other metal proteinases. Biochem J. 1974;139:359–68.
18. Murphy G, Cawston TE, Reynolds JJ. An inhibitor of collagenase from human amniotic fluid. Biochem J. 1981;195:167–70.
19. Pavloff N, Staskus PW, Kishnani NS et al. A new inhibitor of metalloproteinases from chicken – ChIMP-3 – a 3rd member of the TIMP family. J Biol Chem. 1992;267:17321–6.
20. Stetler-Stevenson WG, Krutzsch HC, Liotta LA. Tissue inhibitor of metalloproteinase (TIMP-2). J Biol Chem. 1989;264:17374–8.
21. Goldberg GI, Marmer BL, Grant GA et al. Human 72-kilodalton type IV collagenase forms a complex with a tissue inhibitor of metalloproteases designated TIMP-2. Proc Natl Acad Sci USA. 1989;86:8207–11.
22. Overall CM, Wrana JL, Sodek J. Transcriptional and post-transcriptional regulation of 72-kDa gelatinase/type IV collagenase by transforming growth factor-beta1 in human fibroblasts. J Biol Chem. 1991;266:14064–71.
23. Stetler-Stevenson WG, Brown PD, Onisto M et al. Tissue inhibitor of metalloproteinases-2 (TIMP-2) mRNA expression in tumor cell lines and human tumor tissues. J Biol Chem. 1990;265:13933–8.
24. Howard EW, Bullen EC, Banda MJ. Regulation of the autoactivation of human 72-kDa progelatinase by tissue inhibitor of metalloproteinases-2*. J Biol Chem. 1991;266:13064–9.
25. Howard EW, Banda MJ. Binding of tissue inhibitor of metalloproteinases 2 to two distinct sites on human 72-kDa gelatinase. J Biol Chem. 1991;266:17972–7.
26. Fridman R, Fuerst TR, Bird RE et al. Domain structure of human 72-kDa gelatinase type-IV, collagenase characterization of proteolytic activity and identification of the tissue inhibitor of metalloproteinase-2 (TIMP-2) binding regions. J Biol Chem. 1992;267: 15398–405.
27. De Clerck YA, Yean T-S, Lu HS et al. Inhibition of autoproteolytic activation of interstitial procollagenase by recombinant metalloproteinase inhibitor MI/TIMP-2. J Biol Chem. 1991;266:3893–9.
28. Goldberg GI, Strongin A, Collier IE et al. Interaction of 82-kDa type-IV collagenase with the tissue inhibitor of metalloproteinases prevents dimerization, complex formation with interstitial collagenase, and activation of the proenzyme with stromelysin. J Biol Chem. 1992;267:4583–91.
29. Alcorn JM, Sheffield MF, Sweatman J et al. The expression of the matrix metalloproteinase transin but not collagenase is increased in regenerating rat liver. Hepatology. 1992;16:140A.

30. Hahn EG, Wick G, Pencev D et al. Distribution of basement membrane proteins in normal and fibrotic human liver: collagen type IV laminin and fibronectin. Gut. 1980;21:63–71.
31. Martinez-Hernandez A. The hepatic extracellular matrix. I. Electron immunohistochemical studies in normal rat liver. Lab Invest. 1984;51:57–69.
32. Maher JJ, Friedman SL, Roll FJ et al. Immunolocalization of laminin in normal rat liver and biosynthesis of laminin by hepatic lipocytes in primary culture. Gastroenterology. 1988;94:1053–62.
33. Arenson DM, Friedman SL, Bissell DM. Formation of extracellular matrix in normal rat liver: Lipocytes as a major source of proteoglycan. Gastroenterology. 1988;95:441–7.
34. Bissell DM, Arenson DM, Maher JJ et al. Support of cultured hepatocytes by a laminin-rich gel. J Clin Invest. 1987;79:801–12.
35. Schuetz EG, Li D, Omiecinski CJ et al. Regulation of gene expression in adult rat hepatocytes cultured on a basement membrane matrix. J Cell Physiol. 1988;134:309–23.
36. Friedman SL, Roll FJ, Boyles J et al. Maintenance of differentiated phenotype of cultured rat hepatic lipocytes by basement membrane matrix. J Biol Chem. 1989;264:10756–62.
37. Liotta LA, Abe S, Gehron-Robey P et al. Preferential digestion of basement membrane collagen by an enzyme derived from a metastatic murine tumour. Proc Natl Acad Sci USA. 1979;76:2268–72.
38. Murphy G, McAlpine CG, Poll CT et al. Purification and characterisation of a bone metalloproteinase that degrades gelatin and types IV and V collagen. Biochim Biophys Acta. 1985;831:49–58.
39. Collier IE, Wilhelm SM, Eisen AZ et al. H-ras oncogene-transformed human bronchial epithelial cells (TBE-1) secrete a single metalloprotease capable of degrading basement membrane collagen. J Biol Chem. 1988;263:6579–87.
40. Arthur MJP, Friedman SL, Roll FJ et al. Lipocytes from normal rat liver release a neutral metalloproteinase that degrades basement membrane (type IV) collagen. J Clin Invest. 1989;84:1076–85.
41. Arthur MJP, Jackson CL, Friedman SL. Release of type IV collagenase by human lipocytes. In: Wisse E, Knook DL and McCuskey RS, editors. Cells of the hepatic sinusoid, Vol. 3. Leiden: Kupffer Cell Foundation; 1991:161–3.
42. Arthur MJP, Stanley A, Iredale JP et al. Secretion of 72 kDa type IV collagenase/gelatinase by cultured human lipocytes: Analysis of gene expression, protein synthesis and proteinase activity. Biochem J. 1992;287:701–7.
43. Burt AD, Robertson JL, Heir J et al. Desmin-containing stellate cells in rat liver; distribution in normal animals and response to experimental acute liver injury. J Pathol. 1986;150: 29–35.
44. Johnson SJ, Hillan KJ, Hines JE et al. Proliferation and phenotypic modulation of perisinusoidal (Ito) cells following acute liver injury: temporal relationship with TGF-beta1 expression. In: Clement B, Guillouzo A, editors. Cellular and molecular aspects of cirrhosis. Montrouge: Colloques INSERM/John Libbey Eurotext; 1992:219–22.
45. Iredale JP, Winwood PJ, Choudhury AK et al. Immunostaining for 95 kD and 72 kD type IV collagenase/gelatinase and tissue inhibitor of metalloproteinases-1 during C. parvum-induced rat liver injury. In: Knook DL, Wisse E, eds. Cells of the hepatic sinusoid. Leyden, Netherlands: Kupffer Cell Foundation; 1993;4:105–108.
46. Iredale JP, Winwood PJ, Green I et al. Immunostaining for the matrix metalloproteinases and tissue inhibitor of metalloproteinase-1 in normal and diseased human liver. J Hepatol. 1993 (submitted).
47. Benyon RC, Iredale JP, Ferris WF et al. Increased expression of mRNA for gelatinase A and TIMP-2 in human fibrotic liver disease. Hepatology. 1993 (In press).
48. Wilhelm SM, Collier IE, Marmer BL et al. SV40-transformed human lung fibroblasts secrete a 82 kDa type IV collagenase which is identical to that secreted by normal human macrophages. J Biol Chem. 1989;264:17213–21.
49. Mainardi CL, Hasty KA. Secretion and glycosylation of rabbit macrophage type V collagenase. Matrix. 1990;10:84–90.
50. Winwood PJ, Kowalski-Saunders P, Green I et al. Kupffer cells release a 95 kD gelatinase. In: Clement B, Guillouzo A, editors. Cellular and molecular aspects of cirrhosis. France: John Libbey Eurotext Ltd/Colloque INSERM; 1992:307–10.
51. Winwood PJ, Schuppan D, Arthur MJP. Partial purification and biochemical characteris-

ation of Kupffer cell-derived 95 kD gelatinase. Hepatology. 1992;16:606.

52. Winwood PJ, Schuppan D, Arthur MJP. Characterisation of rat Kupffer cell-derived 95 kDa type IV collagenase/gelatinase B: A matrix metalloproteinase with activity against types III, IV and V collagens. Hepatology. 1993; (submitted).

53. Winwood PJ, Green I, Hembry RM et al. Release of 95 kD type IV collagenase/gelatinase by human Kupffer cells and its expression in diseased human liver. In: Knook DL, Wisse E, eds. Cells of the hepatic sinusoid. Leyden, Netherlands: Kupffer Cell Foundation; 1993;4:301–303.

54. Winwood PJ, Iredale JP, Kawser CA et al. Secretion of 92 kDa type IV collagenase/gelatinase B by cultured human Kupffer cells. Hepatology. 1993; (submitted).

55. Wilhelm SM, Collier IE, Kronberger A et al. Human skin fibroblast stromelysin; structure, glycosylation, substrate specificity, and differential expression in normal and tumorigenic cells. Proc Natl Acad Sci USA. 1987;84:6725–9.

56. Herbst H, Heinrichs O, Schuppan D et al. Temporal and spatial patterns of transin/stromelysin RNA expression following toxic injury in rat liver. Virchows Archiv B Cell Pathol. 1991;60:295–300.

57. Goldberg GI, Wilhelm SM, Kronberger A et al. Human fibroblast collagenase. J Biol Chem. 1986;261:6600–5.

58. Nagase H, Jackson RC, Brinckerhoff CE et al. A precursor form of latent collagenase produced in a cell free system with mRNA from rabbit synovial cells. J Biol Chem. 1981;256:11951–4.

59. Nagase H, Brinckerhoff CE, Vater CA et al. Biosynthesis and secretion of procollagenase by rabbit synovial fibroblasts. Biochem J. 1983;214:281–8.

60. Fujiwara K, Sakai T, Oda T et al. The presence of collagenase in Kupffer cells of the rat liver. Biochem Biophys Res Commun. 1973;54:531–6.

61. Bhatnagar R, Schade U, Rietschel ET et al. Involvement of prostaglandin E and adenosine 3′5′-monophosphate in lipopolysaccharide-stimulated collagenase release by rat Kupffer cells. Eur J Biochem. 1982;124:2405–9.

62. Emonard H, Guillouzo A, Lapiere ChM et al. Human liver fibroblast capacity for synthesizing interstitial collagenase in vitro. Cell Mol Biol. 1990;36:461–7.

63. Arthur MJP. The role of matrix degradation in liver fibrosis. In: Gressner AM, Ramadori G, editors. Molecular and cell biology of liver fibrogenesis. Lancaster: Kluwer; 1992: 213–27.

64. Milani S, Pinzani M, Casini A et al. Interstitial collagenase gene is differentially expressed in human liver and cultured fat-storing cells. Hepatology. 1992;16:186A.

65. Moshage H, Casini A, Lieber CS. Acetaldehyde selectively stimulates collagen production in cultured rat liver fat-storing cells but not in hepatocytes. Hepatology. 1990;12:511–18.

66. Li JJ, Kim CI, Leo MA et al. Polyunsaturated lecithin prevents acetaldehyde-mediated hepatic collagen accumulation by stimulating collagenase activity in culture lipocytes. Hepatology. 1992;15:373–81.

67. Okazaki I, Maruyama K. Collagenase activity in experimental hepatic fibrosis. Nature. 1974;252:49–50.

68. Perez-Tamayo R, Montfort I, Gonzalez E. Collagenolytic activity in experimental cirrhosis of the liver. Exp Mol Pathol. 1987;47:300–8.

69. Maruyama K, Feinman L, Okazaki I et al. Direct measurement of neutral collagenase activity in homogenates from baboon and human liver. Biochim Biophys Acta. 1981;658: 121–31.

70. Maruyama K, Feinman L, Fainsilber Z et al. Mammalian collagenase increases in early alcoholic liver disease and decreases with cirrhosis. Life Sci. 1982;30:1379–84.

71. Levin EG, Fair DS, Loskutoff DJ. Human hepatoma cell line plasminogen activator. J Lab Clin Med. 1983;102:500–8.

72. Fujii S, Lucore CL, Hopkins WE et al. Induction of synthesis of plasminogen activator inhibitor type-1 by tissue-type plasminogen activator in human hepatic and endothelial cells. Thromb Haemost. 1990;64:412–19.

73. Heaton JH, Gelehrter TD. Cyclic nucleotide regulation of plasminogen activator and plasminogen activator–inhibitor messenger RNAs in rat hepatoma cells. Mol Endocrinol. 1990;4:171–8.

74. Hopkins WE, Westerhausen DR Jr, Sobel BE et al. Transcriptional regulation of plasminogen

activator inhibitor type-1 mRNA in Hep G2 cells by epidermal growth factor. Nucl Acids Res. 1991;19:163–8.
75. Cwikel BJ, Barouski-Miller PA, Coleman PL et al. Dexamethasone induction of an inhibitor of plasminogen activator in HTC hepatoma cells. J Biol Chem. 1984;259:6847–51.
76. Quax PH, van den Hoogen CM, Verheijen JH et al. Endotoxin induction of plasminogen activator and plasminogen activator inhibitor type 1 mRNA in rat tissues in vivo. J Biol Chem. 1990;265:15560–3.
77. Emonard H, Grimaud JA. Plasminogen activator activity increases during reversal of hepatic fibrosis in murine schistosomiasis. Cell Mol Biol. 1990;36:233–8.
78. Emonard H, Grimaud J-A. Active and latent collagenase activity during reversal of hepatic fibrosis in murine schistosomiasis. Hepatology. 1989;10:77–83.
79. Takahashi S, Dunn MA, Seifter S. Liver collagenase in murine schistosomiasis. Gastroenterology. 1980;78:1425–31.
80. Takahashi S, Simpser E. Granuloma collagenase and EDTA-sensitive neutral protease production in hepatic murine schistosomiasis. Hepatology. 1981;1:211–20.
81. Takahashi S, Koda K. Radioimmunoassay of soluble and insoluble collagenases in fibrotic liver. Biochem J. 1984;220:157–64.
82. Truden JL, Boros DL. Detection of alpha-2-macroglobulin, alpha-1-protease inhibitor, and neutral protease-antiprotease complexes within liver granulomas of Schistosoma mansoni-infected mice. Am J Pathol. 1988;130:281–8.
83. Andus T, Ramadori G, Heinrich PC et al. Cultured Ito cells of rat liver express the alpha-2-macroglobulin gene. Eur J Biochem. 1987;168:641–6.
84. Kowalski-Saunders PWJ, Choudhury AK, Strain A et al. Interleukin-1 increases release of 72 kDa type IV collagenase activity but decreases alpha$_2$-macroglobulin synthesis by cultured human hepatic lipocytes. Hepatology. 1992;16:558.
85. Iredale JP, Murphy G, Hembry RM et al. Human hepatic lipocytes synthesize tissue inhibitor of metalloproteinases-1 (TIMP-1): implications for regulation of matrix degradation in liver. J Clin Invest. 1992;90:282–7.

10
Cellular localization and kinetics of matrix-metalloproteinase-3 expression following acute and chronic toxic liver injury in the rat

H. HERBST, T. WEGE, S. MILANI, D. V. NGO, A. M. GRESSNER and D. SCHUPPAN

INTRODUCTION

Liver fibrosis is characterized by quantitative and qualitative changes in the extracellular matrix, in particular resulting in an absolute and relative increase of the interstitial collagen types I and III content of fibrotic and cirrhotic liver[1]. Whereas the quantitative aspect may be conceivable in the light of enhanced *de novo* synthesis of almost all ECM components studied at the levels of RNA and protein, the qualitative changes of ECM require consideration of additional mechanisms. In this contribution, we discuss the expression of transin, the rat homologue to human stromelysin[2]. As a member of the matrix-metalloproteinase (MMP) gene family, transin is also referred to as MMP-3. MMPs are zinc-binding matrix-degrading enzymes, all of which are secreted as inactive proenzyme requiring activation by proteolytic cleavage. Because of the destructive potential, MMP activity is stringently regulated at the levels of gene expression, secretion, zymogen activation, and inhibition of active enzyme[3]. Among MMPs three major groups may be distinguished according to substrate specificity: (i) interstitial collagenases such as MMP-1 which degrade interstitial collagens, (ii) stromelysins (such as MMP-3) which degrade a variety of ECM proteins and proteoglycans including laminin, fibronectin and type IV (basement membrane) collagen, and (iii) gelatinases such as MMP-2 degrading type IV collagen and denatured interstitial collagens[3].

MMP expression is regulated by various cytokines such as IL-1, EGF, FGF, PDGF and transforming growth factor (TGF)-β_1. TGF-β_1 represses expression of MMP-1 and -3, whereas MMP-2 expression is up-regulated[3]. Inhibition of MMP-3 expression by TGF-β1 is mediated via c-*fos*/c-*jun*

(AP-1) binding sites[4]. Following secretion in latent, inactive form, MMPs are activated by proteolytic enzymes such as plasmin which itself is subject to stringent regulation by activators and activator-inhibitors[3]. In contrast to other MMPs, MMP-1 requires a two-step proteolytic activation, involving MMP-3 in addition to plasmin or other proteases[5]. Thus, MMP-3 not only degrades non-collagenous ECM, but it furthermore modulates degradation of interstitial collagens. MMP-3 may therefore be considered a key enzyme of fibrolysis. We used RNA/RNA *in situ* hybridization methods to assess steady-state levels and kinetics of MMP-3 expression at the level of cellular RNA transcripts in rat livers following a single or repeated administration of carbon tetrachloride (CCl_4).

MATERIALS AND METHODS

Female rats were intoxicated with CCl_4 by either a single or several intraperitoneal injections at 4-day intervals. Livers were collected at different time points (0.5, 1, 3, 6, 12, 24, 48 and 72 hours) following a single injection, or 12, 24, and 48 hours after the last one of repeated administrations. *In situ* hybridization was carried out using [^{35}S]-labelled RNA probes for rat MMP-3 and human TGF-β_1. The phenotype of MMP-3 expressing cells was determined by combined immunostaining/*in situ* hybridization using monoclonal antibodies specific for cytokeratin, vimentin, and desmin. MMP-3 expression was also studied in cultured rat lipocytes.

RESULTS

MMP-3 transcripts were detectable after a single injection of CCl_4 within and around the area of toxic damage in hepatocytes from 6 to 24 hours and in a few mesenchymal cells from 24 to 48 hours[6]. Most of these few vimentin-positive cells could be further characterized as desmin-positive cells, i.e. lipocytes. In chronically CCl_4-intoxicated rats MMP-3 transcripts were restricted to hepatocytes and were found to peak at 12 hours, whereas no signal was obtained 24 to 48 hours after the last CCl_4 injection. Isolated lipocytes, on the other hand, showed high steady-state levels of MMP-3 transcripts over extended periods (3 to 7 days) of culture. Beginning 12 to 24 hours after initial intoxication, TGF-β_1 RNA was expressed by mesenchymal, mainly desmin-positive, cells. Elevated TGF-β_1 transcript steady-state levels continued to be present at all subsequent time points after a single or repeated CCl_4 administrations.

DISCUSSION

The balanced deposition and degradation of extracellular matrix (ECM) macromolecules is essential for all structural changes occurring in developing and adult tissues, such as ordered morphogenesis, organ involution, tissue repair, angiogenesis, or tumour invasion. Physiological deposition of ECM requires the programmed expression not only of genes coding for ECM components, but also of genes encoding proteases with specificity for the various forms of collagens, ECM glycoproteins, proteoglycans, and other connective tissue constituents. Unbalanced ECM deposition and degradation, however, may ultimately lead to fibrosis[1].

Whereas cultured lipocytes express MMP-3 RNA at high levels, demonstrating the potential of these cells to express MMP-3, hepatocytes located in areas involved in regeneration following toxic injury appeared to be the major source of this proteinase *in vivo*. As previously shown for early phases of liver regeneration and fibrosis related to CCl_4 intoxication[7,8], expression of the MMP-3 gene is preceded by expression of the c-*jun*/AP-1 and c-*fos* proto-oncogenes and is followed by compensatory growth of hepatocytes and non-parenchymal cells as well as by synthesis of extracellular matrix[8]. Expression of TGF-β_1, which is able to down-regulate MMP-3, proved to be detectable 12 to 24 hours after CCl_4 administration and continued to be expressed at similar steady-state levels during all subsequent time points. Continuous TGF-β_1 expression may thus explain our failure to detect MMP-3 expression by mesenchymal cells of livers obtained from chronically CCl_4-intoxicated animals. On the other hand, hepatocellular MMP-3 expression was apparently not disturbed by increased TGF-β_1 levels. This may be due to the absence or low levels of TGF-β receptors on hepatocytes. The distribution and the relative number of hepatocytes with high levels of MMP-3 RNA showed considerable similarity to the hepatocellular pattern of thymidine incorporation after selective damage to zone III hepatocytes with bromobenzene[9], and with the staining pattern described for the proliferation-associated nuclear antigen detected by the monoclonal antibody Ki-67 in rat liver after CCl_4 administration[8]. The patterns of expression suggest a function for MMP-3 in cellular events preceding cell division such as removal of pericellular matrix. Furthermore, in addition to its intrinsic ECM proteinase activity, the function of MMP-3 as an interstitial collagenase (MMP-1) co-activator[5] appears to be of significance for the regulation of fibrolysis. MMP-3 expression by hepatocytes and non-parenchymal cells may be necessary for the restitution of an ordered ECM framework in the process of tissue repair. Altered expression patterns may then result in uncontrolled ECM deposition, e.g., as seen during the course of chronic intoxication with CCl_4.

It is meanwhile established that the majority of extracellular matrix proteins in fibrotic rat and human livers is synthesized by non-parenchymal cells, whereas the contribution by hepatocytes to the hepatic ECM protein pool is insignificant[1]. As to fibrolysis, all of the interstitial collagenase and gelatinase activities also appear to originate from mesenchymal cells, raising the question as to whether there may be any role for parenchymal cells in the development of fibrosis[1]. The demonstration of significant hepatocellular MMP-3 expression may point to a link between the mesenchymal and parenchymal compartment in the development of fibrosis and, perhaps, cirrhosis. Two major mechanisms influencing fibrolysis by depleting intra-parenchymal MMP-3 levels are conceivable: (i) an indirect pathway involving enhanced TGF-β_1 expression following liver damage resulting in down-regulation of MMP-3 expression by cells carrying TGF-β_1 receptors, and consequently leading to decreased MMP-1 activity, and (ii) diminished MMP-3 expression due to direct toxic damage to potentially MMP-3-expressing hepatocytes. In consequence, not only those ECM components susceptible to direct degradation by MMP-3, but also interstitial collagens, largely type I collagen, may accumulate in the liver lobule due to inadequate fibrolysis and concomitant enlargement of the mesenchymal compartment. Thus, the disruption of a coordinated pattern of MMP-3 expression may significantly contribute to the excessive and irregular ECM deposition in chronic hepatic fibrosis, as it is seen after repeated administration of CCl$_4$ in rats or in the course of chronic active hepatitis in human liver.

Acknowledgements

The authors thank Dr L. M. Matrisian for the generous gift of the transin gene probe, and Dr N. Fausto for a human TGF-β_1 cDNA.

References

1. Schuppan D, Herbst H, Milani S. Matrix, matrix synthesis and molecular networks in hepatic fibrosis. In: Zern MA, Reid LM, editors. Extracellular matrix. Chemistry, biology, and pathobiology with emphasis on the liver. New York: Marcel Dekker; 1993:201–54.
2. Matrisian LM, Glaichenhaus N, Gesnel MC, Breathnach R. Epidermal growth factor and oncogenes induce transcription of the same cellular mRNA in rat fibroblasts. EMBO J. 1985;4:1435–440.
3. Woessner JF. Matrix metalloproteinases and their inhibitors in connective tissue remodeling. FASEB J. 1991;5:2145–54.
4. Kerr LD, Miller DB, Matrisian LM. TGF-β_1 inhibition of transin/stromelysin gene expression is mediated through a fos binding sequence. Cell. 1990;61:267–78.
5. He CS, Wilhelm SM, Pentland AP, Marmer BL, Grant GA, Eisen AZ, Goldberg GI. Tissue cooperation in a proteolytic cascade activating human interstitial collagenase. Proc Natl Acad Sci USA. 1989;86:2632–6.
6. Herbst H, Heinrichs O, Schuppan D, Milani S, Stein H. Temporal and spatial patterns of transin/stromelysin expression following toxic injury in rat liver. Virchows Arch B Cell Pathol. 1991;60:295–300.
7. Milani S, Herbst H, Schuppan D, Stein H, Surrenti C. Transforming growth factors β_1 and β_2 are differentially expressed in chronic liver disease. Am J Pathol. 1991;139:1221–9.
8. Herbst H, Milani S, Schuppan D, Stein H. Temporal and spatial patterns of proto-oncogene expression at early stages of toxic liver injury in the rat. Lab Invest. 1991;65:324–33.
9. Nostrant TT, Miller DL, Appelman HD. Acinar distribution of liver cell regeneration after selective zonal injury in the rat. Gastroenterology. 1978;75:181–6.

Section III
Alcohol and liver
fibrogenesis

11
Alcohol and the liver

C. S. LIEBER

INTRODUCTION

Alcoholic liver disease proceeds in three, progressively severe, stages: fatty liver, alcoholic hepatitis and cirrhosis. In a recent prospective survey[1], it was found that, within 48 months, 30% of those with fatty liver, more than half of those with cirrhosis and two-thirds of those with cirrhosis plus alcoholic hepatitis had died. The demonstration that alcohol exerts some intrinsic hepatotoxicity, independent of nutritional deficiencies, reviewed recently elsewhere[2], led to a broadly based search for the mechanism involved. One of the most fruitful leads was the realization that many of the metabolic and toxic effects of alcohol in the liver can in fact be linked to its metabolism in that organ. Indeed, after it is imbibed, ethanol is readily absorbed from the gastrointestinal tract. Only 2–10% of that absorbed is eliminated through the kidneys and lungs; the rest is oxidized in the body, principally in the liver. Except for the stomach, extrahepatic metabolism of ethanol is small. This relative organ specificity, coupled with the high energy content of ethanol (each gram provides 7.1 kcal) and the lack of effective feedback control of its rate of hepatic metabolism, may result in a displacement of up to 90% of the liver's normal metabolic substrates, and probably explains why ethanol disposal produces striking metabolic imbalances in the liver. At present, except for control of alcohol abuse and liver transplantation (in a few selected subjects), there is no established effective means of prevention or treatment of the condition. The purpose of this review is to analyse how our concepts about cirrhosis have evolved to the present state of knowledge which allows for a more optimistic outlook, in terms of treatment and outcome.

The hepatocyte contains three main pathways for ethanol metabolism, each located in a different subcellular compartment: the alcohol dehydrogenase (ADH) pathway of the cytosol or the soluble fraction of the cell, the microsomal ethanol-oxidizing system located in the endoplasmic reticulum, and catalase located in the peroxisomes (Fig. 1). Each of these pathways produces specific metabolic and toxic disturbances, and all three result in the production of acetaldehyde, a highly toxic metabolite.

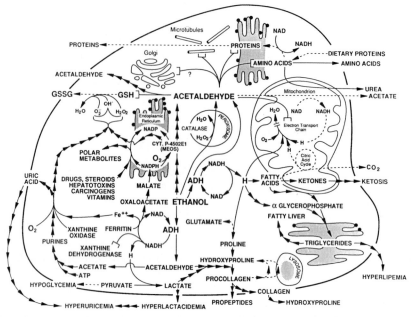

Fig. 1 Oxidation of ethanol in the hepatocyte. Many disturbances in intermediary metabolism and toxic effects can be linked to (1) alcohol dehydrogenase (ADH)-mediated generation of NADH; (2) the induction of the activity of microsomal enzymes, especially P4502E1; and (3) acetaldehyde, the product of ethanol oxidation. NAD, nicotinamide adenine dinucleotide; NADH, reduced NAD; GSH, reduced glutathione; GSSG, oxidized glutathione. The broken lines indicate pathways that are depressed by ethanol, whereas repeated arrows reflect stimulation or activation. The symbol -[denotes interference or binding

THE ALCOHOL DEHYDROGENASE (ADH) PATHWAY

A major pathway for ethanol disposition involves ADH, an enzyme that catalyses the conversion of ethanol to acetaldehyde. The *raison d'être* of this enzyme might be to rid the body of the small amounts of alcohol produced by fermentation in the gut[3]. ADH has a broad substrate specificity, which includes dehydrogenation of steroids[4], oxidation of the intermediary alcohols of the shunt pathway of mevalonate metabolism[5] and omega oxidation of fatty acids[6]; these processes may act as the 'physiological' substrates for ADH.

Multiple forms of ADH

Human ADH is a dimeric zinc metalloenzyme for which several classes have been distinguished[7]. Subunits hybridize within but not between classes. Human liver ADH exists in multiple molecular forms which arise from the association of eight different types of subunits, α, β_1, β_2, β_3, γ_1, γ_2, π and χ, into active dimeric molecules. A genetic model accounts for this multiplicity as products of five gene loci, ADH1 through ADH5[8]. Polymorphism occurs at two loci, ADH2 and ADH3, which encode the β and γ subunits. There are three types of subunit, α, β and γ in class I. Primary structures of all three forms have been established, as well as their overall properties. Each subunit has 374 residues, of which 35 exhibit differences among the α, β and γ chains. Allelic variants occur at the β and γ loci. Corresponding amino acid substitutions have been characterized, and enzymatic differences between the allelic forms are explained by defined exchanges. The subunits of class I are derived from at least three genetic loci[9-11] and constitute the α subunit (the major form expressed in fetal liver), different β subunits, distributed non-identically in various populations (β_1 common in Caucasian populations, β_2 common in Oriental populations and $\beta_{Indianapolis}$ found at least in some African populations[12-14]), and the two allelic types of γ subunit, γ_1 and γ_2 (both of high frequency). Class II isozymes migrate more anodically than class I isozymes and, unlike the latter which generally have low K_m values for ethanol, class II (or π) ADH has a relatively high K_m (34 mmol/l) and a relative insensitivity to 4-methylpyrazole inhibition, with a K_i of 2 mmol/l at pH 7.5[15,16]. Class III (χ ADH) does not participate in the oxidation of ethanol in the liver because of its very low affinity for that substrate; it is not inhibited by 12 mmol/l 4-methylpyrazole[17]. More recently, a new isoenzyme of ADH has been identified in human stomach, so-called σ- or μ-ADH[18,19] (class IV) and a cDNA encoding yet another new form of ADH (class V) in liver and stomach was reported[20].

Hepatic lobular distribution of ADH

Microquantitative measurements of Morrison and Brock[21] had originally revealed that the activity of ADH in the perivenular (pericentral) area of the liver lobule in humans and in female rats was about 1.7 times higher than in the periportal area. By means of modern immunohistochemical techniques, human ADH has again been demonstrated mainly in hepatocytes around the terminal hepatic (central) vein[22], even in cirrhotic livers[23]. Microchemical assays were also performed in microdissected tissue samples from the whole length of the sinusoid[24]: alcohol dehydrogenase activity in men < 50 years of age showed increase in the gradient towards the perivenous zone. Furthermore, alcohol dehydrogenase activity in the livers of women was significantly higher than in men. After the age of 53 in men and 50 in women, the sex specificity of the distribution profiles was no longer apparent.

Effects of excessive hepatic NADH generation

In ADH-mediated oxidation of ethanol, acetaldehyde is produced and hydrogen is transferred from ethanol to the cofactor nicotinamide adenine dinucleotide (NAD), which is converted to its reduced form (NADH) (Fig. 1). The formed acetaldehyde again loses hydrogen and is metabolized to acetate, most of which is released into the blood stream. As a net result, ethanol oxidation generates an excess of reducing equivalents in the liver, primarily as NADH. The large amounts of reducing equivalents overwhelm the hepatocyte's ability to maintain redox homeostasis, and a number of metabolic disorders ensue.

The enhanced NADH/NAD ratio reflects itself in an increased lactate/ pyruvate ratio that results in hyperlacticacidaemia because of both decreased utilization and enhanced production of lactate by the liver. The hyperlactic-acidaemia contributes to the acidosis and also reduces the capacity of the kidney to excrete uric acid, leading to secondary hyperuricaemia[25]. Alcohol-induced ketosis[26] and enhanced purine breakdown[27] may also promote the hyperuricaemia. Hyperuricaemia may be related to the common clinical observation that excessive consumption of alcoholic beverages frequently aggravates or precipitates gouty attacks.

The increased NADH/NAD ratio also raises the concentration of α-glycerophosphate that favours hepatic triglyceride accumulation by trapping fatty acids. In addition, excess NADH may promote fatty acid synthesis[28]. Theoretically, enhanced lipogenesis can be considered a means for disposing of the excess hydrogen. Some hydrogen equivalents are transferred into mitochondria by various 'shuttle' mechanisms. The activity of the citric acid cycle is depressed, partly because of a slowing of the reactions of the cycle that require NAD; the mitochondria will use the hydrogen equivalents originating from ethanol, rather than those derived from the oxidation of fatty acids that normally serve as the main energy source of the liver.

Acute alcohol intoxication does occasionally cause severe hypoglycaemia, which can result in sudden death. As reviewed elsewhere[29], hypoglycaemia is due, in part, to the block of hepatic gluconeogenesis by ethanol, again as a consequence of the increased NADH/NAD ratio in subjects whose glycogen stores are already depleted by starvation or who have pre-existing abnormalities in carbohydrate metabolism. Depending on the conditions, ethanol may accelerate rather than inhibit gluconeogenesis. Indeed, hyperglycaemia may also occur in association with alcoholism. Its mechanism is still obscure, but glucose intolerance may be due, at least in part, to decreased peripheral glucose utilization.

The generation of NADH also interferes with the hepatic metabolism of galactose, serotonin, and other amines and metabolism in favour of the reduced compounds.

Pathological effects in the liver associated with alcohol dehydrogenase-mediated ethanol metabolism

One of the earliest pathological manifestations of alcohol abuse is the excessive accumulation of fat in the liver, resulting in a fatty liver. Theoretically, lipids that accumulate in the liver can originate from three main sources: (1) dietary lipids (which reach the blood stream as chylomicrons), (2) adipose tissue lipids (which are transported to the liver as free fatty acids, FFA), and (3) lipids synthesized in the liver itself. These fatty acids of various sources can accumulate in the liver because of a large number of metabolic disturbances, primarily decreased lipid oxidation in the liver, enhanced hepatic lipogenesis, decreased hepatic release of lipoproteins, increased mobilization of peripheral fat, and enhanced hepatic uptake of circulating lipids. Depending on the experimental conditions, any of the three sources and the various mechanisms can be implicated. Most commonly, the above-described decreased fatty acid oxidation results in the accumulation in the liver of dietary fat[30,31]. In addition to the functional changes that are a direct consequence of the metabolism of ethanol, chronic ethanol abuse results in more persistent changes in the mitochondria. The striking structural changes in the mitochondria[32] are associated with corresponding functional abnormalities, including a decreased capacity to oxidize fatty acids. Thus, decreased fatty acid oxidation, whether as a function of the reduced citric acid cycle activity (secondary to the altered redox potential) or as a consequence of permanent changes in mitochondrial structure, offers the most likely explanation for the deposition of fat in the liver, especially fat derived from the diet. In addition, with stressful amounts of ethanol and/or fasting conditions, some mobilization of fatty acids from adipose tissue may also contribute to the accumulation of lipids in the liver. A characteristic feature of liver injury in the alcoholic is the predominance of steatosis and other lesions in the perivenular (also called centrilobular) zone or zone 3 of the hepatic acinus. The mechanism for this zonal selectivity of the toxic effects involves several distinct and not mutually exclusive mechanisms.

The hypoxia hypothesis originated from the observation that liver slices from rats fed alcohol chronically consume more oxygen than those of controls. It was then postulated that the enhanced consumption of oxygen would increase the gradient of oxygen tensions along the sinusoids to the extent of producing anoxic injury of perivenular hepatocytes[33]. Indeed both in human alcoholics[34] and in animals fed alcohol chronically[35,36], decreases in either hepatic venous oxygen saturation[34] or Po_2[35] and in tissue oxygen tensions[36] have been found during the withdrawal state. However, the changes in hepatic oxygenation found during the withdrawal state disappeared[35,37] or decreased[36] when alcohol was present in the blood. Acute ethanol administration increased splanchnic oxygen consumption in naive baboons, but the consequences of this effect on oxygenation in the perivenular zone were offset by increased blood flow resulting in unchanged hepatic venous oxygen tension[35]. Ethanol in fact induces an increase in portal hepatic blood flow[35,37–40]. In baboons fed alcohol chronically, defective O_2 utilization rather than lack of blood O_2 supply characterized liver injury produced by high concentration of ethanol[40]. We postulated that the low oxygen tensions normally prevailing in perivenular zones could exaggerate the redox shift produced by ethanol[35]. To study the magnitude of such a shift in the baboon, the effects of ethanol on the lactate/pyruvate ratio in hepatic venous blood (an approximation of that in perivenular hepatocytes) were compared with the ratio in total liver. Ethanol increased the lactate/pyruvate ratio and decreased pyruvate more in hepatic venous blood than in total liver. In isolated rat hepatocytes the ethanol-induced redox shift was markedly exaggerated by lowering the oxygen to a tension similar to those found in centrilobular zones. The process was also assessed in the isolated perfused rat liver, by varying the oxygen supply, to produce the oxygen tensions prevailing *in vivo* along the sinusoid[41]. It is noteworthy that hypoxia increases NADH, which in turn inhibits the activity of NAD^+-dependent xanthine dehydrogenase (XD), thereby favouring that of oxygen-dependent xanthine oxidase $(XO)^{42}$ (Fig. 1). It has been postulated that, due to the acetate derived from ethanol, purine metabolites accumulate and could be metabolized via XO. This process may lead to the production of oxygen radicals which can mediate toxic effects towards liver cells, including peroxidation. Physiological substrates for XO, hypoxanthine and xanthine, as well as AMP, significantly increased in the liver after ethanol, together with an enhanced urinary output of allantoin (a final product of xanthine metabolism). Allopurinol pretreatment resulted in 90% inhibition of XO activity, and also significantly decreased ethanol-induced lipid peroxidation[42].

Zonal distribution of some enzymes can influence the selective perivenular toxicity. As discussed subsequently, proliferation of the smooth endoplasmic reticulum after chronic ethanol consumption is maximal in the perivenular zone, with associated enzyme induction and related effects. Furthermore, human ADH has now been demonstrated mainly in hepatocytes around the terminal hepatic venule (see above). Thus, a presumably higher level of ethanol metabolism in the perivenular zone could contribute to the increased hepatotoxicity of ethanol, for instance by providing (together with the 'induced' microsomal pathway; see below) an increased amount of the toxic metabolite acetaldehyde[43]. One must, however, also take into account that after chronic ethanol consumption, unlike the activity of the microsomal ethanol-oxidizing system (MEOS), which is induced, that of ADH may not change, or even decreases[44-46]. Alcoholics may display decreased hepatic ADH activity even in the absence of liver damage[47].

Inhibition of protein synthesis has been observed after addition of ethanol to various preparations *in vitro*[48,49]. *In vivo* the acute effects of ethanol on protein synthesis have been less consistent. The perivenular zone of the hepatic lobule, which is already somewhat hypoxic in the normal state, may represent an area of exaggerated toxicity[41]; the striking exaggeration of the ethanol-induced redox changes in this zone may be sufficient to impair protein synthesis.

The bulk of hepatic ADH is present in the hepatocytes, but traces are also found in lipocytes[50]. Their functional significance was unclear until Flisiak *et al.*[51] showed that acetaldehyde derived from ADH-mediated ethanol metabolism significantly increases prostanoid production in these cells.

Extrahepatic tissues contain isozymes of ADH with a much lower affinity for ethanol than the hepatic isozymes. As a consequence, at the levels of ethanol achieved in the blood, these extrahepatic enzymes are inactive; therefore extrahepatic metabolism of ethanol is negligible, with the exception of the gastric one.

Gastric ADH

At least three different forms of ADH exist in the stomach, with either high or low K_m values for ethanol[52]. Because of the extraordinary high gastric ethanol concentration after alcohol ingestion, even the gastric ADH with the high K_m for ethanol becomes active, and significant gastric ethanol metabolism ensues[53,54]. Ethnic variability is possibly involved, since 80% of Japanese were found to lack one of the gastric isozymes[55]. As mentioned above, one major isozyme requires a relatively high ethanol concentration for optimal activity. Therefore, as expected, the concentration of alcoholic beverages affects the amount metabolized[56] and consequently, in the rat, which has only the high K_m enzyme, relatively high concentrations are required for significant first-pass metabolism to be observed[56]. Accordingly, when only 2.5% alcohol was used, not much gastric metabolism was measurable[57].

First-pass metabolism decreases the bioavailability of ethanol and represents a 'protective barrier' against systemic effects, at least when ethanol is consumed in small 'social drinking' amounts. This 'gastric barrier' disappears after gastrectomy[58] and may be lost, in part, in the alcoholic[59,60], because of a decrease in gastric ADH activity. Similar effects may also result from gastric ADH inhibition by some commonly used drugs. For instance, aspirin[61], or H_2-blockers, such as cimetidine and ranitidine, were found to inhibit gastric ADH activity *in vitro*[62,63] and to result in increased blood levels *in vivo*[62,64]. This interaction is particularly striking at low doses of alcohol, as described by Caballeria *et al.*[62] and Hernandez-Munoz *et al.*[52]. Whether the H_2-blocker effect on blood alcohol can be demonstrated with higher doses of ethanol has been the subject of controversy[65], but various groups have reported such a positive interaction[64,66]. Women also have a lower gastric ADH activity than men[60], at least below the age of 50[67]. As a consequence, for a given intake their blood ethanol levels are higher, an increase that is compounded by differences in body composition (more fat, less water in women) and, on the average, a lower body weight. The higher blood ethanol level, in turn, may contribute to the greater susceptibility of women to alcohol.

ROLE OF CATALASE

The hepatocyte contains catalase primarily in the peroxisomes and mitochondria. Small amounts are also found in isolated microsomes, but in the latter fraction catalase is considered to be a contaminant added during isolation rather than a component of the membrane of the endoplasmic reticulum itself[68].

Catalase is capable of oxidizing ethanol *in vitro* in the presence of an H_2O_2-generating system[69] (Fig. 1). However, under physiological conditions catalase appears to play no major role in ethanol metabolism, and cannot account quantitatively for the ADH-independent pathway.

It has been proposed that the catalase contribution might be enhanced if significant amounts of H_2O_2 become available through β-oxidation of fatty acids such as octanoate, palmitate and oleate in peroxisomes[70]. However, it should be pointed out that the peroxisomal enzymes do not oxidize short-chain fatty acids such as octanoate, and that this phenomenon was observed only in the absence of ADH activity. Otherwise the rate of ethanol metabolism is reduced by adding fatty acids[71], and β-oxidation of fatty acids is inhibited by NADH produced from ethanol metabolism via ADH[71]. Various other results also indicated that peroxisomal fatty acid oxidation does not play a significant role in ethanol metabolism[72]. Furthermore, when fatty acids were used[70] to stimulate ethanol oxidation, this effect was very sensitive to inhibition by aminotriazole (AT), a catalase inhibitor. Therefore, if this mechanism were to play an important role *in vivo*, one would expect a significant inhibition of ethanol metabolism after AT administration *in vivo*, when physiological amounts of fatty acids and other substrates for H_2O_2 generations are present. A number of studies, however, have shown that AT treatment *in vivo* has little, if any, effect on ethanol oxidation *in vivo*. Studies by Takagi et al.[73] and Kato et al.[74] have confirmed this relative lack of effect of AT on ethanol metabolism *in vivo*, while verifying its inhibitory effect on catalase-mediated ethanol peroxidation *in vitro*.

METABOLISM OF ALCOHOL VIA THE MICROSOMAL ETHANOL-OXIDIZING SYSTEM AND ITS INTERACTIONS WITH OTHER DRUGS AND HEPATOTOXIC AGENTS

Characterization of the microsomal ethanol-oxidizing system and its role in ethanol metabolism

Liver microsomes were found to be the site for a distinct and adaptive system of ethanol oxidation[45,75], named the microsomal ethanol-oxidizing system (MEOS). It was concluded that MEOS was distinct from ADH and catalase and dependent on cytochrome P450 because: (a) isolation of a P450-containing fraction from liver microsomes which, although devoid of any ADH or catalase activity, could still oxidize ethanol as well as higher aliphatic alcohols (e.g. butanol which is not a substrate for catalase)[76,77] and (b) reconstitution of ethanol-oxidizing activity using NADPH-cytochrome P450 reductase, phospholipid, and either partially purified or highly purified microsomal P450 from untreated[78] or phenobarbital-treated[79] rats. That chronic ethanol consumption results in the induction of a unique P450 was shown by Ohnishi and Lieber[78] using a liver microsomal P450 fraction isolated from ethanol-treated rats. An ethanol-inducible form of P450, purified from rabbit liver microsomes[80], catalysed ethanol oxidation at rates much higher than other P450 isozymes, and also had an enhanced capacity to oxidize 1-butanol, 1-pentanol and aniline[81], acetaminophen[82], CCl_4[81], acetone[83,84], and N-nitrosodimethylamine (NDMA)[85]. Similar results have been obtained with cytochrome P450j, a major hepatic P450 isozyme purified from ethanol- or isoniazid-treated rats[86,87]. Others have also provided evidence for the existence of a P450j-like isozyme in humans[88,89]. We have succeeded in obtaining the purified human protein (now called CYP2E1 or 2E1) in a catalytically active form, with a high turnover rate for ethanol and other specific substrates[90]. Using antibodies against this 2E1, and the Western blot technique, a 5–10-fold induction was found in biopsies of recently

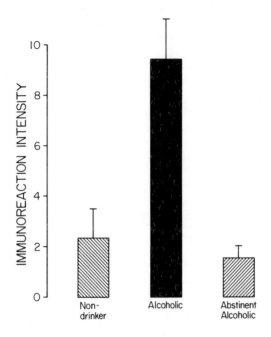

Fig. 2 Hepatic P4502E1 levels in alcoholics and non-drinkers. P4502E1 was quantitated by scanning of Western blots of percutaneous liver biopsies, using anti-2E1 antibodies (data from ref. 91)

drinking subjects (Fig. 2)[91]. Compounds other than ethanol (e.g. acetone) can also serve as 2E1 inducers, but 2E1 can be induced after short-term and relatively light consumption of ethanol, in the absence of increased acetonaemia or hepatic steatosis[92]. MEOS has a relatively high K_m for ethanol (8–10 mmol/l compared with 0.2–2 mmol/l for ADH) and thus normally ADH accounts for the bulk of ethanol oxidation at low blood ethanol concentration (Fig. 3A), but not necessarily at high ethanol levels (Fig. 3B), especially during long-term use of alcohol (Fig. 3C), in view of the inducibility of the MEOS[45,75].

Although data obtained with inhibitors are suggestive of MEOS involvement[45,93–95], they cannot be considered conclusive, since the inhibitors are not sufficiently specific. However, a mutant deermouse strain that lacks the hepatic low K_m ADH (ADH$^-$) nevertheless actively oxidizes ethanol[96–100], and studies with stable isotopes indicated that this effect is mediated principally by the MEOS[100].

It was suggested that 50% or more of ethanol elimination in ADH$^-$ deermice was caused by a mitochondrial dehydrogenase[101,102]. But this was not confirmed[103,104]. Next, it was postulated that gastric mucosal ADH could account for the previously reported isotopic characteristics of ethanol oxidation in ADH$^-$ deermice, and that it catalysed ethanol elimination in the ADH$^-$ strain[105]. Other studies showed, however, that when ethanol is

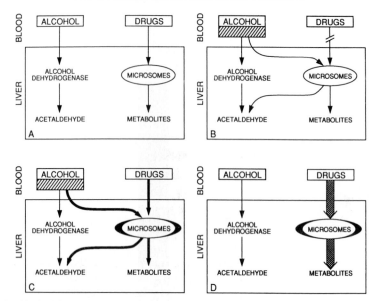

Fig. 3 Alcohol is metabolized by alcohol dehydrogenase, and drugs by microsomes (**A**). Microsomal drug metabolism is inhibited in the presence of high concentrations of ethanol, in part through competition for a common microsomal detoxification process (**B**). Microsomal induction after long-term alcohol consumption contributes to accelerated ethanol metabolism at high blood ethanol levels (**C**). Increased drug metabolism and activation of xenobiotics to toxic metabolites (due to microsomal induction) persist after cessation of long-term alcohol consumption (**D**). Hatching indicates high blood alcohol levels (from ref. 259)

given parenterally, the microsomal ethanol-oxidizing system rather than gastric ADH is a major pathway of ethanol oxidation in ADH⁻ deermice, while both pathways contribute significantly to the metabolism of orally administered ethanol[106].

Interactions with drugs, including drug tolerance

Increases in the metabolism of warfarin, phenytoin, tolbutamide, propranolol, and rifampin have been linked to long-term ethanol consumption[108,109]. Ethanol administration to volunteers under metabolic-ward conditions resulted in a striking increase in the rate of blood clearance of meprobamate and pentobarbital[107]. The metabolic drug tolerance persists several days to weeks after the cessation of alcohol abuse, and the duration of recovery varies with each drug[110].

Contrasting with the induction effect of long-term consumption of ethanol, after short-term administration, inhibition of hepatic drug metabolism is seen[29] (Fig. 3B). Accordingly, whereas long-term ethanol consumption leads to increased hepatic microsomal metabolism of methadone and decreased levels in the brain and liver, short-term administration has the opposite effect: it inhibits microsomal demethylation of methadone and enhances brain and liver concentrations of the drug[111]. These effects may be of clinical relevance, since approximately 50% of the patients taking methadone are alcohol abusers. The combination of ethanol with tranquillizers and barbiturates also results in increased drug concentrations in the blood, sometimes to dangerously high levels[29]. One mechanism of interaction is direct competition for a common metabolic process involving cytochrome P450[29].

Increased xenobiotic toxicity and carcinogenicity in alcoholics; interactions with vitamin A

On occasion the metabolites produced in the microsomes are more toxic than the precursor compound and, therefore, the induction produced by ethanol augments the toxicity of a number of agents. This pertains particularly to those substrates for which the alcohol-inducible 2E1, when compared with other P450s, displays an enhanced capacity for conversion to hepatotoxic metabolites. Indeed, much of the medical significance of MEOS and the ethanol-inducible 2E1 results not only from the oxidation of ethanol but also from the unusual and unique capacity of 2E1 to activate many xenobiotic compounds to toxic metabolites. This pertains for instance to carbon tetrachloride (CCl_4). It is known that CCl_4 exerts its toxicity after conversion to an active compound in the microsomes, and alcohol pretreatment remarkably stimulates[112] the toxicity of CCl_4, with perivenular predominance, which can be explained by the selective presence and induction of 2E1 in that zone of the liver[91]. A large number of other organic compounds were found to display such a selective injurious action in the liver, as well as other tissues, of the alcoholic. These include industrial solvents and anaesthetics such as bromobenzene[113], vinylidene chloride[114], enflurane[115] and halothane, especially when the metabolism is rendered reductive[116]. Ethanol treatment also aggravated haemopoietic toxicity[117] and markedly increased the activity of microsomal low K_m benzene metabolizing enzymes[118]; indeed 2E1 is a benzene hydroxylase which is induced also in the bone marrow[119]; this may be of relevance to the toxicity in that tissue.

Enhanced metabolism (and toxicity) pertains also to a variety of prescribed drugs, including isoniazid and phenylbutazone[120].

The same mechanism of hepatotoxicity also applies to some 'over-the-counter' medications. Among alcoholic patients, hepatic injury associated with acetaminophen (paracetamol, N-acetyl-p-aminophenol), has appeared with a pattern of use of repetitive intake for headaches, including those associated with withdrawal symptoms, dental pain, or the pain of pancreatitis leading in some to high daily doses.

There is an association between alcohol misuse and an increased incidence of upper alimentary and respiratory tract cancers[121]. Many factors have been incriminated, one of which is the effect of ethanol on enzyme systems involved in the cytochrome P450-dependent activation of carcinogens. This effect has been demonstrated with the use of microsomes derived from a variety of tissues, including the liver (the principal site of xenobiotic metabolism)[122,123], the lungs[122,124] and intestines[125,126] (the chief portals of entry for tobacco smoke and dietary carcinogens, respectively), and the oesophagus[123] (where ethanol consumption is a major risk factor in the development of cancer). Alcoholics are commonly heavy smokers, and a synergistic effect of alcohol consumption and smoking on cancer development has been described, as reviewed elsewhere[121]. Long-term ethanol consumption was found to enhance the mutagenicity of tobacco-derived products[121], and benzoflavone (a tobacco-like inducer) has also been shown to increase a liver cytochrome (1A2) that is structurally different but catalytically similar to 2E1[127].

Alcohol may influence carcinogenesis in other ways[128], one of which involves vitamin A. Indeed, ethanol administration in animals has been shown to depress hepatic levels of vitamin A, even when given with diets containing large amounts of vitamin A[129], reflecting in part accelerated microsomal degradation of the vitamin. New hepatic pathways of microsomal retinol metabolism, inducible by either ethanol or drug administration, have been discovered[130,131]. Furthermore, reconstituted systems with purified forms of cytochrome P450 have been used to show that retinoic acid[132] and retinol[130] can serve as substrates for microsomal oxidation, also in human liver microsomes. Immunoblots performed with a monospecific antibody directed against human P4502C8 revealed that appreciable amounts of this enzyme were present in human liver microsomes. The same antibody significantly inhibited retinol metabolism in liver microsomes and in a system reconstituted with P4502C8. The latter also converted retinoic acid to polar metabolites[133]. When ethanol and phenobarbital were combined, a marked potentiation of the hepatic vitamin A depletion was observed[134]. Since alcohol abuse is often associated clinically with overuse of other drugs, and since drug use may also be associated with severe hepatic vitamin A depletion[135], this potentiation may be meaningful in terms of vitamin A depletion in an appreciable section of the population.

Hepatic vitamin A depletion is associated with lysosomal lesions[136], decreased detoxification of NDMA[137], and probably scores of other adverse effects. Excess of vitamin A is also hepatotoxic[138]. Long-term ethanol consumption enhances this effect, resulting in striking morphological and functional alterations of the mitochondria[139], along with hepatic necrosis and fibrosis[140]. Hypervitaminosis A itself can induce fibrosis and even cirrhosis, as reviewed elsewhere[138], but this is an unusual occurrence, necessitating very large amounts of vitamin A (in excess of 50–100 times the daily requirement) given over prolonged periods. A smaller vitamin A supplementation (e.g. five times the normal intake) has, by itself, no detectable adverse effects but, when combined with alcohol, it results in striking leakage of the mitochondrial enzyme glutamine dehydrogenase into the blood stream[139] as well as potentiation of fibrogenesis[140]. Thus, in heavy drinkers, there is a narrowed therapeutic window for vitamin A, and injudicious supplementation might hasten rather than alleviate the liver disease process. Unlike for retinoids, the toxicity of which is well established, this is not the case for β-carotene. Detailed studies are still lacking, but there is at present a consensus that no obvious β-carotene toxicity has been apparent. It must be noted, however, that the possible interaction between β-carotene and liver disease, alcohol and/or other drugs is virtually uncharted at this time, but cannot be excluded *a priori*, especially since, in subhuman primates, enhanced toxicity of β-carotene in the presence of ethanol has been observed recently[141]. Thus caution must be exercised with β-carotene, in view of the possible existence of a defect in utilization and/or excretion associated with liver injury and/or alcohol abuse[142].

Ethanol also affects the microsomal metabolism of exogenous and endogenous steroids, as discussed elsewhere[29]. Furthermore, ethanol alters the metabolism of structurally related compounds, such as vitamin D[143]. This and other micronutrients, such as vitamin E[144] may serve as substrates for the microsomal enzymes; therefore the induction of the microsomal oxidative activities may alter vitamin requirements.

NON-OXIDATIVE METABOLISM OF ETHANOL

The possible pathogenic role of a non-oxidative pathway of ethanol metabolism to form fatty acid ethyl esters was raised by Laposata and Lange[145]. The capacity of ethanol to form ethyl esters *in vivo* had been demonstrated by Goodman and Deykin[146] and also by Lange[147], who purified the enzyme[148]. Laposata and Lange[145] found that, compared to controls in acutely intoxicated subjects, concentrations of fatty acid ethyl esters were significantly higher in pancreas, liver, heart, and adipose tissue. Since this non-oxidative ethanol metabolism occurs in humans in the organs most commonly injured by alcohol abuse, and since some of these organs lack oxidative ethanol metabolism, Laposata and Lange[145] postulated that fatty acid ethyl esters may have a role in the production of alcohol-induced injury. Further experiments are needed to verify the possible role of this mechanism in the pathogenesis of liver injury.

TOXIC EFFECTS OF ACETALDEHYDE

Acetaldehyde is the first major 'specific' oxidation product of ethanol by all three pathways discussed above. In addition to the exogenous ethanol there are endogenous sources of acetaldehyde such as deoxypentosephosphate aldolases, pyruvate dehydrogenase and phosphorylphosphoethanolamine phosphorylase activities, as well as the capacity of commensal microorganisms to produce both ethanol and acetaldehyde from sugars[149]. Another putative source of acetaldehyde is provided by the cleavage of threonine to acetaldehyde and glycine by a threonine aldolase in the hepatic cytosol. Although this is believed to represent minor pathways in the normal degradation of threonine[150], it is conceivable that its relative role may be enhanced if liver injury were to interfere with the major pathways, namely the mitochondrial threonine dehydrogenase and the cytosolic threonine dehydratase, as suggested by recent findings[151].

Chronic ethanol consumption results in a significant reduction of the capacity of rat mitochondria to oxidize acetaldehyde[152]. The decreased capacity of mitochondria of alcohol-fed subjects to oxidize acetaldehyde, associated with unaltered or even enhanced rates of ethanol oxidation (and therefore acetaldehyde generation) because of MEOS induction (see above) results in an imbalance between production and disposition of acetaldehyde which contributes to the elevated acetaldehyde levels observed after chronic ethanol consumption in humans[153], and in baboons[154]; the latter was associated with a tremendous increase of acetaldehyde in hepatic venous blood[40]. Acetaldehyde is released from the liver, travels reversibly bound in plasma and erythrocytes[155], is taken up by extrahepatic tissues and affects many of them, but the most startling changes caused by acetaldehyde involve the liver itself.

Promotion of lipid peroxidation; interaction with cysteine, glutathione, iron and vitamin E

The capacity of acetaldehyde to cause lipid peroxidation in the liver has been demonstrated in isolated perfused livers[156]. *In vitro*, metabolism of acetaldehyde via xanthine oxidase[157] or aldehyde oxidase[158] may generate free radicals, but the concentration of acetaldehyde required is much too high for this to be of significance *in vivo*. Iron overload may also play a role. Iron overload in the alcoholic, as well as iron deficiency, have been reviewed elsewhere, in conjunction with other mineral abnormalities[159].

Binding of acetaldehyde with cysteine and/or glutathione (GSH) may contribute to a depression of liver glutathione[160]. Rats fed ethanol chronically have significantly increased rates of GSH turnover without an increased oxidation[161,162]. Acute ethanol administration inhibits GSH synthesis and produces an increased loss from the liver[163]. GSH transferase activity[164] is decreased by acute ethanol administration, and GSH peroxidase after chronic treatment[162]. Glutathione is selectively depleted in the mitochondria[165] and may contribute to the striking alcohol-induced alterations of that organelle. Glutathione offers one of the mechanisms for the scavenging of toxic free radicals[166]. Consistent with the interaction of GSH with free radical formation is the observation of a significant increase in α-amino-*n*-butyric acid after ethanol administration, both in humans and in the baboon[167]. Although GSH depletion is not necessarily sufficient to cause lipid peroxidation, it is generally agreed that it may favour the peroxidation produced by other factors. GSH is important in the protection of cells against electrophilic drug injury in general, and against reactive oxygen species in particular; it has been shown to spare and potentiate vitamin E[168] (see below).

For several decades, protein, methionine and choline deficiencies have been implicated in the pathogenesis of liver injury. In growing rats, deficiencies in dietary protein and lipotropic factors (choline and methionine) can produce a fatty liver[169] and it has been reported that ethanol increases choline requirements in the rat[170], possibly by enhancing choline oxidation[171]. Primates, however, are far less susceptible to protein and lipotropic deficiency than are rodents[172]. Clinically, choline treatment of patients suffering from alcoholic liver injury has been found to be ineffective in the face of continued alcohol abuse[173-176]. Furthermore, massive supplementation with choline has failed to prevent the fatty liver produced by alcohol in volunteer subjects[177]. This is not surprising since, unlike rat liver, human liver contains very little choline oxidase activity, which may explain the species differences with regard to choline deficiency. Moreover, fatty liver as well as fibrosis (including cirrhosis) developed in baboons despite liberal amounts of methionine[178] and massive supplementation with choline, even to the point of toxicity[179]. However, in addition to its possible role as a lipotrope, methionine also exerts a more specific effect as a selective precursor of cysteine which is a component of the tripeptide glutathione, a key substance for the protection of the liver from xenobiotic and free radical-mediated toxic injury. Moreover, methionine and its activated form, S-adenosyl-L-methionine (SAMe) plays an essential role in phospholipid metabolism and the maintenance of membrane structure and function[180]. Methionine supplementation has been considered for the treatment of liver diseases, especially the alcoholic varieties, but some difficulties have been encountered. Indeed, excess methionine was shown to have some adverse effects[181], including a decrease in hepatic ATP[182]. Whereas in some patients with alcoholic liver disease circulating methionine levels are normal[183], in others elevated concentrations have been reported[183-185]. Furthermore, Kinsell et al.[186] have observed a delay in the clearance of plasma methionine after its systemic administration to patients with liver damage. Similarly, Horowitz et al.[187] reported that the blood clearance of methionine after an oral load of this amino acid was slowed. Since about half the methionine is metabolized by the liver, the above observations suggest impaired hepatic metabolism of this amino acid in patients with alcoholic liver disease. Indeed, Duce et al.[188] reported a decrease in SAMe synthetase and phospholipid methyltransferase activities in cirrhotic livers. Furthermore, long-term alcohol consumption was found to be associated with enhanced methionine utilization and depletion[189]. As a consequence, SAMe depletion, as well as its decreased availability, can be expected. This has been verified in an experimental study which revealed that long-term ethanol consumption is associated with a significant depletion of hepatic SAMe. In baboons, long-term ethanol consumptioon (50% of energy as part of a totally liquid diet) resulted in a significant reduction of the hepatic SAMe concentration[190]. Potentially, such SAMe depletion may have a number of adverse effects, discussed by J. M. Mato elsewhere in these Proceedings.

Experimentally, the GSH depletion could be corrected, in part, by the administration of the active form of methionine, namely SAMe[191], with an associated attenuation of hepatotoxicity of ethanol, as evidenced by a decreased leakage of hepatic enzymes into the blood stream, including that of glutamic dehydrogenase, a mitochondrial enzyme. These findings in the non-human primates were consistent with the observations that SAMe restores the ethanol-induced glutathione depletion in rats[192,193] and increases hepatic glutathione in patients with liver disease[193]. Additional beneficial clinical effects are reviewed by others at this meeting.

Antioxidant protective mechanisms involve both enzymatic and non-enzymatic defence systems[194]. Impairments in such defence systems have been reported in alcoholics, including alterations of ascorbic acid[195], gluta-thione (see above), selenium[196-198] and vitamin E[196,199-201]. These changes could be due to direct effects of ethanol or to the malnutrition associated with alcoholism. Furthermore, these defence systems are mutually interrelated, and α-tocopherol, the major antioxidant in the membrane, is viewed as the 'last line' of defence against membrane lipid peroxidation[202,203]. Bjórneboe et al.[204] reported a reduced hepatic α-tocopherol content after chronic ethanol feeding in rats receiving adequate amounts of vitamin E, as well as in the blood of alcoholics[205]. Hepatic lipid peroxidation is significantly increased after chronic ethanol feeding in rats receiving a low vitamin E diet[144], indicating that dietary vitamin E is an important determinant of hepatic lipid peroxidation induced by chronic ethanol feeding. The lowest hepatic α-tocopherol was found in rats receiving a combination of low vitamin E and ethanol: both low dietary vitamin E and ethanol feeding significantly reduced hepatic α-tocopherol content; the latter, in part, because of increased conversion of α-tocopherol to α-tocopherylquinone[144]. In patients with cirrhosis, diminished hepatic vitamin E levels have been observed[142].

Acetaldehyde–protein adducts and effects on enzyme activities, including repair of nucleoproteins

Protein adduct formation is another mode of acetaldehyde toxicity. Nomura and Lieber[206] reported covalent binding of acetaldehyde to liver proteins. Acetaldehyde binds covalently to 2E1[207], other hepatic macromolecules[208], circulating proteins (serum albumin[209], and haemoglobin[210]). Of interest is the binding of acetaldehyde to tubulin, the constituent protein of microtubules. Acetaldehyde has a high affinity for sulphydryl groups, and its binding to these, as well as to lysine, may alter the capacity of tubulin to polymerize. One of the key functions of microtubules is to promote the intracellular transport of proteins and their secretion. Long-term alcohol feeding seriously delays the secretion of proteins from the liver into the plasma, with a corresponding hepatic retention[211]. The increases in lipid, protein, water, and electrolytes result in enlargement of the hepatocytes. Acetaldehyde adducts may serve as neoantigens, generating an immune response in mice[212] and in humans[213-215].

Another mode of acetaldehyde toxicity involves interference with enzyme activities[216], possibly secondary to its binding with critical functional groups. Minute concentrations of acetaldehyde (as low as $0.05 \mu mol/l$) were found to impair the repair of alkylated nucleoproteins[217]. Increased oxygen radical generation by ethanol-induced microsomes (see above) may participate in this enzyme inactivation[218].

Alcohol-induced disorders of phospholipids and collagen metabolism; production of membrane alterations and cirrhosis

Baboon studies suggested that perivenular fibrosis is a common and early warning sign of impending cirrhosis if drinking continues[219]. Similar conclusions were derived from clinical studies in alcoholics[220].

The accumulation of hepatic collagen during the development of cirrhosis could theoretically be accomplished by increased synthesis, decreased degradation, or both. The role of increased collagen synthesis was suggested by increased activity of hepatic peptidylproline hydroxylase in rats and primates and increased incorporation of proline ^{14}C into hepatic collagen in rat liver slices[221]. Increased hepatic peptidylproline hydroxylase activity was also found in patients with alcoholic cirrhosis[222], hepatitis[223], and in all stages of alcoholic liver disease[224]. The role of increased collagen synthesis has been confirmed indirectly in humans by autoradiographic techniques utilizing liver biopsies[225]. In baboons given ethanol that developed significant fibrosis, type I procollagen mRNA content was significantly increased (per liver RNA) as determined by hybridization analysis[226]. Whereas there is still some discussion about the relative contributions of hepatocytes and lipocytes in the production of collagen in the liver, lipocytes are 'activated' after chronic alcohol consumption and appear to play a major role[227,228]. Normal lipocytes, when isolated and cultured on plastic surfaces, undergo spontaneous transformation into transitional-like cells, thereby mimicking *in vitro* the condition that prevails *in vivo* after chronic alcohol consumption[229]. These cells in culture produce collagen[229]. When acetaldehyde is added to these cells they respond with a further increase in collagen accumulation[229], with increased mRNA for collagen[230]. Other aldehydes, such as malonaldehyde resulting from lipid peroxidation, as well as other peroxidation products, may also stimulate collagen production, as discussed by others at this meeting. Acetaldehyde also stimulates collagen synthesis in cultured myofibroblasts[231], and a similar effect was observed for lactate. These cells were shown to proliferate in the perivenular zones of the liver after chronic alcohol consumption, and are similar to activated lipocytes, but can be differentiated by ultrastructural and cytochemical characteristics, as discussed by K. Mak *et al.* in these proceedings.

Collagen accumulation not only reflects enhanced synthesis, but results from an imbalance between collagen degradation and collagen production. Thus, cirrhosis might, in part, represent a relative failure of collagen degradation to keep pace with synthesis. Interestingly, polyunsaturated lecithin may affect this balance. Indeed, addition of polyunsaturated lecithin to transformed lipocytes was found to prevent the acetaldehyde-mediated increase in collagen accumulation, possibly by stimulation of collagenase activity[232]. The active ingredient was identified as dilinoleoylphosphatidylcholine[233]. The role of collagenase was shown indirectly in humans by the correlation of the development of alcoholic fibrosis with increased activity of the circulating tissue inhibitor of metalloproteinase (TIMP)[234]. Indeed serum TIMP was significantly increased in alcoholic cirrhosis and may not only play a role in its pathogenesis through inhibition of collagenase activity,

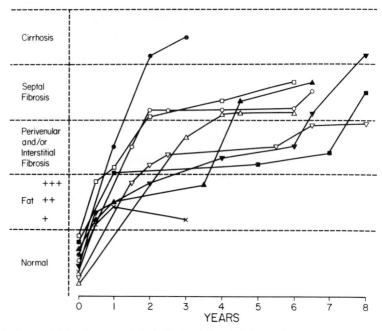

Fig. 4 Sequential development of alcoholic liver injury in baboons fed ethanol with a normal diet. Liver morphology in animals pair-fed control diet remained normal (not shown) (from ref. 235)

but also can serve as a marker of precirrhotic and cirrhotic states, since this test was more sensitive in detecting either PVF or SFC and offered better discrimination from fatty liver than serum PIIIP.

The stimulation of collagenase activity[234] may explain, at least in part, why polyunsaturated lecithin attenuates the development of fibrosis, including cirrhosis after chronic alcohol administration[235], an effect confirmed using more purified lecithin extracts, which identified dilinoleoylphosphatidyl-choline as the active ingredient of the polyunsaturated lecithin[233]. In these studies the control livers remained normal, whereas the baboons fed alcohol without phosphatidylcholine developed septal fibrosis or cirrhosis (Fig. 4), with transformation of most of the hepatic lipocytes to collagen-producing transitional cells. By contrast, none of the animals fed alcohol with phos-phatidylcholine developed septal fibrosis or cirrhosis[235], and less than half of their lipocytes were transformed, as discussed in greater detail by Mak *et al.* at this meeting.

Polyunsaturated phosphatidylcholine may improve the liver in other ways. Ethanol also results in a decrease of liver phospholipids, especially of phosphatidylcholine (PC); both can be corrected by PC supplementation[233]. The total phospholipid content of the mitochondrial membranes is decreased, with a significant reduction in the levels of phosphatidylcholine[236] and associated striking morphological changes[237]. The alterations in the phospho-lipid composition of the mitochondrial membranes appear responsible for some of the depression of cytochrome oxidase activity produced by chronic ethanol consumption[236]. This, in turn, may be the cause, at least in part, for the biochemical alterations observed in the hepatic mitochondria of baboons fed ethanol[237]. The mechanism whereby chronic ethanol consumption alters phospholipids has not been clarified, but may be related, at least in part, to decreased phospholipid methyltransferase activity described in cirrhotic liver[188]. That this is not simply secondary to the cirrhosis, but may in fact be a primary defect related to alcohol, is suggested by the observation that the enzyme activity is already decreased prior to the development of cirrhosis[238]. Administration of polyunsaturated lecithin was shown to correct this enzyme deficiency[238] and the hepatic phospholipid and phosphatidylcholine deficiency produced by alcohol[233]. Polyunsaturated lecithin contains choline, and choline deficiency has been incriminated in the pathogenesis of liver injury for several decades (see above). However, fatty liver as well as fibrosis (including cirrhosis) developed in baboons despite massive supplementation with choline[179]. Thus, the beneficial effect of polyunsaturated phospholipids cannot be attributed simply to their choline content, but may be due perhaps to their high bioavailability and selective incorporation into liver membranes[239], and their effect on hepatic lipocytes (see above).

ROLE OF IMMUNOLOGICAL FACTORS, CYTOKINES AND HEPATITIS VIRUSES

Derangements of immune systems are present in alcoholic liver disease, but there is still some debate whether they represent a consequence or a cause of the liver injury. Whereas studies by Spinozzi et al.[240] suggest an alteration of T-lymphocyte activation pathways in alcoholic liver disease (even in the absence of evidence of malnutrition or hepatic cirrhosis), studies of Müller et al.[241] reported no difference in lymphocyte subsets between controls and patients with alcohol-induced fatty liver; abnormalities were seen only in patients with cirrhosis.

Alcoholism and viral hepatitis can occur in the same patients, but in many subjects with alcoholic cirrhosis there is no evidence for antecedent viral hepatitis. However, hepatitis C is commonly associated, and may play an important role[242]. Indeed, in alcoholic patients, portal and/or lobular inflammation is strongly associated with HCV antibody, even in the absence of HCV risk factors[243], and there is increasing evidence for the involvement of viruses in the pathogenesis of chronic hepatitis in alcoholics. It has been proposed that tumour necrosis factor, a mediator of endotoxic shock and sepsis, also plays a role in alcoholic hepatitis.

Experimentally, acute administration of alcohol enhances endotoxin hepatotoxicity when the dose of endotoxin is small, but the effect of alcohol is masked when larger doses of endotoxin are given[244]. Circulating tumour necrosis factor (TNF)-α, and interleukin-1 remained elevated for up to 6 months after the diagnosis of alcoholic hepatitis, whereas interleukin-6 normalized in parallel with clinical recovery[245]. Concentrations of all three cytokines correlated with biochemical parameters of liver injury. Sheron et *al.*[246] also found that the cytokine interleukin-6 is activated in severe alcoholic hepatitis, and postulated that this may mediate hepatic or extrahepatic tissue damage. On the one hand, TNF appears to be a proximal mediator of multiple types of experimental injury and TNF activity is elevated in alcoholic liver disease, as are the levels of certain other cytokines[247]. On the other hand, low physiological amounts of cytokines appear to be important for liver regeneration (and perhaps are beneficial to the organism as a whole). The challenge is now to acquire sufficient knowledge to conserve the positive growth-enhancing effects of cytokines while attenuating their cytotoxic effects.

EFFECT OF GENDER AND GENETICS

The average cirrhogenic doses, as well as the threshold doses, are lower in females than males: a daily intake of alcohol of 40–60 g in men but only 20 g in women resulted in a statistically significant increase in the incidence of cirrhosis in a well-nourished population[248]. There is also evidence that the progression to more severe liver injury is accelerated in women: incidence of chronic advanced liver disease is higher among women than among men for a similar history of alcohol abuse[249-251]. Gender differences in ethanol metabolism, not only in the liver but also in the stomach[60], may be contributory. Thus, gender must be recognized as one of the factors that determines severity of alcoholic liver injury. Individual differences in rates of ethanol metabolism appear, in part, to be genetically controlled, and the possible role of heredity for the development of alcoholism in humans has been emphasized[252]. In patients with chronic alcoholic liver disease the HLA-B8 was more prevalent in patients with alcoholic cirrhosis than in controls or in patients with fatty liver or minimal fibrosis[253]. Another difference was the absence of HLA-A28 in the cirrhotic patients[254]. The cirrhotics with HLA-B8 had been drinking for a shorter period of time than patients with comparable clinical and histological diseases but without HLA-B8[255]. These results suggested the hypothesis that genetic factors may be implicated in alcohol-induced liver damage, and particularly its progression to cirrhosis. These data, however, have not been confirmed[256-258].

SUMMARY AND CONCLUSIONS

Until three decades ago, liver disease of the alcoholic was attributed exclusively to dietary deficiencies. Since then, however, our understanding of the impact of alcoholism on nutritional status has undergone a progressive evolution, as discussed in detail elsewhere[29]. Alcohol, because of its high energy content, was at first perceived to act exclusively as 'empty calories' displacing other nutrients in the diet, and causing primary malnutrition through decreased intake of essential nutrients. With improvement in the overall nutrition of the population, the role of primary malnutrition waned, and secondary malnutrition was emphasized as a result of a better understanding of maldigestion and malabsorption caused by chronic alcohol consumption and various diseases associated with alcoholism. At the same time the concept of the direct toxicity of alcohol came to the forefront as an explanation for the widespread cellular injury. Some of the hepatotoxicity was found to result from the metabolic disturbances associated with the oxidation of ethanol via the liver alcohol dehydrogenase (ADH) pathway and the redox changes produced by NADH generation, which in turn affects the metabolism of lipids, carbohydrates, proteins and purines. Exaggeration of the redox change by the relative hypoxia which prevails physiologically in the perivenular zone contributes to the exacerbation of the ethanol-induced lesions in zone III. In addition to ADH, ethanol can be oxidized by liver microsomes: studies over the past 20 years have culminated in the molecular elucidation of the ethanol-inducible cytochrome P4502E1 (2E1) which contributes not only to ethanol metabolism and tolerance, but also to the hepatic perivenular toxicity of various xenobiotics, since 2E is selectively present and induced in the perivenular zone. Their activation by 2E1 now provides an understanding for the increased susceptibility of the heavy drinker to the toxicity of industrial solvents, anaesthetic agents, commonly prescribed drugs, over-the-counter analgesics, chemical carcinogens and even nutritional factors such as vitamin A. Ethanol not only causes vitamin A depletion, but it also enhances its hepatotoxicity. Furthermore, induction of the microsomal pathway contributes to increased acetaldehyde generation, with formation of protein adducts, resulting in antibody production, enzyme inactivation, decreased DNA repair; it is also associated with a striking impairment of the capacity of the liver to utilize oxygen. Moreover, acetaldehyde promotes glutathione depletion, free-radical-mediated toxicity and lipid peroxidation. In addition, acetaldehyde affects hepatic collagen synthesis: both *in vivo* and *in vitro* (in cultured myofibroblasts and lipocytes) ethanol and/or its metabolite acetaldehyde were found to increase collagen accumulation and mRNA levels for collagen.

This better understanding of the biochemical alterations produced by ethanol in the body provides insight into processes whereby ethanol alters both the activation and degradation of key nutrients. In turn, nutritional factors were shown to strikingly affect the detoxification of noxious agents. 'Supernutrients', such as S-adenosyl-L-methionine and polyunsaturated lecithin, were found to significantly offset some of the toxic or fibrotic manifestations. Thus, the originally opposed notions of nutritional versus toxic effects of ethanol have now been bridged and – at cellular, biochemical, and molecular levels – nutritional and toxic effects of ethanol have converged, yielding better understanding of the pathology generated by ethanol, with resulting improved prospects for therapy.

Acknowledgements

Original studies reviewed here were supported, in part, by DHHS grants AA03508, AA05934, AA07275, DK 32810 and the Department of Veterans Affairs. We wish to thank Mrs J. Cohen and Ms R. Cabell for skilful typing of the manuscript.

References

1. Chedid A, Mendenhall CL, Gartside P et al. Prognostic factors in alcoholic liver disease. Am J Gastroenterol. 1991;82:210–16.
2. Lieber CS, DeCarli LM. Hepatotoxicity of ethanol. J Hepatol. 1991;12:394–401.
3. Krebs HA, Perkins JR. The physiological role of liver alcohol dehydrogenase. Biochem J. 1970;118:635–44.
4. Okuda K, Takigawa N. Rat liver 5β-cholestane-3α,7α,12α 26-tetrol dehydrogenase as a liver alcohol dehydrogenase. Biochim Biophys Acta. 1970;22:141–8.
5. Keung W-M. Human liver alcohol dehydrogenases catalyze the oxidation of the intermediary alcohols of the shunt pathway of mevalonate metabolism. Biochem. Biophys Res Commun. 1991;174:701–7.
6. Bjorkhem I. On the role of alcohol dehydrogenase in β-oxidation of fatty acids. Eur J Biochem. 1972;30:441–51.
7. Jörnvall H, Hoog J-O, Bahr-Lindstrom H et al. Mammalian alcohol dehydrogenases of separate classes: Intermediates between different enzymes and intraclass isozymes. Proc Natl Acad Sci USA. 1987;84:2580–4.
8. Bosron WF, Li T-K. Catalytic properties of human liver alcohol dehydrogenase isoenzymes. Enzyme. 1987;37:19–28.
9. Smith M, Hopkinson DA, Harris H. Developmental changes and polymorphism in human alcohol dehydrogenase. Ann Hum Genet (Lond). 1971;34:251–71.
10. von Bahr-Lindstrom H, von Wog J-O, Heden L-O et al. cDNA and protein structure for the α subunit of human liver alcohol dehydrogenase. Biochemistry. 1986;25:2465–70.
11. Duester G, Smith M, Bilanchone V et al. Molecular analysis of the human class I alcohol dehydrogenase gene family and nucleotide sequence of the gene encoding the β subunit. J Biol Chem. 1986;261:2027–33.
12. von Wartburg JP, Papenberg J, Aebi H. An atypical human alcohol dehydrogenase. Can J Biochem. 1965;43:889–98.
13. Jörnvall H, Hempel J, Vallee BL et al. Human liver alcohol dehydrogenase: amino acid substitution in the β2β2 Oriental isozyme explains functional properties, establishes an active site structure, and parallels mutational exchanges in the yeast enzyme. Proc Natl Acad Sci USA. 1984;81:3024–8.
14. Bosron WF, Magnes LJ, Li T-K. Human liver alcohol dehydrogenase: ADH Indianapolis results from genetic polymorphism at the ADH2 gene locus. Biochem Genet. 1983;21: 735–44.
15. Li T-K, Magnes LJ. Identification of a distinctive molecular form of alcohol dehydrogenase in human livers with high activity. Biochem Biophys Res Commun. 1975;63:202–8.
16. Bosron WF, Li T-K, Dafeldecker WP et al. Human liver π-alcohol dehydrogenase: kinetic and molecular properties. Biochemistry. 1979;18:1101–5.
17. Pares X, Vallee BL. New human liver alcohol dehydrogenase forms with unique kinetic characteristics. Biochem Biophys Res Commun. 1989;98:122–30.
18. Yin S-J, Wang M-F, Liao C-S et al. Identification of a human stomach alcohol dehydrogenase with distinctive kinetic properties. Biochem Int. 1990;22:829–35.
19. Moreno A, Parés X. Purification and characterization of a new alcohol dehydrogenase from human stomach. J Biochem. 1991;266:1128–33.
20. Yasunami M, Chen C-S, Yoshida A. A human alcohol dehydrogenase gene (ADH6) encoding an additional class of isozyme. Proc Natl Acad Sci USA. 1991;88:7610–14.
21. Morrison GR, Brock FE. Quantitative measurement of alcohol dehydrogenase activity within the liver lobule of rats after prolonged alcohol ingestion. J Nutr. 1967;92:186–292.
22. Beuhler R, Hess M, von Wartburg J-P. Immunohistochemical localization of human liver alcohol dehydrogenase in liver tissue, cultured fibroblasts and hela cells. Am J Pathol. 1982;108:89–99.
23. Sokal EM, Colette C, Buts JP. Continuous increase of alcohol dehydrogenase activity along the liver plate in normal and cirrhotic human livers. Hepatology. 1993;17:202–5.
24. Maly IP, Sasse D. The intra-acinar distribution patterns of alcohol-dehydrogenase activity in the liver of juvenile, castrated and testosterone-treated rats. Biochem H Seyler. 1987;368:315–21.
25. Lieber CS, Jones DP, Losowsky MS et al. Interrelation of uric acid and ethanol metabolism

ALCOHOL AND THE LIVER

in man. J Clin Invest. 1962;41:1863–70.
26. Lefèvre A, Adler H, Lieber CS. Effect of ethanol on ketone metabolism. J Clin Invest. 1970;49:1775–82.
27. Faller J, Fox IH. Evidence for increased urate production by activation of adenine nucleotide turnover. N Engl J Med. 1982;307:1598–602.
28. Lieber CS, Pignon J-P. Ethanol and lipids. In: Fruchart JC, Shepherd J, editors. Human plasma lipoproteins: chemistry, physiology and pathology. Berlin–New York, Walder De Gruyter; 1989:245–80.
29. Lieber CS. Medical and nutritional complications of alcoholism: mechanisms and management. New York: Plenum Press; 1992.
30. Lieber CS, Spritz N, DeCarli LM. Role of dietary, adipose and endogenously synthesized fatty acids in the pathogenesis of the alcoholic fatty liver. J Clin Invest. 1966;45:51–62.
31. Lieber CS, Spritz N. Effects of prolonged ethanol intake in man: role of dietary, adipose, and endogenously synthesized fatty acids in the pathogenesis of the alcoholic fatty liver. J Clin Invest. 1966;45:1400–11.
32. Lane BP, Lieber CS. Ultrastructural alterations in human hepatocytes following ingestion of ethanol with adequate diets. Am J Pathol. 1966;49:593–603.
33. Israel Y, Kalant H, Orrego H et al. Experimental alcohol-induced hepatic necrosis: Suppression by propylthiouracil. Proc Natl Acad Sci USA. 1975;72:1137–41.
34. Kessler BJ, Lieber JB, Bronfin GJ et al. The hepatic blood flow and splanchnic oxygen consumption in alcohol fatty liver. J Clin Invest. 1954;33:1338–45.
35. Jauhonen P, Baraona E, Miyakawa H et al. Mechanism for selective perivenular hepatotoxicity of ethanol. Alcoholism: Clin Exp Res. 1982;6:350–7.
36. Sato N, Kamada T, Kawano S et al. Effect of acute and chronic ethanol consumption on hepatic tissue oxygen tension in rats. Pharmacol Biochem Behav. 1983;18:443–7.
37. Shaw S, Heller E, Friedman H et al. Increased hepatic oxygenation following ethanol administration in the baboon. Proc Soc Exp Biol Med. 1977;156:509–13.
38. Stein SW, Lieber CS, Cherrick GR et al. The effect of ethanol upon systemic hepatic blood flow in man. Am J Clin Nutr. 1963;13:68–74.
39. Carmichael FJ, Saldivia V, Israel Y et al. Ethanol-induced increase in portal hepatic blood flow: interference by anesthetic agents. Hepatology. 1987;97:89–94.
40. Lieber CS, Baraona E, Hernández-Muñoz R et al. Impaired oxygen utilization: A new mechanism for the hepatotoxicity of ethanol in sub-human primates. J Clin Invest. 1989;83:1682–90.
41. Jauhonen P, Baraona E, Lieber CS et al. Dependence of ethanol-induced redox shift on hepatic oxygen tensions prevailing in vivo. Alcohol. 1985;2:163–7.
42. Kato S, Kawase T, Alderman J et al. Role of xanthine oxidase in ethanol-induced lipid peroxidation in rats. Gastroenterology. 1990;98:203–10.
43. Lieber CS. Alcohol and the liver: metabolism of ethanol, metabolic effects and pathogenesis of injury. Acta Med Scand Suppl. 1985;703:11–55.
44. Brighenti L, Pancaldi G. Effetto della somministrazione di alcool etilico su alcune attivita enzimatiche del fegato di ratto. Boll Soc It Biol Sper. 1970;46:1–5.
45. Lieber CS, DeCarli LM. Hepatic microsomal ethanol oxidizing system: In vitro characteristics and adaptive properties in vivo. J Biol Chem. 1970;245:2505–12.
46. Salaspuro MP, Shaw S, Jayatilleke E et al. Attenuation of the ethanol induced hepatic redox change after chronic alcohol consumption in baboons: metabolic consequences in vivo and in vitro. Hepatology. 1980;1:33–8.
47. Ugarte G, Pino ME, Insunza I. Hepatic alcohol dehydrogenase in alcoholic addicts with and without hepatic damage. Am J Dig Dis. 1967;12:589–92.
48. Rothschild MA, Oratz M, Mongelli J et al. Alcohol induced depression of albumin synthesis: reversal by tryptophan. J Clin Invest. 1971;50:1812–18.
49. Jeejeebhoy KN, Bruce-Robertson A, Ho J et al. The effect of ethanol on albumin and fibrinogen synthesis in vivo and in hepatocyte suspension. In: Rothschild MA, Oratz M, Schrieber S, editors. Alcohol and abnormal protein synthesis. New York: Pergamon Press, 1975:373–91.
50. Yamauchi M, Potter JJ, Mezey E. Characteristics of alcohol dehydrogenase in fat-storing (Ito) cells of rat liver. Gastroenterology. 1988;94:163–9.
51. Flisiak R, Baraona E, Li J et al. Effects of ethanol on prostanoid production by fat-storing

cells. Hepatology. 1993;18:153–9.

52. Hernández-Muñoz R, Caballeria J, Baraona E et al. Human gastric alcohol dehydrogenase: Its inhibition by H_2-receptor antagonists, and its effect on the bioavailability of ethanol. Alcoholism: Clin Exp Res. 1990;14:946–50.

53. Julkunen RJK, DiPadova C, Lieber CS. First pass metabolism of ethanol a gastrointestinal barrier against the systemic toxicity of ethanol. Life Sci. 1985;37:567–73.

54. Julkunen RJK, Tannenbaum L, Baraona E et al. First pass metabolism of ethanol: an important determinant of blood levels after alcohol consumption. Alcohol. 1985;2:437–41.

55. Baraona E, Yokoyama A, Ishii H et al. Lack of alcohol dehydrogenase isoenzyme activities in the stomach of Japanese subjects. Life Sci. 1991;49:1929–34.

56. Roine RP, Gentry RT, Lim Jr RT et al. Effect of concentration of ingested ethanol on blood alcohol levels. Alcoholism: Clin Exp Res. 1991;15:734–8.

57. Smith T, DeMaster EG, Furne JK et al. First-pass gastric mucosal metabolism of ethanol is negligible in the rat. J Clin Invest. 1992;89:1801–6.

58. Caballeria J, Frezza M, Hernandez-Munoz R et al. The gastric origin of the first pass metabolism of ethanol in man: effect of gastrectomy. Gastroenterology. 1989;97:1205–9.

59. Di Padova C, Worner TM, Julkunen RJK et al. Effects of fasting and chronic alcohol consumption on the first pass metabolism of ethanol. Gastroenterology. 1987;92:1169–73.

60. Frezza M, Di Padova C, Pozzato G et al. High blood alcohol levels in women: Role of decreased gastric alcohol dehydrogenase activity and first pass metabolism. N Engl J Med. 1990;322:95–9.

61. Roine R, Gentry RT, Hernández-Muñoz R et al. Aspirin increases blood alcohol concentrations in human after ingestion of ethanol. JAMA. 1990;264:2406–8.

62. Caballeria J, Baraona E, Rodamilans M et al. Effects of cimetidine on gastric alcohol dehydrogenase activity and blood ethanol levels. Gastroenterology. 1989;96:388–92.

63. Caballeria J, Baraona E, Deulofeu R et al. Effects of H_2-receptor antagonists on gastric alcohol dehydrogenase activity. Dig Dis Sci. 1991;36:1673–97.

64. Di Padova C, Roine R, Frezza M et al. Effects of ranitidine on blood alcohol levels after ethanol ingestion: comparison with other H_2-receptor antagonists. JAMA. 1992;267: 83–6.

65. Roine RP, Hernández-Muñoz R, Gentry RT et al. H_2-antagonists and blood alcohol levels. Dig Dis Sci. 1993;38:572–3.

66. Seitz HK, Veith S, Czygan P et al. In vivo interactions between H_2-receptor antagonists and ethanol metabolism in man and in rats. Hepatology. 1984;4:1231–4.

67. Seitz HK, Egerer G, Simanowski UA. High blood alcohol levels in women. N Engl J Med. 1990;323:58.

68. Redman CM, Grab DJ, Irukulla R. The intracellular pathway of newly formed rat liver catalase. Arch Biochem Biophys. 1972;152:496–501.

69. Keilin D, Hartree EF. Properties of catalase catalysis of coupled oxidation of alcohols. Biochem J. 1945;39:293–301.

70. Handler JA, Thurman RG. Fatty acid-dependent ethanol metabolism. Biochem Biophys Res Commun. 1985;133:44–51.

71. Williamson J, Scholz R, Browning ET et al. Metabolic effects of ethanol in perfused rat liver. J Biol Chem. 1969;25:5044–54.

72. Inatomi N, Kato S, Ito D et al. Role of peroxisomal fatty acid beta-oxidation in ethanol metabolism. Biochem Biophys Res Commun. 1989;163:418–23.

73. Takagi T, Alderman J, Gellert J et al. Assessment of the role of non-ADH ethanol oxidation in vivo and in hepatocytes from deermice. Biochem Pharmacol. 1986;35:3601–6.

74. Kato S, Alderman J, Lieber CS. Respective roles of the microsomal ethanol oxidizing system (MEOS) and catalase in ethanol metabolism by deermice lacking alcohol dehydrogenase. Arch Biochem Biophys. 1987;254:586–91.

75. Lieber CS, DeCarli LM. Ethanol oxidation by hepatic microsomes: adaptive increase after ethanol feeding. Science. 1968;162:917–18.

76. Teschke R, Hasumura Y, Joly JG et al. Microsomal ethanol-oxidizing system (MEOS): purification and properties of a rat liver system free of catalase and alcohol dehydrogenase. Biochem Biophys Res Commun. 1972;49:1187–93.

77. Teschke R, Hasumura Y, Lieber CS. Hepatic microsomal alcohol oxidizing system Solubilization, isolation and characterization. Arch Biochem Biophys. 1974;163:404–15.

78. Ohnishi K, Lieber CS. Reconstitution of the microsomal ethanol-oxidizing system: qualitative and quantitative changes of cytochrome P-450 after chronic ethanol consumption. J Biol Chem. 1977;252:7124–31.
79. Miwa GT, Levin W, Thomas PE et al. The direct oxidation of ethanol by catalase- and alcohol dehydrogenase-free reconstituted system containing cytochrome P-450. Arch Biochem Biophys. 1978;187:464–75.
80. Koop DR, Morgan ET, Tarr GE et al. Purification and characterization of a unique isozyme of cytochrome P-450 from liver microsomes of ethanol-treated rabbits. J Biol Chem. 1982;257:8472–80.
81. Morgan ET, Koop DR, Coon MJ. Catalytic activity of cytochrome P-450 isozyme 3a isolated from liver microsomes of ethanol-treated rabbits. J Biol Chem. 1982;257: 13951–7.
82. Morgan ET, Koop DR, Coon MJ. Comparison of six rabbit liver cytochrome P-450 isozymes in formation of a reactive metabolite of acetaminophen. Biochem Biophys Res Commun. 1983;112:8–13.
83. Ingelman-Sundberg M, Johansson I. Mechanisms of hydroxyl radical formation and ethanol oxidation by ethanol-inducible and other forms of rabbit liver microsomal cytochromes P-450. J Biol Chem. 1984;259:6447–58.
84. Koop DR, Casazza JP. Identification of ethanol-inducible P-450 isozyme 3a as the acetone and acetol monooxygenase of rabbit microsomes. J Biol Chem. 1985;260:13607–12.
85. Yang CS, Tu YY, Koop DR et al. Metabolism of nitrosamines by purified rabbit liver cytochrome P-450 isozymes. Cancer Res. 1985;45:1140–5.
86. Ryan DE, Ramathan L, Iida S et al. Characterization of a major form of rat hepatic microsomal cytochrome P-450 induced by isoniazid. J Biol Chem. 1985;260:6385–93.
87. Ryan DE, Koop DR, Thomas PE et al. Evidence that isoniazid and ethanol induced the same microsomal cytochrome P-450 in rat liver, and isozyme homologous to rabbit liver cytochrome P-450 isozymes 3a. Arch Biochem Biophys. 1986;246:633–44.
88. Wrighton SA, Campanile C, Thomas PE et al. Identification of a human liver cytochrome P-450 homologous to the major isosafrole-inducible cytochrome P-450 in the rat. Mol Pharmacol. 1986;29:405–10.
89. Song BJ, Gelboin HV, Park SS et al. Complementary DNA and protein sequences of ethanol-inducible rat and human cytochrome P-450s. J Biol Chem. 1986;261:16689–97.
90. Lasker JM, Raucy J, Kubota S et al. Purification and characterization of human liver cytochrome P-450-ALC. Biochem Biophys Res Commun. 1987;148:232–8.
91. Tsutsumi M, Lasker JM, Shimizu M et al. The intralobular distribution of ethanol-inducible P450IIE1 in rat and human liver. Hepatology. 1989;10:437–46.
92. Lieber CS, Lasker JM, DeCarli LM et al. Role of acetone, dietary fat, and total energy intake in the induction of the hepatic microsomal ethanol oxidizing system. J Pharmacol Exp Ther. 1988;247:791–5.
93. Lieber CS, DeCarli LM. The role of the hepatic microsomal ethanol oxidizing system (MEOS) for ethanol metabolism in vivo. J Pharmacol Exp Ther. 1972;181:279–87.
94. Teschke R, Hasumura Y, Lieber CS. Hepatic ethanol metabolism: respective roles of alcohol dehydrogenase, the microsomal ethanol oxidizing system and catalase. Arch Biochem Biophys. 1976;175:635–43.
95. Matsuzaki S, Gordon E, Lieber CS. Increased alcohol dehydrogenase independent ethanol oxidation at high ethanol concentrations in isolated rat hepatocytes: the effect of chronic ethanol feedings. J Pharmacol Exp Ther. 1981;217:133–7.
96. Burnett KG, Felder MR. Ethanol metabolism in peromyscus genetically deficient in alcohol dehydrogenase. Biochem Pharmacol. 1980;128:1–8.
97. Shigeta Y, Nomura F, Iida S et al. Ethanol metabolism in vivo by the microsomal ethanol oxidizing system in deermice lacking alcohol dehydrogenase (ADH). Biochem Pharmacol. 1984;33:807–14.
98. Kato S, Alderman J, Lieber CS. Ethanol metabolism in alcohol dehydrogenase deficient deermice is mediated by the microsomal ethanol oxidizing system, not by catalase. Alcohol Alcoholism. 1987(Suppl 1):231–4.
99. Kato S, Alderman J, Lieber CS. In vivo role of the microsomal ethanol oxidizing system in ethanol metabolism by deermice lacking alcohol dehydrogenase. Biochem Pharmacol. 1988;37:2706–8.

100. Alderman J, Takagi T, Lieber CS. Ethanol metabolizing pathways in deermice: estimation of flux calculated from isotope effects. J Biol Chem. 1987;262:7497–503.
101. Ingelman-Sundberg M, Norsten C, Ekström G et al. Ethanol effects and metabolism. A study using stable isotopes. In: Kuriyama K, Takada A, Ishii H, editors. Biomedical and social aspects of alcohol and alcoholism. Amsterdam: Excerpta Medica; 1988:119–22.
102. Norsten C, Cronholm T, Ekstrom G et al. Dehydrogenase-dependent ethanol metabolism in deermice (Peromyscus maniculatus) lacking cytosolic alcohol dehydrogenase. J Biol Chem. 1989;264:5593–7.
103. Inatomi N, Ito D, Lieber CS. Ethanol oxidation by deermice mitochondria under physiologic conditions. Alcoholism: Clin Exp Res. 1990;14:130–3.
104. Cronholm T, Norsten-Hoog C, Ekstrom G et al. Oxidoreduction of butanol in deermice (Peromyscus maniculatus) lacking hepatic cytosolic alcohol dehydrogenase. Eur J Biochem. 1992;204:353–7.
105. Cronholm T, Norsten-Hoog C, Ekstrom G et al. Role of extrahepatic alcohol dehydrogenase (ADH) in the metabolism of ethanol and butanol in deer mice. Alcohol Alcoholism. 1992;27:35.
106. Ito D, Lieber CS. Ethanol metabolism in deermice: role of extrahepatic alcohol dehydrogenase. Alcoholism: Clin Exp Res. 1993;17:919–25.
107. Misra PS, Lefèvre A, Ishii H et al. Increase of ethanol meprobamate and pentobarbital metabolism after chronic ethanol administration in man and in rats. Am J Med. 1971;51:346–51.
108. Kater RMH, Tobon F, Iber FL. Increased rate of tolbutamide metabolism in alcoholic patients. JAMA. 1969;207:363–5.
109. Pritchard JF, Schneck DW. Effects of ethanol and phenobarbital on the metabolism of propanolol by 9000g rat liver supernatant. Biochem Pharmacol. 1977;26:2453–4.
110. Hetu C, Joly J-G. Differences in the duration of the enhancement of liver mixed-function oxidase activities in ethanol-fed rats after withdrawal. Biochem Pharmacol. 1985;34:1211–16.
111. Borowsky SA, Lieber CS. Interaction of methadone and ethanol metabolism. J Pharmacol Exp Ther. 1978;207:123–9.
112. Hasumura Y, Teschke R, Lieber CS. Increased carbon tetrachloride hepatotoxicity, and its mechanism, after chronic ethanol consumption. Gastroenterology. 1974;66:415–22.
113. Hetu C, Dumont A, Joly J-G. Effect of chronic ethanol administration on bromobenzene liver toxicity in the rat. Toxicol Appl Pharmacol. 1983;67:166–7.
114. Siegers CP, Heidbuchel K, Younes M. Influence of alcohol, dithiocard and (+)-catechin on the hepatotoxicity and metabolism of vinylidene chloride in rats. J Appl Toxicol. 1983;3:90–5.
115. Tsutsumi R, Leo MA, Kim C et al. Interaction of ethanol with enflurane metabolism and toxicity: role of P450IIE1. Alcoholism: Clin Exp Res. 1990;14:174–9.
116. Takagi T, Ishii H, Takahashi H et al. Potentiation of halothane hepatotoxicity by chronic ethanol administration in rat: An animal model of halothane hepatitis. Pharmacol Biochem Behav. 1983;18(Suppl 1):461–5.
117. Nakajima T, Okuyama S, Yonekura I et al. Effects of ethanol and phenobarbital administration on the metabolism and toxicity of benzene. Chem Biol Interact. 1985;55:23–38.
118. Nakajima TM, Okino T, Sato A. Kinetic studies on benzene metabolism in rat liver – possible presence of three forms of benzene metabolizing enzymes in the liver. Biochem Pharmacol. 1987;36:2799–804.
119. Schnier GG, Laethem CL, Koop DR. Identification and induction of cytochromes P450, P450IIE1 and P450IA1 in rabbit bone marrow. J Pharmacol Exp Ther. 1989;251:790–6.
120. Beskid M, Bialck J, Dzieniszewski J et al. Effect of combined phenylbutazone and ethanol administration on rat liver. Exp Pathol. 1980;18:487–91.
121. Lieber CS, Garro A, Leo MA et al. Alcohol and cancer. Hepatology. 1986;6:1005–19.
122. Garro AJ, Seitz HK, Lieber CS. Enhancement of dimethylnitrosamine metabolism and activation to a mutagen following chronic ethanol consumption. Cancer Res. 1981;41:120–4.
123. Farinati F, Zhou Z, Bellah J et al. Effect of chronic ethanol consumption on activation of nitrosopyrrolidine to a mutagen by rat upper alimentary tract, lung and hepatic tissue. Drug Metab Dispos. 1985;13:210–14.

124. Seitz HK, Garro AJ, Lieber CS. Enhanced pulmonary and intestinal activation of procarcinogens and mutagens after chronic ethanol consumption in the rat. Eur J Clin Invest. 1981;11:33–8.
125. Seitz HK, Czygan P, Waldherr K et al. Ethanol and intestinal carcinogenesis in the rat. Alcohol. 1985;2:491–4.
126. Shimizu M, Lasker JM, Tsutsumi M et al. Immunohistochemical localization of ethanol-inducible P450IIE1 in the rat alimentary tract. Gastroenterology. 1990;99:1044–53.
127. Lasker JM, Tsutsumi M, Bloswick BP et al. Characterization of a benzoflavone (BF)-inducible hamster liver cytochrome P-450 isozyme catalytically similar to cytochrome P-450-ALC. Hepatology. 1987;7:432 (abstract).
128. Garro AJ, Lieber CS. Alcohol and cancer. Annu Rev Pharmacol Toxicol. 1990;30:219–49.
129. Sato M, Lieber CS. Hepatic vitamin A depletion after chronic ethanol consumption in baboons and rats. J Nutr. 1981;111:2015–23.
130. Leo MA, Lieber CS. New pathway for retinol metabolism in liver microsomes. J Biochem. 1985;260:5228–31.
131. Leo MA, Kim CI, Lieber CS. NAD$^+$-dependent retinol dehydrogenase in liver microsomes. Arch Biochem Biophys. 1987;259:241–9.
132. Leo MA, Iida S, Lieber CS. Retinoic acid metabolism by a system reconstituted with cytochrome P-450. Arch Biochem Biophys. 1984;234:305–12.
133. Leo MA, Lasker JM, Raucy JL et al. Metabolism of retinol and retinoic acid by human liver cytochrome P450IIC8. Arch Biochem Biophys. 1989;269:305–12.
134. Leo MA, Lowe N, Lieber CS. Potentiation of ethanol-induced hepatic vitamin A depletion by phenobarbital and butylated hydroxytoluene. J Nutr. 1987;117:70–6.
135. Leo MA, Lowe N, Lieber CS. Decreased hepatic vitamin A after drug administration in humans and in rats. Am J Clin Nutr. 1984;40:1131–6.
136. Leo MA, Sato M, Lieber CS. Effect of hepatic vitamin A depletion on the liver in men and rats. Gastroenterology. 1983;84:562–72.
137. Leo MA, Lowe N, Lieber CS. Interaction of drugs and retinol. Biochem Pharmacol. 1986;35:3949–53.
138. Leo MA, Lieber CS. Hypervitaminosis A: a liver lover's lament. Hepatology. 1988;8:412–17.
139. Leo MA, Arai M, Sato M et al. Hepatotoxicity of vitamin A and ethanol in the rat. Gastroenterology. 1982;82:194–205.
140. Leo MA, Leiber CS. Hepatic fibrosis after long term administration of ethanol and moderate vitamin A supplementation in the rat. Hepatology. 1983;2:1–11.
141. Leo MA, Kim CI, Lowe N et al. Interaction of ethanol with β-carotene: delayed blood clearance and enhanced hepatotoxicity. Hepatology. 1992;15:883–91.
142. Leo MA, Rosman A, Lieber CS. Differential depletion of carotenoids and tocopherol in liver diseases. Hepatology. 1993;17:977–86.
143. Gascon-Barré M. Interrelationships between vitamin D2 and 25-hydroxyl-vitamin D3 during chronic ethanol administration in the rat. Metabolism. 1982;31:67–72.
144. Kawase T, Kato S, Lieber CS. Lipid peroxidation and antioxidant defense systems in rat liver after chronic ethanol feeding. Hepatology. 1989;10:815–21.
145. Laposata EA, Lange LG. Presence of nonoxidative ethanol metabolism in human organs commonly damaged by ethanol abuse. Science. 1986;231:497–9.
146. Goodman DW, Deykin D. Fatty acid ethyl ester formation during ethanol metabolism in vivo. Proc Soc Exp Biol. 1963;113:65–7.
147. Lange LG. Nonoxidative ethanol metabolism: formation of fatty acid ethyl esters by cholesterol esterase. Proc Natl Acad Sci. 1959;79:3954–7.
148. Mogelson S, Lange LG. Nonoxidative ethanol metabolism in rabbit myocardium: purification to homogeneity of fatty acyl ethyl ester synthase. Biochemistry. 1984;23:4075–81.
149. Baraona E, Julkunen R, Tannenbaum L et al. Role of intestinal bacterial overgrowth in ethanol production and metabolism in rats. Gastroenterology. 1986;90:103–10.
150. Bird MI, Nunn PB. Metabolic homeostasis of L-threonine in the normally-fed rat. Biochem J. 1983;214:687–94.
151. Ma X-L, Baraona E, Hernández R et al. High levels of acetaldehyde in non-alcoholic liver injury after threonine or ethanol administration. Hepatology. 1989;10:933–40.

152. Hasumura Y, Teschke R, Lieber CS. Acetaldehyde oxidation by hepatic mitochondria: its decrease after chronic ethanol consumption. Science. 1975;189:727–9.
153. Di Padova C, Worner TM, Julkunen RJK et al. Effects of fasting and chronic alcohol consumption on the first pass metabolism of ethanol. Gastroenterology. 1987;92:1169–73.
154. Pikkarainen PH, Gordon ER, Lebsack ME et al. Determinants of plasma free acetaldehyde level during the oxidation of ethanol: effects of chronic ethanol feeding. Biochem Pharmacol. 1981;30:799–802.
155. Baraona E, Di Padova C, Tabasco J et al. Transport of acetaldehyde in red blood cells. Alcohol Alcoholism. 1987(Suppl 1):203–6.
156. Müller A, Sies H. Role of alcohol dehydrogenase activity and of acetaldehyde in ethanol-induced ethane and pentane production by isolated perfused rat liver. Biochem J. 1982;206:153–6.
157. Shaw S, Jayetilleke E, Herbert V et al. Cleavage of folates during ethanol metabolism. Role of acetaldehyde xanthine oxidase-generated superoxide. Biochem J. 1989;257:277–80.
158. Shaw S, Jayatilleke E. The role of aldehyde oxidase in ethanol-induced hepatic lipid peroxidation in the rat. Biochem J. 1990;268:579–83.
159. Lieber CS. The influence of alcohol on nutritional status. Nutr Rev. 1988;46:241–5.
160. Shaw S, Jayatilleke E, Ross WA et al. Ethanol-induced lipid peroxidation: potentiation by long-term alcohol feeding and attenuation by methionine. J Lab Clin Med. 1981;98:417–24.
161. Vendemiale G, Jayatilleke E, Shaw S et al. Depression of biliary glutathione excretion by chronic ethanol feeding in the rat. Life Sci. 1984;34:1065–73.
162. Morton S, Mitchell MC. Effects of chronic ethanol feeding on glutathione turnover in the rat. Biochem Pharmacol. 1985;34:1559–63.
163. Speisky H, MacDonald A, Giles G et al. Increased loss and decreased synthesis of hepatic glutathione after acute ethanol administration. Biochem J. 1985;225:565.
164. Kocak-Toker N, Uysal M, Aykac G et al. Influence of acute ethanol administration on hepatic glutathione peroxidase and glutathione transferase activities in the rat. Pharmacol Res Commun. 1985;17:233–9.
165. Hirano T, Kaplowitz N, Tsukamoto H et al. Hepatic mitochondrial glutathione depletion and progression of experimental alcoholic liver disease in rats. Hepatology. 1992;6:1423–7.
166. Lieber CS. Alcohol, liver injury and protein metabolism. Pharmacol Biochem Behav. 1980;13(Suppl 1):17–30.
167. Shaw S, Lieber CS. Increased hepatic production of alpha-amino-n-butyric acid after chronic alcohol consumption in rats and baboons. Gastroenterology. 1980;78:108–13.
168. Barclay LR. The cooperative antioxidant role of glutathione with a lipid-soluble and a water-soluble antioxidant during peroxidation of liposomes initiated in the aqueous phase and in the lipid phase. J Biol Chem. 1988;263:16138–42.
169. Best CH, Hartroft WS, Lucas CC et al. Liver damage produced by feeding alcohol or sugar and its prevention by choline. Br Med J. 1941;2:1001–6.
170. Klatskin G, Hrchl WA, Coon HO. The effect of alcohol on the choline requirement. I. Changes in the rat's liver following prolonged ingestion of alcohol. J Exp Med. 1954;100:605–14.
171. Thompson JA, Reitz RC. Studies on the acute and chronic effects of ethanol ingestion on choline oxidation. Ann NY Acad Sci. 1976;273:194–204.
172. Hoffbauer FW, Zaki FG. Choline deficiency in baboon and rat compared. Arch Pathol. 1965;79:364–9.
173. Olson RE. Nutrition in alcoholism. In: Wohl MG, Goodhart RS, editors. Modern nutrition in health and disease, 3rd edn. Philadelphia: Lea & Febiger; 1964:779–95.
174. Phillips GR, Davidson CS. Acute hepatic insufficiency of the chronic alcoholic. Arch Intern Med. 1954;94:585–603.
175. Post JJ, Benton H, Breakstone R et al. The effects of diet and choline on fatty infiltration of the human liver. Gastroenterology. 1952;20:403–10.
176. Volwiler W, Jones CM, Mallory TB. Criteria for the measurement of results of treatment in fatty cirrhosis. Gastroenterology. 1948;11:164–82.
177. Rubin E, Lieber CS. Alcohol induced hepatic injury in nonalcoholic volunteers. N Engl J Med. 1968;278:869–76.

178. Lieber CS, DeCarli LM. An experimental model of alcohol feeding and liver injury in the baboon. J Med Primatol. 1974;3:153–64.
179. Lieber CS, Leo MA, Mak KM et al. Choline fails to prevent liver fibrosis in ethanol-fed baboons but causes toxicity. Hepatology. 1985;5:561–75.
180. Mato JM. Progress in protein–lipid interactions, Vol. 2. New York: Elsevier; 1986:267.
181. Finkelstein JD, Martin JJ. Methionine metabolism in mammals: adaption to methionine excess. J Biol Chem. 1986;261:1582–7.
182. Hardwick DF, Applegarth DA, Cockcroft DM et al. Pathogenesis of methionine-induced toxicity. Metabolism. 1970;19:381–91.
183. Fischer JE, Yoshimura N, Aguirre A et al. Plasma amino acids in patients with hepatic encephalopathy. Am J Surg. 1974;127:40–7.
184. Iber FL, Rosen H, Stanley MA et al. The plasma amino acids in patients with liver failure. J Lab Clin Med. 1957;50:417–25.
185. Montanari A, Simoni I, Valisa D et al. Free amino acids in plasma and skeletal muscle of patients with liver cirrhosis. Hepatology. 1988;8:1034–9.
186. Kinsell L, Harper HA, Barton HC et al. Rate of disappearance from plasma of intravenously administered methionine in patients with liver damage. Science. 1947;106:589–94.
187. Horowitz JH, Rypins EB, Henderson JM et al. Evidence for impairment of transsulfuration pathway in cirrhosis. Gastroenterology. 1981;81:668–75.
188. Duce AM, Ortizz P, Cabrero C et al. S-adenosoyl-L-methionine synthetase and phospholipid methyltransferase are inhibited in human cirrhosis. Hepatology. 1988;8:65–8.
189. Finkelstein JD, Cello JP, Kyle WE. Ethanol-induced changes in methionine metabolism in rat liver. Biochem Biophys Res Commun. 1974;61:475–81.
190. Lieber CS, Casini A, DeCarli LM et al. S-adenosyl-L-methionine attenuates alcohol-induced liver injury in the baboon. Hepatology. 1990;11:165–72.
191. Feo F, Pascale R, Garcea R et al. Effect of the variations of S-adenosyl-L-methionine liver content on fat accumulation and ethanol metabolism in ethanol-intoxicated rats. Toxicol Appl Pharmacol. 1986;83:331–41.
192. Paredes SR, Kozicki PA, Fukuda H et al. S-adenosyl-L-methionine: its effects on aminolevulinate dehydratase and glutathione in acute ethanol intoxication. Alcohol. 1987;4:81–5.
193. Vendemiale G, Altomare E, Trizio T et al. Effects of oral S-adenosyl-L-methionine on hepatic glutathione in patients with liver disease. Scand J Gastroenterol. 1989;24:407–15.
194. Tribble DL, Au TY, Jones DP. The pathological significance of lipid peroxidation in oxidative cell injury. Hepatology. 1987;7:377–87.
195. Bonjour JP. Vitamins and alcoholism. Int J Vit Nutr Res. 1979;49:434–41.
196. Tanner AR, Bantock I, Hinks L et al. Depressed selenium and vitamin E levels in an alcoholic population: possible relationship to hepatic injury through increased lipid peroxidation. Dig Dis Sci. 1986;31:1307–12.
197. Dworkin B, Rosenthal W, Jankowski R et al. Low blood selenium levels in alcoholics with and without advanced liver disease. Dig Dis Sci. 1985;30:838–44.
198. Korepal H, Kumpulainen J, Luoma PV et al. Decreased serum selenium in alcoholics as related to liver structure and function. Am J Clin Nutr. 1985;42:147–51.
199. Losowsky MS, Leonard PJ. Evidence of vitamin E deficiency in patients with malabsorption or alcoholism and the effect of therapy. Gut. 1967;8:539.
200. Yoshikawa Y, Takemura S, Kondo M. α-Tocopherol level in liver diseases. Acta Vitaminol Enzymol. 1982;4:311–18.
201. Bjórneboe GEA, Johnsen J, Bjórneboe A et al. Effect of heavy alcohol consumption on serum concentration of fat soluble vitamins and selenium. Alcohol Alcoholism. 1987;1(Suppl):533–7.
202. McCay PB. Vitamin E interaction with free radical and ascorbate. Annu Rev Nutr. 1985;5:323–40.
203. Niki E. Interaction of ascorbate and α-tocopherol. Ann NY Acad Sci. 1987;493:186–99.
204. Bjórneboe GEA, Bjórneboe A, Hagen BF et al. Reduced hepatic α-tocopherol content after long-term administration of ethanol to rats. Biochem Biophys Acta. 1987;918:236–41.
205. Bjórneboe GEA, Johnsen J, Bjórneboe A et al. Some aspects of antioxidant status in blood from alcoholics. Alcoholism Clin Exp Res. 1988;12:806–10.

206. Nomura F, Lieber CS. Binding of acetaldehyde to rat liver microsomes: enhancement after chronic alcohol consumption. Biochem Biophys Res Commun. 1981;100:131–7.
207. Behrens UJ, Hoerner M, Lasker JM et al. Formation of acetaldehyde adducts with ethanol-inducible P450IIE1 in vivo. Biochem Biophys Res Commun. 1988;154:584–90.
208. Lin RC, Smith RS, Lumeng L. Detection of a protein–acetaldehyde adduct in the liver of rats fed alcohol chronically. J Clin Invest. 1988;81:615–19.
209. Donohue TM Jr, Tuma DJ, Sorrell MF. Acetaldehyde adducts with proteins: binding of [^{14}C] acetaldehyde to serum albumin. Arch Biochem Biophys. 1983;220:239–46.
210. Stevens VJ, Fantl WJ, Newman CB et al. Acetaldehyde adducts with hemoglobin. J Clin Invest. 1981;67:361–9.
211. Baraona E, Leo MA, Borowsky SA et al. Pathogenesis of alcohol-induced accumulation of protein in the liver. J Clin Invest. 1977;60:546–54.
212. Israel Y, Hurwitz E, Niëmalä O et al. Monoclonal and polyclonal antibodies against acetaldehyde-containing epitopes in acetaldehyde–protein adducts. Proc Natl Acad Sci USA. 1986;83:7923–7.
213. Hoerner M, Behrens UJ, Worner T et al. Humoral immune response to acetaldehyde adducts in alcoholic patients. Res Commun Chem Pathol Pharmacol. 1986;54:3–12.
214. Hoerner M, Behrens UJ, Worner TM et al. The role of alcoholism and liver disease in the appearance of serum antibodies against acetaldehyde adducts. Hepatology. 1988;8: 569–74.
215. Niemala O, Klajner F, Orrego H et al. Antibodies against acetaldehyde-modified protein epitopes in human alcoholics. Hepatology. 1987;7:1210–14.
216. Solomon LR. Evidence for the generation of transaminase inhibitor(s) during ethanol metabolism by rat liver homogenates a potential mechanism for alcohol toxicity. Biochem Med Metabol Biol. 1987;38:9–18.
217. Espina N, Lima V, Lieber CS et al. In vitro and in vivo inhibitor effect of ethanol and acetaldehyde on O^6 methylguanine transferase. Carcinogenesis. 1988;9:761–6.
218. Dicker E, Cederbaum AI. Increased oxygen radical-dependent inactivation of metabolic enzymes by liver microsomes after chronic ethanol consumption. FASEB J. 1988;2: 2901–6.
219. Van Waes L, Lieber CS. Early perivenular sclerosis in alcoholic fatty liver: an index of progressive liver injury. Gastroenterology. 1977;73:646–50.
220. Worner TM, Lieber CS. Perivenular fibrosis as precursor lesion of cirrhosis. JAMA. 1985;254:627–30.
221. Feinman L, Lieber CS. Hepatic collagen metabolism: effect of alcohol consumption in rats and baboons. Science. 1972;176:795.
222. Patrick RS. Alcohol as a stimulus to hepatic fibrogenesis. J Alcoholism. 1973;8:13–27.
223. Mezey E, Potter JJ, Iber FL et al. Hepatic collagen proline hydroxylase activity in alcoholic hepatitis: effect of d-penicillamine. J Lab Clin Med. 1979;93:92–100.
224. Mann SW, Fuller GC, Rodil JV et al. Hepatic prolyl hydroxylase and collagen synthesis in patients with alcoholic liver disease. Gut. 1979;20:825–32.
225. Chen TSN, Leevy CM. Collagen biosynthesis in liver disease of the alcoholic. J Lab Clin Med. 1975;85:103–12.
226. Zern MA, Leo MA, Giambrone MA et al. Increased type I procollagen mRNA levels and in vitro protein synthesis in the baboon model of chronic alcoholic liver disease. Gastroenterology. 1985;89:1123–31.
227. Mak KM, Leo MA, Lieber CS. Alcoholic liver injury in baboons: transformation of lipocytes to transitional cells. Gastroenterology. 1984;87:188–200.
228. Mak KI, Lieber CS. Lipocytes and transitional cells in alcoholic liver disease: a morphometric study. Hepatology. 1988;8:1027–33.
229. Moshage H, Casini A, Lieber CS. Acetaldehyde stimulates collagen production in cultured rat liver fat-storing cells but not in hepatocytes. Hepatology. 1990;12:511–18.
230. Casini A, Cunningham M, Rojkind M et al. Acetaldehyde increases procollagen type I and fibronectin gene transcription in cultured rat fat-storing cells through a protein synthesis-dependent mechanism. Hepatology. 1991;13:758–65.
231. Savolainen E-R, Leo MA, Timpl R et al. Acetaldehyde and lactate stimulate collagen synthesis of cultured baboon liver myofibroblasts. Gastroenterology. 1984;87:777–87.
232. Li J-J, Kim C-I, Leo MA et al. Polyunsaturated lecithin prevents acetaldehyde-mediated

hepatic collagen accumulation by stimulating collagenase activity in cultured lipocytes. Hepatology. 1992;15:373–81.

233. Lieber CS, Robins S, Li J-J et al. Phosphatidylcholine protects against fibrosis and cirrhosis in the baboon. Gastroenterology. 1994 (in press).

234. Li J-J, Rosman AS, Leo MA, Nagai Y et al. Tissue inhibitor of metalloproteinase (TIMP) is increased in the serum of precirrhotic and cirrhotic alcoholics, and can serve as a marker of fibrosis. Gastroenterology. 1993;104:a939(abstract).

235. Lieber CS, DeCarli LM, Mak KM et al. Attenuation of alcohol-induced hepatic fibrosis by polyunsaturated lecithin. Hepatology. 1990;12:1390–8.

236. Arai M, Gordon ER, Lieber CS. Decreased cytochrome oxidase activity in hepatic mitochondria after chronic ethanol consumption and the possible role of decreased cytochrome aa$_3$ content and changes in phospholipids. Biochem Biophys Acta. 1984;797:320–7.

237. Arai M, Leo MA, Nakano M et al. Biochemical and morphological alterations of baboon hepatic mitochondria after chronic ethanol consumption. Hepatology. 1984;4:165–74.

238. Lieber CS, Leo MA, Robins S et al. Ethanol decreases hepatic phosphatidyl methyltransferase activity whereas phosphatidylcholine increases it, with protection against cirrhosis. FASEB J. Part II, 1993;7:A842.

239. Lekim D, Graf E. Tierexperimentelle Studien zur Pharmakokinetik der 'essentiellen' Phospholipide (EPL). Drug Res – Arzneim-Forsch. 1976;26:1772–82.

240. Spinozzi F, Bertotto A, Rondoni F et al. T-lymphocyte activation pathways in alcoholic liver disease. Immunology. 1991;73:140–6.

241. Müller C, Wolf H, Gottlicher J et al. Helper-inducer and suppressor-inducer lymphocyte subsets in alcoholic cirrhosis. Scand J Gastroenterol. 1991;26:295–301.

242. Parés A, Barrera JM, Caballeria J et al. Hepatitis C virus antibodies in chronic alcoholic patients: association with severity of liver injury. Hepatology. 1990;12:1295–9.

243. Rosman AS, Paronetto F, Galvin K et al. Hepatitis C virus antibody in alcoholic patients: Association with the presence of portal and/or lobular hepatitis. Arch Intern Med. 1993;153:965–9.

244. Shibayama Y, Asaka S, Nakata K. Endotoxin hepatotoxicity augmented by ethanol. Exp Mol Pathol. 1991;55:196–301.

245. Khoruts A, Stahnke L, McClain CJ et al. Circulating tumor necrosis factor, interleukin-1 and interleukin-6 concentrations in chronic alcoholic patients. Hepatology. 1991;13: 267–76.

246. Sheron N, Bird G, Goka J et al. Elevated plasma interleukin-6 and increased severity and mortality in alcoholic hepatitis. Clin Exp Immunol. 1991;84:449–53.

247. McClain C, Hill D, Schmidt J et al. Cytokines and alcoholic liver disease. Semin Liver Dis. 1993;13:170–82.

248. Peguignot G, Tuyns AJ, Berta JL. Ascitic cirrhosis in relation to alcohol consumption. Int J Epidemiol. 1978;7:113–20.

249. Morgan MY, Sherlock S. Sex-related differences among 100 patients with alcoholic liver disease. Br Med J. 1977;1:939–41.

250. Maier KP, Haag SG, Peskar BM et al. Verlaufsformen alkoholischer Lebererkrankungen. Klin Wochenschr. 1979;57:311–17.

251. Nakamura S, Takezawa Y, Sato T et al. Alcoholic liver disease in women. Tohoku J Exp Med. 1979;129:351–5.

252. Goodwin DW. Is alcoholism hereditary? Arch Gen Psychiatry. 1971;25:545–9.

253. Bailey RJ, Krasner N, Eddleston ALWF et al. Histocompatibility antigens, autoantibodies, and immunoglobulins in alcoholic liver disease. Br Med J. 1976;2:727–9.

254. Morgan M, Ross MGR, Ng CM et al. HLA-B8 immunoglobulins, and antibody responses in alcohol-related liver disease. J Clin Pathol. 1980;33:488–92.

255. Saunders JB, Haines A, Portman B et al. Accelerated development of alcoholic cirrhosis in patients with HLA-B8. Lancet. 1982;1:1381–4.

256. Scott BB, Rajah SM, Losowsky MD. Histocompatibility antigens in chronic liver disease. Gastroenterology. 1977;72:122–5.

257. Bell H, Nordhagen R. Association between HLA-BW40 and alcoholic liver disease with cirrhosis. Br Med J. 1978;1:822.

258. Gluud C, Aldershvile J, Dietrichson O et al. Human leucocyte antigens in patients with

alcoholic liver cirrhosis. Scand J Gastroenterol. 1980;15:337–41.
259. Lieber CS. Biochemical and molecular basis for alcohol-induced injury to liver and other tissues. N Engl N Med. 1988;319:1639–50.

12
Transformation of fat-storing cells into transitional cells in alcoholic liver fibrosis

K. M. MAK, M. A. LEO and C. S. LIEBER

INTRODUCTION

Hepatic fat-storing cells (Ito cells, lipocytes) are the principal cells residing in the space of Disse between the sinusoidal endothelium and hepatocytes, and have been considered to have the greatest potential for fibrogenesis. In liver fibrosis, fat-storing cells undergo striking changes from an apparently quiescent appearance to an activated morphology accompanying the onset and progression of fibrosis. This phenotypic change, characterized by diminished lipid droplets and increased rough endoplasmic reticulum (RER) with dilated cisternae, has come to be known as transformation[1,2] or activation[3,4] of fat-storing cells. Indeed, it was first proposed by Kent et al.[1] in 1976 that, in association with CCl_4-induced hepatic fibrosis in the rat, stimulation of fat-storing cells may result in their transformation to fibroblasts which, in turn, may promote fibrosis. The transformation of fat-storing cells to fibrogenic cells is accompanied by an increased appearance of cells with ultrastructural features intermediate between fat-storing cells and fibroblasts. Such transitional forms were named transitional cells. Subsequently, transitional cells were also observed in the fibrotic tissue of the liver of rats fed a moderate amount of vitamin A with an ethanol diet[5], baboons after alcohol consumption[2] and alcoholics[3,6-8]. We will review here some earlier and recent data on the transformational changes of fat-storing cells into transitional cells in alcoholic liver fibrosis of baboons and humans, and the effect of polyunsaturated lecithin on the process of fat-storing cell transformation induced by ethanol.

ULTRASTRUCTURE OF FAT-STORING CELLS

Fat-storing cells contain characteristically from a single to as many as 20 lipid droplets in the cytoplasm. The diameters of the lipid droplets range from 1 to 10 μm and they are either free in the cytoplasm or membrane-bound. They are storage sites for hepatic vitamin A. In control baboons, 97% of the cells have a lipid droplet volume greater than 20% of the cell volume, as determined by morphometry. Therefore, cells are considered arbitrarily to be fat-storing cells when the volume of lipid droplets is greater than 20% of the cell volume; conversely, cells are considered to be transitional cells when the volume of lipid droplets is less than 20% of the cell volume[2].

The nuclei of fat-storing cells appear heterochromatic and are often deformed into various shapes by the lipid droplets. In most apparently quiescent fat-storing cells the RER is randomly distributed in the cytoplasm as short, narrowed cisternae. However, there are also fat-storing cells that contain fairly dilated RER enclosing a fibrillar or flocculent material in their channels, indicative of synthetic activity. In the fat-storing cells, mitochondria are small and few in number. The cytocentre consists of the Golgi apparatus and a single pair of centrioles; the latter sometimes appear in the form of a basal body with a single cilium protruding from the cell surface. Fat-storing cells contain few lysosomes that are often in close association with the membrane-bound lipid droplets, suggesting lysosomal degradation of these lipid droplets[9]. In the peripheral cytoplasm of the cells there are pinocytic vesicles, sometimes arranged in rows; the function of these organelles is not known.

Intermediate-sized filaments are difficult to visualize, but microfilaments are common and are either loosely arranged in the cytoplasm or gathered in small bundles in the peripheral cytoplasm of the cell. Few dense bodies are present in association with the microfilaments in close proximity to the plasma membrane. The microfilaments are more easily discernible in the cell processes which extend from the cell bodies into the Disse space along the endothelial lining of the sinusoids. Because of the microfilament content and the close proximity of the cell processes to the sinusoids, it has been suggested that fat-storing cells may regulate the flow of the blood in the liver lobules. Indeed, Pinzani et al.[10] demonstrated the contractile potential of human fat-storing cells in culture, and proposed that fat-storing cells are analogous to contractile pericytes of the capillary and post-capillary venule.

Cell junctions of the adherens type are seen between fat-storing cells and hepatocytes. This linkage between fat-storing cells and parenchymal cells may contribute to the spatial organization of the fat-storing cells in the space of Disse. Fat-storing cells are not surrounded by a basal lamina. In the extracellular space immediately surrounding the fat-storing cells, both coarse banded collagen fibres and fine fibrils are present, and sometimes these appear to be attached to the plasma membrane of the cells. The morphological features of the RER and the spatial relationship of the collagen fibres to the fat-storing cells suggest that the latter possess a capacity for collagen production. This correlates well with the immunohistochemical demonstration of collagen types I, III and IV and other extracellular matrices in human fat-storing cells[11].

TRANSFORMATION OF FAT-STORING CELLS TO TRANSITIONAL CELLS

Alcohol consumption induces striking changes of fat-storing cells. The number of 'normal' fat-storing cells as seen by light microscopy on plastic sections stained with toluidine blue is significantly decreased in fatty liver and at various stages of liver fibrosis[2,3,7]. This is associated with a decreased hepatic vitamin A content. Because one relies largely on the presence of lipid droplets in the cytoplasm for the detection of fat-storing cells by light microscopy, the reduction in the number of fat-storing cells may, at least in part, reflect an impairment in their detection due to the appearance of transitional cells that display fewer as well as smaller lipid droplets. By ultrastructural analysis of baboons fed alcohol, only 48% of the cells were found to be fat-storing cells, whereas 52% are transitional cells defined by a volume of lipid droplets of less than 20% of the cell volume[2]. Moreover, there is an increase in the appearance of transitional cells accompanying the progression of fibrosis in the liver up to 81–83% (Tables 2 and 3). Concurrently there is a corresponding decrease in the number of fat-storing cells[2,3,8]. This, together with the observation that transitional cells maintain virtually all the characteristic organelles seen in fat-storing cells (Figs 1 and 2), support the contention that the appearance of transitional cells represents transformed fat-storing cells. However, transitional cells are distinguished from fat-storing cells by their relative paucity of cytoplasmic lipid droplets (less than 20% of the cell volume).

Morphometric analysis of baboons and human livers showed that transitional cells are smaller than fat-storing cells, and this is primarily due to the smaller lipid droplet compartment of the cells. The RER in transitional cells is better developed and occupies a greater area of the cell than that in fat-storing cells. More collagen fibres are seen surrounding the transitional cells than fat-storing cells. Like fat-storing cells, the appearance of the nuclei of transitional cells is variable, depending on the number of lipid droplets in the cells. Like fat-storing cells, transitional cells are not surrounded by a basal lamina.

TRANSITIONAL CELLS, PERISINUSOIDAL FIBROSIS, AND ALTERATIONS OF ENDOTHELIAL FENESTRATIONS

In the process of alcoholic liver fibrosis, transitional cells produce extracellular matrix (ECM) in the space of Disse, leading to perisinusoidal fibrosis. Concurrently, there is a striking change in the morphology of the endothelial fenestrations. In baboons fed ethanol chronically, the number of endothelial fenestrations and porosity of the endothelium (fractional area occupied by fenestrations) decrease with the progression of liver fibrosis, as determined by scanning electron microscopy[12]. In alcoholics the loss of fenestrations correlates with the collagenization of the Disse space and the formation of subendothelial basal laminas in acinar zone 3[13,14]. These findings raise the possibility that perisinusoidal ECM may directly affect the formation of

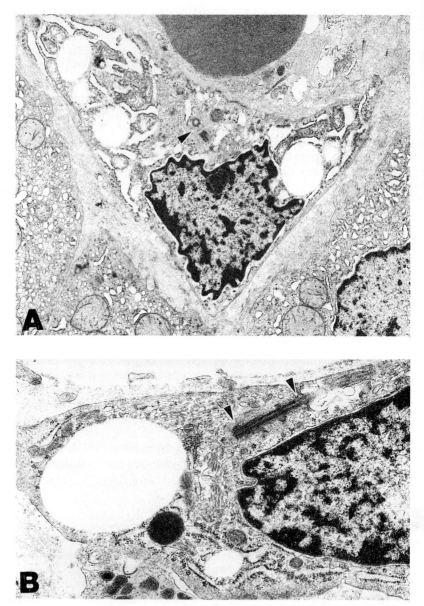

Fig. 1 **A**: Transitional cell in the space of Disse from an ethanol-fed baboon showing paired centrioles (arrowhead) in juxtaposition to the Golgi apparatus, constituting the cytocentre of the cell. Note that the cell possesses few small lipid droplets and dilated RER. In **B**, a single cilium (arrowheads) protruding from the cell surface is demonstrated. (A × 10 000; B × 20 000)

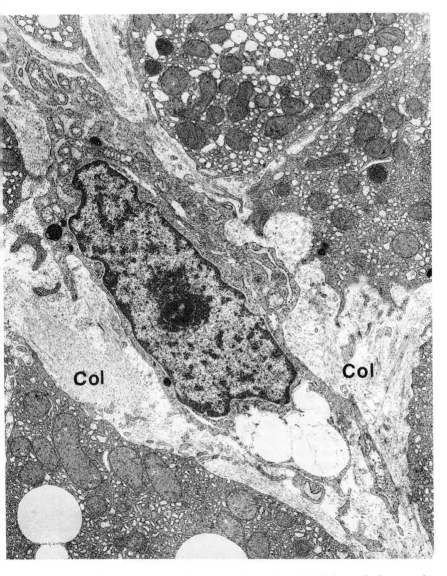

Fig. 2 Transitional cell in a small fibrous scar of an ethanol-fed baboon. Such a scar is probably formed by excess deposition of collagens in the perisinusoidal space with obliteration of the sinusoid. The cell shows paucity of lipid droplets and a well-developed RER and Golgi apparatus. Note both coarse and fine collagen fibrils (Col) in the extracellular space surrounding the cell (× 10 000)

endothelial fenestrations. This was examined by McQuire et al.[15], using rat liver endothelial cells cultured on different ECM proteins. Physiologically derived basement membrane of the amnion was found to support fenestral formation, whereas interstitial collagen (types I and III) does not, suggesting that the formation of endothelial fenestrations requires the support of a complex matrix. The accumulation of interstitial collagens in the perisinusoidal space may contribute, in part, to the loss of fenestrations associated with hepatic fibrosis. An alternative hypothesis is that ethanol or one of its metabolites directly decreases the fenestral number and sinusoidal porosity without involvement of fibrosis. In support of this view is the observation by Horn et al.[14] in alcoholics that there is a slight but significant loss of fenestrations and porosity in acinar zones 1 and 3 of liver without histological evidence of fibrosis. Furthermore, hormones (serotonin and noradrenalin), oxygen tension, sinusoidal pressure[16] and even alcohol administration to rats[17] can alter sinusoidal fenestral morphology independently of fibrosis. Whatever the mechanisms involved, the reduction in the porosity of sinusoidal endothelium after ethanol consumption is most likely accompanied by a disturbance in exchanges of solutes and particles between the sinusoidal blood and liver parenchyma across the Disse space, and may thereby contribute to the pathogenesis of alcoholic liver injury.

TRANSITIONAL CELLS AND COLLAGEN PHAGOCYTOSIS

Transitional cells are present in the perisinusoidal space, fibrous scar and septa. In septal connective tissue, transitional cells are ubiquitous among macrophages and other mononuclear cells with diverse ultrastructural features (Fig. 3). Typical myofibroblasts are rarely encountered. In alcohol-fed baboons, septal transitional cells display not only dilated RER and increased number of lysosomes, but also, albeit infrequently, intracellular collagen fibrils within membranous channels of the cell cytoplasm (Fig. 4). The appearance of intracellular collagen has been reported by others in the fibroblasts of the foot pad of rats[18], vitamin A-containing cells in the liver and intestine of lampreys[19], cultured human gingival fibroblasts[20] and, more recently, in septal cells of septal connective tissue in the liver of rats induced by porcine serum[21]. Intracellular collagen is considered to represent phagocytosed fibrils, and phagocytosis of collagen has been regarded as a main pathway of collagen degradation[20]. Thus, transitional cells may contribute to the digestion and turnover of collagens of septal tissue.

TRANSITIONAL CELLS AND MYOFIBROBLASTS

Another population of mesenchymal cells that has the potential for collagen production consist of the myofibroblasts which are localized in the wall of the terminal hepatic venules in normal and fibrotic livers of baboons and humans[22,23]. Myofibroblasts are also present in the portal space of baboons[24] and diseased human livers[25,26]. Myofibroblasts characteristically contain abundant microfilaments that are disposed in bundles in parallel to the long axis of the cells, and these are associated with conspicuous dense bodies (Fig. 5). There are numerous easily discernible pinocytic vesicles beneath the plasma membrane. The presence of a single cilium protruding from the cell

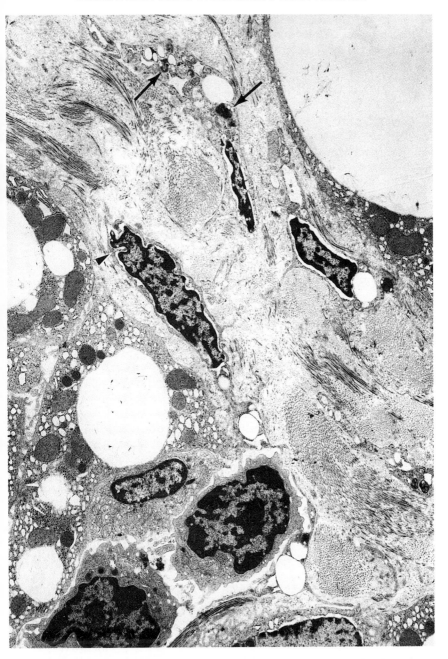

Fig. 3 Transitional cells in a fibrous septum of an ethanol-fed baboon. The cells show one or two small lipid droplets, characteristic of transitional cells, and an increased number of lysosomes (arrows). The nucleus (arrowhead) of one transitional cell appears slightly convoluted. Mononuclear cells are also present (bottom of figure) (× 6250)

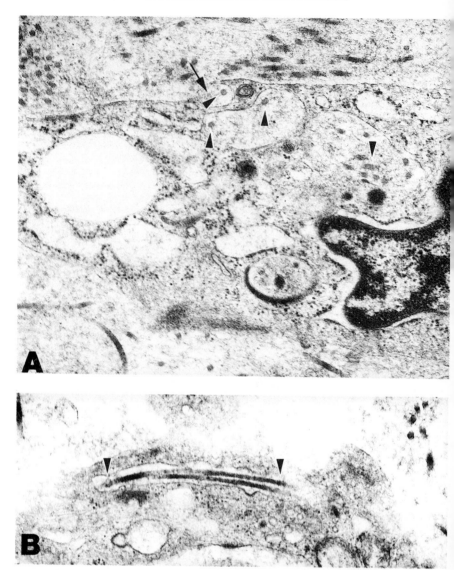

Fig. 4A: Intracellular collagen fibrils (arrowhead) within membranous channels of a septal transitional cell of an ethanol-fed baboon. The fibrils show similar width and diameter as those of extracellular fibrils. The arrow points to a vacuole apparently in communication with the extracellular space. **B**: Another view of intracellular collagen fibrils (arrowhead) revealing the characteristic bandings of the collagen. (A × 40 000; B × 40 000)

surface has also been described[26]. Although microfilaments, dense bodies, and pinocytic vesicles are also present in transitional cells, they are far fewer in number and less readily discernible compared to those of myofibroblasts. Moreover, myofibroblasts rarely contain lipid droplets and consistently

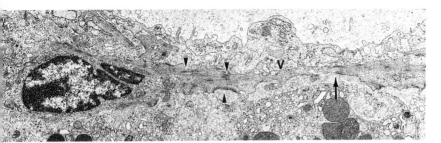

Fig. 5 Myofibroblasts from an ethanol-fed baboon showing abundant cytoplasmic microfilaments with conspicuous dense bodies (arrowheads) and numerous pinocytic vesicles (V) at the cell periphery. The nucleus appears convoluted. Part of the cell surface is covered by a basal lamina (arrow) (× 6400)

Table 1 Comparative ultrastructural features of fat-storing cells, transitional cells, fibroblasts and myofibroblasts

	Fat-storing cells	Transitional cells	Fibroblasts	Myofibroblasts
Lipid droplets	+ +	+	±	±
Microfilaments and dense bodies	+	+	−	+ +
Pinocytic vesicles	+	+	±	+ +
Endoplasmic reticulum	+	+ +	+ +	+ +
Basal lamina	−	−	−	+
Convoluted nucleus	−	±	−	+

±, Variably present; +, present; + +, marked; −, absent

reveal a convoluted nucleus and an extracellular basal lamina, and the combination of these features serve to distinguish them from transitional cells (Table 1). Nevertheless, the ultrastructural features of transitional cells, in particular those of septal connective tissue, resemble more a myofibroblastic phenotype than a fibroblastic one, and transitional cells may alternatively be called myofibroblast-like cells. Whether transitional cells can evolve into myofibroblasts remains speculative at present. The application of cytoskeletal proteins as differentiation markers may aid in elucidating the relationship between these cells.

In the rat, desmin expression may be useful in distinguishing fat-storing cells from myofibroblasts[27], but in baboons and humans, fat-storing cells do not stain with the desmin antibodies. In diseased liver including alcoholic liver fibrosis, Schmitt-Graff et al.[28] and Nouchi et al.[29] consider the appearance of α-smooth muscle actin (α-SMA) (a smooth muscle differentiation marker[30]) in fat-storing cells to be an expression of their activation, leading to transformation of fat-storing cells to a myofibroblastic phenotype[31]. Similarly, in experimental liver injury of the rat, activated fat-storing cells co-express desmin and α-SMA, and the acquisition of fat-storing cells of α-SMA represents their transformation to myofibroblasts during liver injury[32-34]. By immunohistochemistry at the light microscope level we also

Table 2 Effects of polyunsaturated lecithin (PUL) on fat-storing cell transformation to transitional cells in the baboon, expressed as a percentage of total fat-storing cells

Control diet	Control diet + PUL	Ethanol	Ethanol + PUL	Ethanol after PUL withdrawal
8% (26)	4% (26)	81%[a] (49)	55% (53)	83%[a] (61)

Number of cells evaluated is indicated in parentheses.
[a]Significantly different from ethanol + PUL ($p < 0.01$) by χ^2 test.
Data from ref. 35.

observed in human liver the appearance of α-SMA in perisinusoidal fat-storing cells, cells in fibrous scars and septa, in association with the progression of alcoholic liver fibrosis (unpublished observation), in agreement with the observations of others[28,29].

EFFECTS OF PHOSPHATIDYLCHOLINE ON FAT-STORING CELL TRANSFORMATION

We have recently shown that polyunsaturated lecithin (PUL) extracted from soybeans and containing 55–60% of phosphatidylcholine (PC) protects against alcoholic fibrosis and cirrhosis in baboons[35]. To assess the mechanism involved in the protection against fibrosis we have studied fat-storing cell transformation, because it is now apparent that their transformation into transitional cells plays a major role in hepatic fibrosis (see above). In baboons that had septal fibrosis after ethanol feeding (seven of nine baboons), an expected increase was noted in the appearance of transitional cells (81% vs 8% in controls) (Table 2). Septal fibrosis did not develop in any animals fed ethanol with the lecithin. They did not progress beyond the stage of perivenular fibrosis, sometimes associated with pericellular and perisinusoidal fibrosis, and had a significantly lesser transformation of fat-storing cells to transitional cells (55% vs 81% in ethanol-fed baboons). Furthermore, when three of these animals were taken off lecithin, but continued on the same amount of the ethanol-containing diet, they rapidly progressed to cirrhosis (within 18–21 months), and this was accompanied by an increase of transformation of their fat-storing cells to transitional cells (85% after PUL withdrawal vs 55% before withdrawal). The change of fat-storing cells into transitional cells induced by ethanol was slowed down in the presence of PUL. In view of the putative role of transitional cells in the process of fibrogenesis, it is conceivable that the slowing by PUL of the ethanol-induced fibrosis may be a consequence of the blocking effect of PUL on the transformation of the fat-storing cells.

To assess whether PC was the active agent in the protection by PUL against alcoholic fibrosis in baboons, we used a diet supplemented with a more purified lecithin extract, containing 94–96% of PC[36]. Whereas ten of 12 baboons fed ethanol developed septal fibrosis or cirrhosis, none of the eight animals fed ethanol with PC developed septal fibrosis or cirrhosis,

Table 3 Effects of ethanol and/or phosphatidylcholine (PC) on fat-storing cell transformation to transitional cells in the baboon, expressed as a percentage of total fat-storing cells

Control diet	Control diet + PC	Ethanol	Ethanol + PC
3 ± 2%	5 ± 2%	81 ± 3%	48 ± 9%[a]

[a]$p < 0.01$ when compared to ethanol.
Data from ref. 36.

indicating that PC was indeed the protective compound. The transformation of fat-storing cells to transitional cells in ethanol-fed baboons was decreased from 81% to 48% after feeding of the PC-enriched diet (Table 3). The corresponding values in controls and animals fed PC without ethanol were 3% and 5%, respectively. PC also prevented the associated hepatic phospholipid depletion by ethanol and increased collagen breakdown, as shown in fat-storing cells in culture enriched with purified dilinoleoylphosphatidylcholine (18:2–18:2 PC), as discussed in greater detail elsewhere in these proceedings (Chapter 13).

In summary, fat-storing cells play a major role in alcoholic liver fibrosis after their transformation into transitional cells. Transitional cells bear features that resemble a myofibroblastic phenotype and may alternatively be called myofibroblast-like cells. Production of interstitial collagen by transitional cells may contribute, in part, to the decreased porosity of sinusoidal endothelium associated with hepatic fibrosis. Alternatively, ethanol may directly change the fenestral morphology without involvement of fibrosis. Transitional cells not only produce collagen, but also, albeit infrequently, display phagocytosis of extracellular collagen, suggesting that they may contribute to the turnover of fibrous tissue. Phosphatidylcholine protects against the ethanol-induced liver fibrosis and cirrhosis in the baboon, and strikingly decreases the associated transformation of fat-storing cells into transitional cells.

Acknowledgements

This study was supported, in part, by DHHS grants AA 03508, AA 09497, and the Department of Veterans Affairs. The authors thank Mr C. Din and P. Aryeh Cohen for excellent technical help and for preparation of the manuscript.

References

1. Kent G, Gay S, Inouye T et al. Vitamin A-containing lipocytes and formation of type III collagen in liver injury. Proc Natl Acad Sci USA. 1976;73:3719–22.
2. Mak KM, Leo MA, Lieber CS. Alcoholic injury in baboons: Transformation of lipocytes to transitional cells. Gastroenterology. 1984;87:188–200.
3. Horn T, Junge J, Christofferson P. Early alcoholic liver injury: activation of lipocytes in

acinar zone 3 and correlation to degree of collagen formation in the Disse space. J Hepatol. 1986;3:333–40.

4. French SW, Takahashi H, Wong K et al. Ito cell activation induced by chronic ethanol feeding in the presence of different dietary fats. Alcohol Alcoholism. 1991;Suppl 1:357–61.
5. Leo MA, Lieber CS. Hepatic fibrosis after long-term administration of ethanol and moderate vitamin A supplementation in the rat. Hepatology. 1983;3:1–11.
6. Minato Y, Hasumura Y, Takeuchi J. The role of fat-storing cells in Disse space fibrogenesis in alcoholic liver disease. Hepatology. 1983;3:559–66.
7. Okanoue T, Burbige EJ, French SW. The role of the Ito cell in perivenular and intralobular fibrosis in alcoholic hepatitis. Arch Pathol Lab Med. 1983;107:459–63.
8. Mak KM, Lieber CS. Lipocytes and transitional cells in alcoholic liver disease: a morphometric study. Hepatology. 1988;8:1027–33.
9. Geerts A, Bouwens L, Wisse E. Ultrastructure and function of hepatic fat-storing and pit cells. J Electron Microsc Tech. 1990;14:247–56.
10. Pinzani M, Failli P, Ruocco C et al. Fat-storing cells as liver-specific pericytes. Spatial dynamics of agonist-stimulated intracellular calcium transients. J Clin Invest. 1992;90:642–6.
11. Clement B, Grimaud JA, Campion JP et al. Cell types involved in collagen and fibronectin production in normal and fibrotic human liver. Hepatology. 1986;6:225–34.
12. Mak KM, Lieber CS. Alterations in endothelial fenestrations in liver sinusoids of baboon fed alcohol: a scanning electron microscopic study. Hepatology. 1984;4:386–91.
13. Horn T, Jung J, Christoffersen P. Early alcoholic liver injury: changes of the Disse space in acinar zone 3. Liver. 1985;5:301–10.
14. Horn T, Christofferson P, Henriksen JH. Alcoholic liver injury: defenestration in noncirrhotic livers — a scanning electron microscopic study. Hepatology. 1987;7:77–82.
15. McGuire RF, Bissell DM, Boyles J et al. Role of extracellular matrix in regulating fenestrations of sinusoidal endothelial cells isolated from rat liver. Hepatology. 1992;15:989–97.
16. Wisse E, De Zanger RB, Charles K et al. The liver sieve: considerations concerning the structure and function of endothelial fenestrae, the sinusoidal wall and the space of Disse. Hepatology. 1985;5:683–92.
17. Fraser R, Bowler LM, Day WA. Damage of rat liver sinusoidal endothelium by ethanol. Pathology. 1980;12:371–6.
18. Marchi F, Leblond CP. Collagen biogenesis and assembly into fibrils as shown by ultrastructural and ^{3}H-proline radioautographic studies on the fibroblasts of the rat foot pad. Am J Anat. 1983;168:167–97.
19. Wake K, Kamino T, Ueki Y et al. Endocytosis and degradation of collagen fibrils by vitamin A-containing cells in the liver and intestine of the lamprey. Proc 11th Congress on Electron Microscopy. J Electron Microsc. 1986;35(Suppl):1941–4.
20. Knowles GC, McKeown M, Sodek J et al. Mechanism of collagen phagocytosis by human gingival fibroblasts: Importance of collagen structure in cell recognition and internalization. J Cell Sci. 1991;98:551–8.
21. Bhunchet E, Wake K. Role of mesenchymal cell populations in porcine serum-induced rat liver fibrosis. Hepatology. 1992;16:1452–73.
22. Nakano M, Lieber CS. Ultrastructure of initial stages of perivenular fibrosis in alcohol-fed baboons. Am J Pathol. 1982;106:145–55.
23. Nakano M, Worner TS, Lieber CS. Perivenular fibrosis in alcoholic liver injury: Ultrastructure and histologic progression. Gastroenterology. 1982;83:777–85.
24. Mak KM, Lieber CS. Portal fibroblasts and myofibroblasts in baboons after long-term alcohol consumption. Arch Pathol Lab Med. 1986;110:513–16.
25. Grimaud JA, Borojevic R. Myofibroblasts in hepatic schistosomal fibrosis. Experientia. 1977;33:890–2.
26. Callea F, Mebis J, Desmet VJ. Myofibroblasts in focal nodular hyperplasia of the liver. Virch Arch A Pathol Anat. 1982;396:155–66.
27. Takase S, Leo MA, Nouchi T et al. Desmin distinguishes cultured fat-storing cells from myofibroblasts, smooth muscle cells and fibroblasts in the rat. J Hepatol. 1988;6:267–76.
28. Schmitt-Graff A, Kruger S, Bochard F et al. Modulation of alpha smooth muscle actin and desmin expression in perisinusoidal cells of normal and diseased human livers. Am J Pathol.

1991;138:1233–42.

29. Nouchi T, Tanaka Y, Tsukada T et al. Appearance of alpha-smooth-muscle-actin-positive cells in hepatic fibrosis. Liver. 1991;11:100–5.

30. Skalli O, Schurch W, Seemayer T et al. Myofibroblasts from diverse pathologic settings are heterogeneous in their content of actin isoforms and intermediate filament proteins. Lab Invest. 1989;60:275–85.

31. Schmitt-Graff A, Gabbiani G. Modulation of fibroblastic cytoskeletal features during wound healing and fibrosis. International Falk Symposium. 'Molecular and Cell Biology of Liver Fibrogenesis', Marburg, 22–23 January 1992:99–106.

32. Ramadori G, Veit T, Schwogler S et al. Expression of the gene of the smooth muscle-actin isoform in rat liver and in rat fat-storing (Ito) cells. Virch Arch B Cell Pathol. 1990;59: 349–57.

33. Tanaka Y, Nouchi T, Yamane M et al. Phenotypic modulation in lipocytes in experimental liver fibrosis. J. Pathol. 1991;164:273–8.

34. Rockey DC, Boyles JK, Gabbiani G et al. Rat hepatic lipocytes express smooth muscle actin upon activation in vivo and in culture. J Submicrosc Cytol Pathol. 1992;24:193–203.

35. Lieber CS, DeCarli LM, Mak KM et al. Attenuation of alcohol-induced hepatic fibrosis by polyunsaturated lecithin. Hepatology. 1990;12:1390–8.

36. Lieber CS, Robins S, Li J-J et al. Phosphatidylcholine protects against fibrosis cirrhosis in the baboon. Gastroenterology. (in press).

13
Effects of ethanol and acetaldehyde on extracellular matrix gene regulation in fat-storing cells

A. CASINI

INTRODUCTION

The extracellular matrix (ECM) of the liver is composed of several collagenous and non-collagenous components and contains small amounts of proteoglycans. Type I and type III are the most abundant collagens in animal and human liver; they account for about 80% of the total liver collagen[1-4]. Collagens type IV and V are also present in the liver where they represent about 10% and 7–10%, respectively[5-7]. Among the non-collagenous proteins laminin, a component of all liver membrane basement, and fibronectin are the most represented[5,6,8].

The deposition of collagen in the Disse space and around the hepatocytes is an important morphological feature of alcohol-induced liver injury. However, mechanisms responsible for the increased collagen deposition are still under debate. Alcohol-induced liver fibrosis may occur in the absence of inflammation, both in baboons[9,10] and in humans[11]. These observations therefore suggest that mechanisms other than such inflammation can induce the hepatic fibrosis.

Fat-storing cells (FSC, also known as hepatic lipocytes, Ito cells or perisinusoidal stellate cells) reside in the space of Disse and have been considered to play an important role in the development of ethanol-induced liver fibrosis[12,13]. FSC can transform into 'activated' transitional cells in experimental[14,15] and human[16] alcoholic liver injury.

Conflicting results have been reported with regard to the liver cells responsible for the increased collagen deposition and the synthesis of different ECM components. It has not yet been clarified whether hepatocytes are involved[17-20] or not[21-24] in hepatic collagen synthesis and accumulation. In particular, no definitive data exist about the possible involvement of hepatocytes in alcohol-induced liver fibrogenesis.

The lack of any stimulatory effect of ethanol on collagen production in cultures of human skin and lung fibroblasts[25,26] and baboon liver myofibroblasts[27] suggests that ethanol *per se* does not directly induce liver fibrogenesis. On the other hand, acetaldehyde and lactate can stimulate collagen production in baboon liver myofibroblasts[27] and in human skin fibroblasts[25]. Moreover, a stimulatory effect of acetaldehyde on procollagen type I gene transcription in cultured skin fibroblasts has been reported[28]. However, all these interesting studies on ethanol and acetaldehyde were done in 'non-liver-specific' experimental models. Therefore, additional studies were needed to evaluate the role of ethanol and acetaldehyde in alcoholic fibrosis. First, does ethanol and/or acetaldehyde stimulate collagen production by liver FSC? Second, the gene expression of collagen and other ECM components should be examined in FSC treated with ethanol or acetaldehyde (rather than in fibroblasts) and the role of lipid peroxidation and acetaldehyde-protein adduct formation explored.

ETHANOL, ACETALDEHYDE AND MATRIX SYNTHESIS BY FSC AND HEPATOCYTES

In a first group of experiments we used FSC isolated from rats after collagenase–pronase digestion of the liver and centrifugation over a 11.4% (wt/vol) Nycodenz gradient[29]. Cells were then washed and cultured in Dulbecco's modified Eagle's medium containing 10% fetal calf serum, 2 mmol/l L-glutamine and antibiotics. Subcultures were obtained by trypsinization. Cells were identified by their typical phase-contrast light microscopic appearance and the constant positive immunofluorescence staining for desmin that was maintained even after the first and second passages *in vitro*[30,31].

In order to verify whether hepatocytes were involved in liver collagen synthesis we isolated them from rat livers by a two-step perfusion method using collagenase, as described by Seglen[32]. Hepatocytes were then cultured in serum-free, hormonally defined Williams E medium[30]. Collagen type I, III, IV and laminin were determined in culture media and cell layers by an ELISA method[30] adapted from Rennard *et al.*[33]. Rabbit anti-laminin and anti-collagen type I, III and IV antibodies were kindly provided by Dr D. Schuppan, Department of Gastroenterology, Klinikum Steglitz, Free University of Berlin, Berlin, Germany.

Primary, as well as passage 1 and 2, FSC cultures produced significant amounts of both type I and III collagen (950 and 395 ng/μg cellular DNA/24 h, respectively), whereas the production of collagen type IV and laminin was lower (1 and 8 ng/μg DNA/24 h, respectively); primary cultures of hepatocytes synthesized significant amounts only of collagen type III (58 ng/μg DNA/24 h), whereas collagen type I, type IV and laminin were undetectable[30].

Addition of ethanol had no effect on collagen or laminin production in FSC cultures. In contrast, acetaldehyde significantly enhanced collagen type I production 2.5-fold but did not modify the FSC production of collagen type III and laminin[30]. Neither ethanol nor acetaldehyde significantly modified collagen type III production in the primary cultures of hepatocytes.

Since the FSC collagenolytic activity was not decreased in the cell media after acetaldehyde exposure (98 ± 9% of controls), the enhancement of collagen accumulation appeared to have been caused by an active production by FSC. Significant amounts of collagen type III and smaller amounts of collagen IV and laminin were synthesized by FSC, but only type I collagen accumulation was enhanced by acetaldehyde. In the same experimental model ethanol itself did not significantly affect the production of collagens and laminin. These *in vitro* findings confirm previous *in vivo* studies which reported that alcohol-induced liver fibrosis is associated with 'activation' of lipocytes to 'transitional' cells surrounded by collagen fibres and characterized by a depletion of lipid droplets, hypertrophy of the rough endoplasmic reticulum and increased capacity of collagen synthesis, both in baboons[15] and humans[14]. The ethanol concentration that we used (50 mmol/l) corresponds to the blood level of baboons fed ethanol chronically[34]. The concentrations of acetaldehyde maintained in the cultures (85–40 µmol/l) were slightly higher than the hepatic venous blood levels observed in baboons given alcohol[35]; however, it is known that acetaldehyde concentrations in the liver are higher than those observed in the blood[36]; therefore, amounts used in the cell culture media are close to the intracellular hepatic acetaldehyde levels.

In our *in vitro* model collagen production by hepatocytes was limited to type III and was much less extensive than that of FSC. These data are in agreement with other reports[21-24] that stressed the role of non-parenchymal cells, particularly FSC, as the principal collagen-producing cells of the liver, and demonstrated that type I collagen is the most abundant type[22].

The first group of experiments therefore suggests that acetaldehyde (a metabolite of ethanol), but not ethanol itself, plays a key role in the development of alcohol-induced liver fibrosis, and that FSC are the target of the acetaldehyde-mediated increased collagen synthesis.

EFFECT OF ACETALDEHYDE ON MATRIX GENE EXPRESSION BY FSC

The mechanisms of the increased collagen production induced by acetaldehyde are not yet established. In particular, the question arose whether acetaldehyde exerts its stimulatory effect at the level of gene expression. To verify this hypothesis, FSC were cultured with acetaldehyde and the total cellular RNA extracted at different times (3, 6, 12 and 24 h). Total RNA was then electrophoresed on an agarose/formaldehyde gel and the steady-state mRNA levels were measured by Northern blot hybridization according to standard techniques[37]. Specific cDNA probes for rat pro $\alpha_1(I)$ collagen, rat total fibronectin (FN) and human transforming growth factor β_1 (TGF-β_1) were used[38].

Acetaldehyde increased the FSC levels of procollagen I and FN mRNAs up to 24 h with a peak (3-fold) at 6 h of incubation; in contrast, no increase in TGF-β_1 mRNA was observed at 6 h, whereas a slight increase (1.5-fold) was evident at 24 h[38]. Transcription run-on assays showed that acetaldehyde increased both procollagen type I and FN gene transcription 3-fold. The effect of acetaldehyde required the formation of newly synthesized protein intermediates because it had no effect when administered to FSC at the same time as a protein synthesis inhibitor (cycloheximide); however, when this substance was given 15 min after the acetaldehyde procollagen type I and FN mRNA increased, showing that the required proteins are synthesized within the first 15 min of acetaldehyde administration[38].

Regulation of collagen gene expression is dependent upon interactions between protein factors, also known as transcriptional factors or activating proteins, and regulatory DNA sequences (promoter) that bind the proteins[39-47]. The FN promoter also contains multiple protein-binding regulatory elements, including a cAMP-responsive element and a Sp1 site[48,49]. Prevention of the acetaldehyde effect by cycloheximide may thus be due to inhibition of the DNA-binding protein synthesis.

MECHANISMS OF THE ACETALDEHYDE-INDUCED STIMULATION OF MATRIX SYNTHESIS BY FSC

Acetaldehyde can be metabolized by FSC because its concentration in media dropped with time but remained high when the cells were cultured in the presence of cyanamide, an aldehyde dehydrogenase inhibitor[38]. Metabolism of acetaldehyde may affect the redox state of the cell by increasing the NADH/NAD ratio[50]. Since lactate, which also increases the NADH/NAD ratio, has been shown to increase collagen synthesis in different experimental models[27,51], the question arose whether a change in the redox state is responsible at least in part for the acetaldehyde effect. However, in our experiment we did not find any effect of lactate on collagen and FN gene expression even at very high concentrations[38]. Moreover, acetaldehyde was effective even in the presence of cyanamide, an inhibitor of aldehyde dehydrogenase. It thus appears unlikely that the acetaldehyde effect on the gene expression of ECM components is mediated through a change in the intracellular redox state. An alternative hypothesis is that the acetaldehyde effect may be due to the formation of acetaldehyde–protein adducts.

Acetaldehyde adducts with proteins

Acetaldehyde may condense with amino groups of several proteins (as a Schiff's base) and react with thiol groups of proteins or thiol compounds, thus forming the acetaldehyde–protein adducts[52,53]. Experiments with methylene blue, a reducing equivalent scavenger that blocked the stimulatory effect of acetaldehyde on matrix synthesis by FSC[38], are consistent with this hypothesis. It has been reported that reducing equivalents enhance the formation of acetaldehyde adducts and the proportion of stable adducts *in vitro*[54]. To confirm this hypothesis we repeated some experiments with acetaldehyde in the presence of two inhibitors of adduct formation: pyridoxal-phosphate and *p*-hydroxy-mercuribenzoate[52]. These two compounds strongly reduced the formation of acetaldehyde adducts in FSC cultures (measured as TCA-precipitable [^{14}C]acetaldehyde) and blocked the stimulatory effect of acet-aldehyde on collagen and FN synthesis by acting at the level of gene transcription[55]. These data therefore suggest that acetaldehyde could exert its stimulatory activity on procollagen I and FN synthesis through the formation of adducts with proteins. However, different mechanisms of the acetaldehyde-induced collagen accumulation, other than the formation of adducts with proteins, might be involved.

LIPID PEROXIDATION AND MATRIX SYNTHESIS BY FSC

Ethanol and aldehydes easily induce the formation of reactive oxygen species (ROS) with consequent lipid peroxidation phenomena in the liver. There are several reports indicating that lipid peroxidation may contribute to the development of liver fibrosis.

Exposure of FSC, recently isolated and purified from normal human livers[56], to the pro-oxidant system ascorbate/iron results in early induction of lipid peroxidation (monitored by malondialdehyde and fluorescent aldehyde/protein adduct production), and in a significant increase of the constitutive expression of procollagen type I mRNA paralleled by the accumulation of the protein in the cell culture media[57]. This stimulatory effect is strongly reduced by pretreatment of FSC with antioxidants (vitamin E or diphenyl-phenylendiamine).

These findings indicate that oxidative reaction may directly influence the synthesis of collagen by FSC, thus contributing to the accumulation of matrix within the liver.

CULTURED FSC: A GOOD TOOL FOR STUDYING ALCOHOLIC LIVER FIBROSIS

It has been reported that rat FSC cultured on plastic change their phenotype with a decrease in fat droplets and increase in rough endoplasmic reticulum; this 'transformation' parallels an increase of collagen production and a higher procollagen type I and FN gene expression[58,59]. A very similar phenotype modification has been recently described in human FSC cultured on plastic[56]. The above-mentioned differentiation does not occur when FSC are cultured on gel matrices[60]. When the alcohol-induced liver injury occurs FSC modify their phenotype and transform into 'transitional cells'[15] which resemble the FSC cultured on plastic. Therefore, the *in vitro* model mimics what happens *in vivo* when lipocytes are activated and produce increasing amounts of collagen after chronic alcohol intake.

CONCLUSIONS

All the above-mentioned studies indicate that FSC are the principal effectors of hepatic fibrosis and stress the role of acetaldehyde in the induction of alcoholic liver fibrosis. Acetaldehyde is able to increase the gene transcription of ECM components in 'activated' FSC and this stimulatory effect is possibly due to the formation of adducts. Moreover, we showed[38] that acetaldehyde can increase the gene expression of TGF-β_1, a cytokine that plays a key role in the induction of tissue fibrosis. However, different mechanisms of alcohol-induced matrix synthesis, other than the formation of acetaldehyde adducts, have to be considered; in particular, the lipoperoxidation injury due to ethanol and, maybe, to acetaldehyde itself. The study of Parola and co-workers[57] suggests that lipid peroxidation induced by ROS may contribute to the development of alcoholic liver fibrosis.

What we have not established yet is whether the responsiveness of FSC to acetaldehyde depends on their 'activation'. In other words, can acetaldehyde directly stimulate matrix synthesis in the 'resting' FSC and induce their activation? Shiratori and co-workers[61] found no effect of acetaldehyde on collagen production by FSC in early primary cultures. Acetaldehyde may have been ineffective in that model because lipocytes were not 'primed' by prolonged primary or passaged cultures and thus unresponsive to acetaldehyde. Furthermore, these authors reported that, unlike cells from normal liver, collagen production by FSC activated *in vivo* by CCl$_4$ treatment was stimulated *in vitro* by acetaldehyde. Kupffer cells might play a key role in the activation of FSC after chronic alcohol feeding, as recently suggested by Matsuoka and co-workers[62]. According to that study TGF-β_1 might be the Kupffer cell mediator that activates lipocytes and makes them responsive to acetaldehyde. Acetaldehyde could maintain this 'activation state' by the induction of TGF-β_1 synthesis in FSC, in a sort of autocrine loop. Recent studies, however, suggest that lipoperoxidative events could directly stimulate the expression of PDGF receptors in the 'resting' FSC, thus activating these cells[63]. If this is true, ethanol might initiate the transformation of 'resting' FSC into the 'activated' phenotype (myofibroblast-like); acetaldehyde on one hand, and lipoperoxidative phenomena on the other, would maintain the activation of FSC and stimulate the synthesis of matrix in addition to cytokines.

References

1. Seyer JM. Interstitial collagen polymorphism in rat liver with CCl$_4$-induced cirrhosis. Biochem Biophys Acta. 1980;629:490–8.
2. Rojkind M, Rojkind MH, Cordero-Hernandez J. *In vivo* collagen synthesis and deposition in fibrotic and regenerating rat livers. Collagen Rel Res. 1983;3:335–47.
3. Seyer JM, Hutcheson ET, Kang AH. Collagen polymorphism in normal and cirrhotic human liver. J Clin Invest. 1977;59:241–7.
4. Rojkind M, Giambrome MA, Biempica L. Collagen types in normal and cirrhotic liver. Gastroenterology. 1979;76:710–19.
5. Hahn E, Wick G, Pencev D et al. Distribution of basement membrane proteins in normal and fibrotic human liver: collagen type IV, laminin and fibronectin. Gut. 1980;21:63–71.
6. Martinez-Hernandez A. The hepatic extracellular matrix. I. Electron immunohistochemical studies in normal rat liver. Lab Invest. 1984;51:57–74.
7. Schuppan D, Becker J, Boehm H et al. Immunofluorescent localization of type V collagen as a fibrillar component of interstitial connective tissue of human oral mucosa, artery and liver. Cell Tissue Res. 1986;243:535–43.
8. Abrahamson DR, Caulfield JP. Distribution of laminin within rat and mouse renal, splenic,

intestinal, and hepatic basement membranes identified after the intravenous injection of heterologous antilaminin IgG. Lab Invest. 1985;52:169–81.

9. Lieber CS, DeCarli LM. An experimental model of alcohol feeding and liver injury in the baboon. J Med Primatol. 1974;3:153–63.

10. Popper H, Lieber CS. Histogenesis of alcoholic fibrosis and cirrhosis in baboon. Am J Pathol. 1980;98:695–716.

11. Nakano M, Worner TM, Lieber CS. Perivenular fibrosis in alcoholic liver injury; ultrastructure and histologic progression. Gastroenterology. 1982;83:777–85.

12. Minato Y, Hashamura Y, Takeuchi J. The role of fat-storing cells in Disse space in fibrogenesis in alcoholic liver disease. Hepatology. 1983;3:559–66.

13. French SW, Miyamoto K, Wong K et al. Role of the Ito cell in liver parenchymal fibrosis in rats fed alcohol and a high fat–low protein diet. Am J Pathol. 1988;132:73–85.

14. Mak KM, Lieber CS. Lipocytes and transitional cells in alcoholic liver disease: a morphometric study. Hepatology. 1988;8:1027–33.

15. Mak KM, Leo MA, Lieber CS. Alcoholic liver injury in baboons: transformation of lipocytes to transitional cells. Gastroenterology. 1984;87:188–200.

16. Horn T, Jumge J, Christoffersen P. Early alcoholic liver injury. Activation of lipocytes in acinar zone 3 and correlation to degree of collagen formation in the Disse space. J Hepatol. 1986;3:333–40.

17. Clement B, Grimaud JA, Campion JP et al. Cell types involved in collagen and fibronectin production in normal and fibrotic human liver. Hepatology. 1986;6:225–34.

18. Chojkier M. Hepatocyte collagen production in vivo in normal rats. J Clin Invest. 1986;78:333–9.

19. Chojkier M, Lyche K, Filip M. Increased production of collagen in vivo by hepatocytes and nonparenchymal cells with carbon tetrachloride-induced hepatic fibrosis. Hepatology. 1988;8:808–14.

20. Chojkier M, Brenner DA, Leffert HL. Vasopressin inhibits type I collagen and albumine gene expression in primary cultures of adult rat hepatocytes. J Biol Chem. 1989;264: 9583–91.

21. De Leeuw AM, McCarthy SP, Geerts A et al. Purified rat liver fat-storing cells in culture divide and contain collagen. Hepatology. 1984;4:392–403.

22. Friedman SL, Roll FJ, Boyles J et al. Hepatic lipocytes: the principal collagen-producing cells of normal rat liver. Proc Natl Acad Sci USA. 1985;82:8681–5.

23. Maher JJ, Bissel DM, Friedman SL et al. Collagen measured in primary cultures of normal rat hepatocytes derives from lipocytes within the monolayer. J Clin Invest. 1988;82:450–9.

24. Milani S, Herbst H, Schuppan D et al. In situ hybridization for procollagen types I, III and IV mRNA in normal and fibrotic rat liver: evidence for predominant expression in nonparenchymal liver cells. Hepatology. 1989;10:84–92.

25. Holt K, Bennett M, Chojkier M. Acetaldehyde stimulates collagen and noncollagen protein production by human fibroblasts. Hepatology. 1984;4:843–8.

26. Thanassi NM, Rokowski RJ, Sheehy J et al. Non-selective decrease of collagen synthesis by cultured fetal lung fibroblasts after non-lethal doses of ethanol. Biochem Pharmacol. 1980;29:2417–24.

27. Savolainen ER, Leo MA, Timpl R et al. Acetaldehyde and lactate stimulate collagen synthesis of cultured baboon liver myofibroblasts. Gastroenterology. 1984;87:777–87.

28. Brenner DA, Chojkier M. Acetaldehyde increases collagen gene transcription in cultured human fibroblasts. J Biol Chem. 1987;262:17690–5.

29. Knook DL, Seffelaar AM, De Leeuw AM. Fat storing cells of the rat liver. Exp Cell Res. 1982;139:468–71.

30. Moshage H, Casini A, Lieber CS. Acetaldehyde selectively stimulates collagen production in cultured rat liver fat-storing cells but not in hepatocytes. Hepatology. 1990;12:511–18.

31. Takase S, Leo MA, Nouchi T et al. Desmin distinguishes fat-storing cells from myofibroblasts, smooth muscle cells and fibroblasts in the rat. J Hepatol. 1988;6:267–76.

32. Seglen PO. Preparation of isolated rat liver cells. In: Prescott DM, editor. Methods of cellular biology. New York: Academic Press; 1976:29–83.

33. Rennard SI, Berg R, Martin GR et al. Enzyme-linked immunoassay (ELISA) for connective tissue components. Anal Biochem. 1980;104:205–14.

34. Jauhonen P, Baraona E, Miyakawa H et al. Mechanism for selective perivenular hepatotoxic-

ity of ethanol. Alcoholism Clin Exp Res. 1982;6:350–7.
35. Baraona E, DiPadova C, Tabasco J et al. Transport of acetaldehyde in red blood cells. Alcohol Alcoholism. 1987;(Suppl. 1):203–6.
36. Baraona E, Matsuda Y, Pikkarainen P et al. Effects of ethanol on hepatic protein secretion and microtubules. Possible mediation by acetaldehyde. In: Galanter M, editor. Currents in alcoholism, Vol. VIII. New York: Grune & Stratton; 1981:421–34.
37. Maniatis T, Fritch EF, Sambrook J. Gel electrophoresis. In: Maniatis T, Fritch EF, Sambrook J, editors. Molecular cloning: a laboratory manual, 1st edn. New York: Cold Spring Harbor Laboratory; 1982:161.
38. Casini A, Cunningham M, Rojkind M et al. Acetaldehyde increases procollagen type I and fibronectin gene transcription in cultured rat fat-storing cells through a protein synthesis-dependent mechanism. Hepatology. 1991;13:758–65.
39. Ramirez F, Di Liberto M. Complex and diversified regulatory programs control the expression of vertebrate collagen genes. FASEB J. 1990;4:1616–23.
40. Brenner DA, Rippe RA, Veloz L. Analysis of the collagen alpha 1(I) promoter. Nucl Acids Res. 1989;17:6055–64.
41. Rippe RA, Lorenzen SI, Brenner DA et al. Regulatory elements in the 5′-flanking region and the first intron contribute to transcriptional control of the mouse alpha 1 type I collagen gene. Mol Cell Biol. 1989;9:2224–7.
42. Schmidt A, Rossi P, de Crombrugghe B. Transcriptional control of the mouse alpha 2(I) collagen gene: functional deletion analysis of the promoter and evidence for cell-specific expression. Mol Cell Biol. 1989;6:347–54.
43. Rossouw CM, Vergeer WP, du Plooy SJ et al. DNA sequences in the first intron of the human pro-alpha 1(I) collagen gene enhance transcription. J Biol Chem. 1987;262:15151–7.
44. Bornstein P, McKay J, Liska DJ et al. Interactions between the promoter and first intron are involved in transcriptional control of alpha 1(I) collagen gene expression. Mol Cell Biol. 1988;8:4851–7.
45. Karsenty G, Golumbek PT, de Crombrugghe B. Point mutations and small substitution mutations in 3 different upstream elements inhibit the activity of the mouse alpha 2(I) collagen promoter. J Biol Chem. 1988;263:13909–15.
46. Hatamochi A, Golumbek PT, Van Schaftingen E et al. A CCAAT DNA binding factor consisting of two different components that are both required for DNA binding. J Biol Chem. 1988;263:5940–7.
47. Maity SN, Golumbek PT, Karsenty G et al. Selective activation of transcription by a novel CCAAT binding factor. Science. 1988;241:582–5.
48. Dean DC, Blakeley MS, Newby RF et al. Forskolin inducibility and tissue-specific expression of the fibronectin promoter. Mol Cell Biol. 1989;9:1498–506.
49. Dean DC, Bowlus CL, Borgeois S. Cloning and analysis of the promoter region of the human fibronectin gene. Proc Natl Acad Sci USA. 1987;84:1876–80.
50. Lieber CS. Metabolic effects produced by alcohol in the liver and other tissues. Adv Intern Med. 1968;14:151–99.
51. Cerbon-Ambriz J, Cerbon J, Gonzalez E et al. Lactate and pyruvate increase the incorporation of [^{3}H]proline into collagen [^{3}H]hydroxyproline in liver slices of CCl$_4$ cirrhotic rats. Lab Invest. 1987;57:392–6.
52. Nomura F, Lieber CS. Binding of acetaldehyde to rat liver microsomes: enhancement after chronic alcohol consumption. Biochem Biophys Res Commun. 1981;100:131–7.
53. Pratt OE, Rooprai HK, Shaw GK et al. The genesis of alcoholic brain tissue injury. Alcohol Alcoholism. 1990;25:217–30.
54. Tuma DJ, Donohue TM Jr, Medina VA et al. Enhancement of acetaldehyde-protein formation by L-ascorbate. Arch Biochem Biophys. 1984;234:377–81.
55. Casini A, Galli G, Salzano R et al. Acetaldehyde, but not lactate and pyruvate, stimulates gene transcription of different extracellular matrix components in fat-storing cell cultures through the formation of acetaldehyde-protein adducts. J Hepatol. 1993 (In press).
56. Casini A, Pinzani M, Milani S et al. Regulation of extracellular matrix synthesis by transforming growth factor-β_1 in human fat-storing cells. Gastroenterology. 1993;105:245–53.
57. Parola M, Pinzani M, Casini A et al. Lipid peroxidation stimulates human liver fat-storing cells to increase procollagen α_1(I) gene expression and synthesis. A possible pro-oxidant

mechanism in liver fibrogenesis. Biochem Biophys Res Commun. 1993;194:1044–50.
58. Geerts A, Vrijsen R, Rauteberg J et al. *In vitro* differentiation of fat storing cells parallels marked increase of collagen synthesis and secretion. J Hepatol. 1989;9:59–68.
59. Weiner FR, Giambrome MA, Czaja MJ et al. Ito-cell gene expression and collagen regulation. Hepatology. 1990;11:111–17.
60. Friedman SL, Roll FJ, Boyles J et al. Maintenance of differentiated phenotype of cultured rat hepatic lipocytes by basement membrane matrix. J Biol Chem. 1989;264:10756–62.
61. Shiratori Y, Ichida T, Kawase T et al. Effect of acetaldehyde on collagen synthesis by fat-storing cells isolated from rats treated with carbontetrachloride. Liver. 1986;6:246–51.
62. Matsuoka M, Zhang MY, Tsukamoto H. Sensitization of hepatic lipocytes by high-fat diet to stimulatory effects of Kupffer cell-derived factors: implication in alcoholic fibrogenesis. Hepatology. 1990;11:173–82.
63. Friedman SL, Wong L, Yamasaki G. Gene expression of cytokine receptors during lipocyte activation. Chapter 18, this volume.

14
Activation of fat-storing cells in alcoholic liver fibrosis: role of Kupffer cells and lipid peroxidation

H. TSUKAMOTO

FSC ACTIVATION IN EXPERIMENTAL ALCOHOLIC LIVER FIBROSIS

Convincing *in vitro* and *in vivo* evidence is available to incriminate fat-storing cells (FSC) as the primary source of excessive extracellular matrices in liver fibrosis[1-5]. It has been proposed that this vitamin A-storing perisinusoidal cell undergoes myofibroblastic activation upon liver injury to play a central role in liver fibrogenesis[6,7]. This proposal has been supported by our previous study[8] which demonstrated three primary changes characteristic of fibroproliferative activation in experimental alcoholic liver fibrogenesis. These are: (1) decreased DNA synthesis; (2) enhanced collagen gene expression; and (3) loss of intracellular vitamin A. Furthermore, this activation was shown to take place in two major phases characterized as the early stage of mitogenic activation accompanied by vitamin A depletion and the late phase of fibrogenic activation (Fig. 1). The former was associated with an 83% decrease in the content of retinyl palmitate, a major retinyl ester in FSC, as well as a reduced level of cellular retinol binding protein[8]. The latter was also confirmed by demonstration of 2–3-fold increases in procollagen $\alpha_1(I)$ and TGF-β_1 gene expression in FSC freshly isolated from rats undergoing this stage of activation (Fig. 2). The enhanced TGF-β_1 mRNA level in these cells supported the autocrine role of this fibrogenic cytokine as demonstrated for *in vitro* activation of FSC[7].

ROLES OF KUPFFER CELL-DERIVED CYTOKINES IN FSC ACTIVATION

Over the past few years there has been an explosive amount of new information with regard to the role of cytokines in modulation of FSC functions. Studies

189

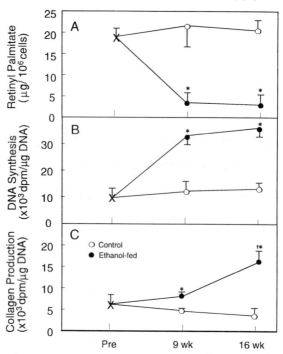

Fig. 1 Changes in fat-storing cell retinyl palmitate content, DNA synthesis, and collagen production during alcoholic liver fibrogenesis. The retinyl palmitate content was determined in freshly isolated fat-storing cells from age-matched chow-fed (Pre), ethanol-fed (●) and pair-fed control (○) rats. DNA synthesis and collagen production were measured *in vitro* using 3-day primary cultures of fat-storing cells from each group. Data are expressed as means ± SD. Note the early (9-week) mitogenic response of fat-storing cells from the ethanol-fed rats which is accompanied by marked vitamin A depletion in these animals. Also note the late fibrogenic response of these fat-storing cells as characterized by a prominent increase in collagen production at 16 weeks. $*p < 0.05$ compared to the data at Pre (data determined in the age-matched chow-fed rats prior to the experiment); $\dagger p < 0.05$ compared to the 9-week data

from other[9-11] and our[12] laboratories have demonstrated that cytokines can be potent mediators to induce phenotypic changes known to occur during activation of FSC. Kupffer cells, resident macrophages in the liver, have been examined by Matsuoka *et al.*[13] as a possible effector cell for cytokine-mediated FSC activation in experimental alcoholic liver fibrogenesis. Kupffer cells were isolated from rats developing alcoholic liver fibrosis and cultured in the medium containing 10% serum for collection of conditioned medium. The conditioned medium was subsequently dialysed (molecular cut-off = 12 kDa), concentrated, and added to the culture of autologous FSC to examine effects of Kupffer cell-derived soluble factors on FSC DNA and collagen synthesis. This study revealed that Kupffer cell-conditioned medium established from rats with alcoholic liver fibrosis, *but not* that from control animals, contained factor(s) which induced a 2-fold increase in FSC collagen production. The further characterization of the fibrogenic factors using HPLC gel filtration chromatography and specific antibodies against cytokines

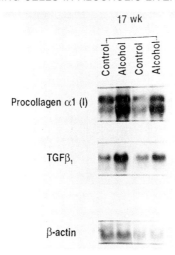

Fig. 2 Enhanced gene expression of procollagen α_1(I) and TGF-β_1 in fat-storing cells from rats with advanced alcoholic liver fibrosis. Total RNA was extracted from freshly isolated fat-storing cells from rats infused with a high-fat diet plus glucose (control) or ethanol (alcohol) for 17 weeks. Twenty micrograms of RNA were size-fractionated by electrophoresis in a denaturing 1.2% agarose gel, transferred to Nytran filters, and hybridized overnight with ^{32}P-labelled cDNA for procollagen α_1(I), TGF-β_1, or β-actin. Visualization of specific transcripts was achieved by overnight (procollagen α_1(I) and β-actin) or 3-day (TGF-β_1) autoradiography of the filters. Note 2–3-fold increases in the levels of both transcripts for procollagen α_1(I) and the concomitant increase in TGF-β_1 mRNA in fat-storing cells isolated from the livers with active alcoholic liver fibrogenesis

demonstrated that a major fibrogenic activity in this conditioned medium was TGF-β[14]. This conclusion was also supported by detection of TGF-β_1 mRNA in cultured Kupffer cells isolated from rats with alcoholic liver fibrosis[14]. Further, Northern blot analysis of RNA of freshly isolated Kupffer cells at both early and late stages of alcoholic liver fibrogenesis, revealed a 75–100% increase in the level of TGF-β_1 mRNA as compared to controls (unpublished data). Interestingly, IL-6 mRNA expression in these freshly isolated Kupffer cells was also shown to be enhanced, and this observation has correlated with the increased level of this cytokine in the conditioned medium established from the alcoholic animals (unpublished data). This acute-phase cytokine has recently been shown to enhance FSC collagen gene expression[15]. It is currently unknown what degree of contribution this cytokine makes to either *in vitro* or *in vivo* fibrogenic stimulation of FSC derived from these animals.

The conditioned medium from alcoholic rats also contained potent mitogenic activity towards FSC as demonstrated by marked enhancement of FSC DNA synthesis *in vitro* by this medium[13]. Our subsequent study showed that the major mitogenic activity derived from Kupffer cell-conditioned medium dialysed with the molecular cut-off of 12 kDa could be blocked with anti-PDGF antibody as shown in Fig. 3. However, if this conditioned medium was dialysed with the molecular cut-off of 3 kDa it produced a greater stimulation of Ito cell DNA synthesis, and this additional

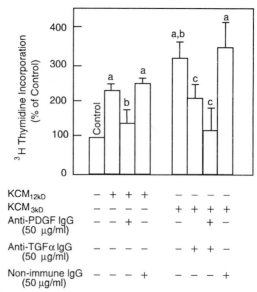

Fig. 3 Kupffer cell-derived fat-storing cell mitogenic activity. Three-day primary cultures of fat-storing cells were exposed for 48 h to Kupffer cell-conditioned media dialysed with molecular cut-off of 12 kDa ($KCM_{12\ kD}$) or 3 kDa ($KCM_{3\ kD}$) which were established from rats fed alcohol and high-fat diet for 10 weeks. Antibodies against human PDGF (R&D Systems), rat TGF-α (Peninsula Lab, Inc.) or non-immune IgG were added to the cultures, and the cells were labelled for the last 18 h with [³H]thymidine (1 μCi/ml) in the serum-supplemented medium. The results were means ± SD from four or five experiments expressed as the percentage of control (cultures added with dialysed unconditioned medium). (**a**) $p < 0.05$ compared to control; (**b**) $p < 0.05$ compared to $KCM_{12\ kD}$; (**c**) $p < 0.05$ compared to $KCM_{3\ kD}$

increase was mostly blocked with anti-TGFα IgG (Fig. 3). These results suggest the release of these mitogenic cytokines into the medium by Kupffer cells from alcoholic rats. However, a possibility still exists that Kupffer cell-derived factors other than PDGF and TGF-α might have induced increased sensitivity and responsiveness of FSC to these cytokines contained in the serum of the media. The analogous mechanism was evidenced by a study by Friedman and Arthur[16] which demonstrated up-regulation of FSC PDGF receptor expression by Kupffer cell-conditioned medium.

ROLE OF LIPID PEROXIDATION IN ALCOHOLIC LIVER FIBROGENESIS

The pathogenetic importance of lipid peroxidation in liver fibrogenesis has been proposed by studies in which increased collagen gene expression was demonstrated *in vitro* by fibroblasts with enhanced lipid peroxidation[17]. This hypothesis has been tested by Kamimura *et al.*, who examined *in vivo* correlation between the degree of hepatic lipid peroxidation and that of liver fibrosis in our model[18]. Lipid peroxidation was assessed in isolated microsomes and mitochondria, known subcellular sites of oxidative stress in

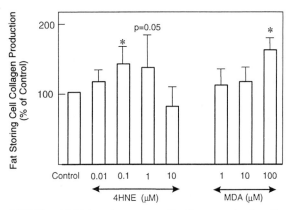

Fig. 4 Effects of 4HNE and MDA on fat-storing cell collagen production. Fat-storing cells in early passages were incubated for 18 h in MEME without serum in the absence or presence of 4HNE (0.01–10 μmol/l) of MDA (1–100 μmol/l). [^{3}H]proline (10 μCi/ml) was used to determine collagen production. *$p < 0.05$ compared to control. Data are means ± SD from four experiments

alcoholic liver injury. Three parameters were used for assessment of lipid peroxidation: malondialdehyde (MDA) equivalent as measured by thiobarbituric acid-reacting substances, conjugated diene formation with absorbance of extracted lipids at 233 nm, and 4-hydroxynonenal (4HNE) measured by TLC and HPLC as 2,4-dinitrophenylhydrazine derivative. All these parameters showed consistent increases at the time when alcoholic liver fibrosis was active. Furthermore, a statistically significant correlation was seen between the hepatic content of hydroxyproline and the level of MDA or 4HNE, supporting the possible mechanistic relationship between lipid peroxidation and alcoholic liver fibrogenesis.

To further define the cause and effect relationship of these two events we have examined direct *in vitro* effects of MDA and 4HNE on FSC collagen gene expression. Various concentrations of MDA (1–100 μmol/l) and 4HNE (0.01–10 μmol/l) were tested for their abilities to modulate collagen production and the mRNA levels of procollagen α_1(I). Both 4HNE and MDA stimulated FSC collagen production approximately by 50%, but the 4HNE concentration required to achieve this effect was 1/1000 of that for MDA (Fig. 4). Higher concentrations of 4HNE (> 10 μmol/l) tended to suppress collagen production. The mRNA levels of procollagen α_1(I) were also elevated by 50–70% following incubation of FSC with 4HNE (0.01 and 0.1 μmol/l) for 6 h (unpublished data). These results supported the direct stimulatory effects of lipid peroxidation aldehydic products on FSC gene expression as previously shown for fibroblasts[17]. Moreover, these concentrations of 4HNE, shown to stimulate FSC collagen gene expression, are well within the range of hepatic 4HNE levels determined *in vivo* in experimental alcoholic liver fibrosis[18].

To further validate the fibrogenic role of lipid peroxidation we have further enhanced hepatic lipid peroxidation in our model of alcoholic liver fibrosis by supplementing the diet with iron, a pro-oxidant, in the form of carbonyl iron (0.25% w/v), and tested whether this would promote alcoholic liver

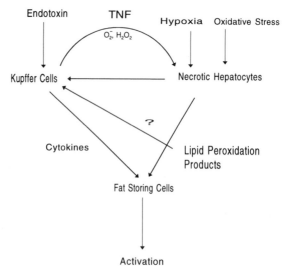

Fig. 5 Fat-storing cell activation in alcoholic liver fibrogenesis

fibrogenesis[19]. This supplementation elevated the hepatic level of non-haem iron in both alcohol-fed and pair-fed control rats by only 2–3-fold. The iron-supplemented controls did not show any signs of either enhanced oxidative stress or hepatic abnormalities. However, the supplementation to alcohol-fed animals resulted in marked potentiation of alcohol-induced hepatic lipid peroxidation and liver fibrosis with subsequent induction of diffuse bridging fibrosis in most of the animals, and micronodular liver cirrhosis in some animals[19]. Thus, iron supplementation, a condition which enhanced alcohol-induced oxidative liver injury, caused marked promotion of alcoholic liver fibrogenesis, providing additional evidence for the hypothetical link between these two events.

CONCLUSIONS

Using the rat model of alcoholic liver fibrosis we identified two major classes of factors believed to be involved in 'activation' of FSC in alcoholic liver fibrogenesis. They are Kupffer cell-derived cytokines and lipid peroxidation aldehydic products. Our findings to date support paracrine mechanisms involving Kupffer cell-derived TGF-β and growth factors (PDGF and TGF-α) for fibrogenic and mitogenic FSC activation in alcoholic liver fibrogenesis. The autocrine role of TGF-β_1 in FSC fibrogenic activation is also supported by enhanced expression of this cytokine in FSC undergoing this phase of activation. Both *in vivo* and *in vitro* evidence support another hypothetical mechanism implicating lipid peroxidation aldehydic products (MDA and 4HNE) in direct induction of FSC collagen gene expression. It is our current working hypothesis that these two mechanisms work in concert to achieve FSC fibroproliferative activation in alcoholic liver fibrogenesis (Fig. 5).

Acknowledgements

The studies described here were supported by a USPHS grant AA06603 and the Department of Veterans Affairs.

References

1. Friedman SL. Cellular sources of collagen and regulation of collagen production in liver. Semin Liver Dis. 1990;10:20–9.
2. Takahara T, Kojima T, Kojima T et al. Collagen production in fat-storing cells after carbon tetrachloride intoxication in the rat. Immunoelectron microscopic observation of type I, type III collagens and prolyl hydroxylase. Lab Invest. 1988;59:509–21.
3. Milani S, Herbst H, Schuppan D et al. Procollagen expression by non-parenchymal rat liver cells in experimental biliary fibrosis. Gastroenterology. 1990;98:175–84.
4. Nakatsukasa H, Nagy P, Evarts RP et al. Cellular distribution of transforming growth factor-B1 and pro-collagen type I, III, and IV transcripts in carbon tetrachloride-induced rat liver fibrosis. J Clin Invest. 1990;85:1833–43.
5. Maher JJ, McGuire RF. Extracellular matrix gene expression increases preferentially in rat lipocytes and sinusoidal endothelial cells during hepatic fibrosis in vivo. J Clin Invest. 1990;86:1641–8.
6. Mak KM, Leo MA, Lieber CS. Alcoholic liver injury in baboons: transformation of lipocytes to transitional cells. Gastroenterology. 1984;87:188–200.
7. Bachem MG, Meyer D, Melchior R et al. Activation of rat liver perisinusoidal lipocytes by transforming growth factors derived from myofibroblast-like cells. Potential mechanism of self perpetuation in liver fibrogenesis. J Clin Invest. 1992;89:19–27.
8. Tsukamoto H, Matsuoka M, Blaner W et al. Ito cell activation during progression of alcoholic liver fibrosis. In: Wisse E, Knook DL, McCuskey RS, editors. Cells of the hepatic sinusoid, Vol. 3. The Netherlands: Kupffer Cell Foundation; 1991:453–6.
9. Pinzani M, Gesualdo L, Sababah GH et al. Effects of platelet-derived growth factor and other polypeptide mitogens on DNA synthesis and growth of cultured rat liver fat-storing cells. J Clin Invest. 1989;4:843–8.
10. Davis BH. Transforming growth factor-beta responsiveness is modulated by the extracellular collagen matrix during hepatic Ito cell culture. J Cell Physiol. 1988;136:547–53.
11. Bachem MG, Riess U, Melchior R et al. Transforming growth factors (TGF alpha and TGF beta 1) stimulate chondroitin sulfate and hyaluronate synthesis in cultured rat liver fat storing cells. FEBS Lett. 1989;257:134–7.
12. Matsuoka M, Pham N-T, Tsukamoto H. Differential effects of interleukin-1-alpha, tumor necrosis factor-alpha, and transforming growth factor-beta-1 on cell proliferation and collagen formation by cultured fat-storing cells. Liver. 1989;9:71–8.
13. Matsuoka M, Zhang M, Tsukamoto H. Sensitization of hepatic lipocytes by high fat diet to stimulatory effects of Kupffer cell-derived factors: implication in alcoholic liver fibrogenesis. Hepatology. 1990;11:173–82.
14. Matsuoka M, Tsukamoto H. Stimulation of hepatic lipocyte collagen production by Kupffer cell-derived transforming growth factor-beta: implication for a pathogenic role in alcoholic liver fibrogenesis. Hepatology. 1990;11:599–605.
15. Greenwel P, Schwartz M, Rojkind M. Cell lines from normal and CCl4-cirrhotic livers differ in their phenotypic expression of cytokines and extracellular matrix components. In: Gressnor AM, Ramadori G, editors. Molecular and cell biology of liver fibrogenesis. Lancaster: Kluwer; 1992:107–14.
16. Friedman SL, Arthur MJP. Activation of cultured rat hepatic lipocytes by Kupffer cell conditioned medium. J Clin Invest. 1989;84:1780–5.
17. Chojkier M, Houglum K, Solis-Herruzo J et al. Stimulation of collagen gene expression by ascorbic acid in cultured human fibroblast. A role for lipid peroxidation? J Biol Chem. 1989;264:16957–62.
18. Kamimura S, Gaal K, Britton RS et al. Increased 4-hydroxynonenal levels in experimental alcoholic liver disease: association of lipid peroxidation with liver fibrogenesis. Hepatology. 1992;16:448–53.
19. Tsukamoto H, Kamimura S, Yeager S et al. Hepatic cirrhosis in rats fed a diet with added alcohol and iron. Hepatology. 1992;16:113A.

Section IV
Cytokines, growth factors and liver fibrosis

15
A role for transforming growth factor-β in hepatic fibrogenesis

F. R. WEINER, S. DEGLI ESPOSTI and M. A. ZERN

INTRODUCTION

Hepatic fibrosis refers to the pathological accumulation of extracellular matrix (ECM) proteins, such as collagen, fibronectin, laminin, proteoglycans, and elastin within the liver[1]. Whereas there are many different causes of hepatic fibrosis, the pathogenesis of hepatic fibrogenesis appears to be similar, regardless of the underlying cause, reflecting the limited repertoire of liver responses to injury. In recent years considerable progress has been made in our understanding of the pathophysiology of liver fibrosis. It is now apparent that the accumulation of ECM associated with hepatic fibrogenesis is due to increased synthesis of its various components[2]. Molecular techniques have revealed that this increase in ECM synthesis generally results from increased transcription of the various ECM genes[3-5]. However, diminished ECM degradation may also play a role in the process of hepatic fibrogenesis[6]. It has also become evident in the past few years that hepatic lipocytes are the major cellular source of ECM synthesis during hepatic fibrogenesis. The participation of lipocytes in this pathological process requires the transformation of these cells from a quiescent state to an activated state[7,8]. Activation of lipocytes during the development of liver fibrosis is associated with their proliferation, enhanced ECM synthesis, morphological changes and their ability to respond to various fibrogenic factors (e.g. acetaldehyde)[3].

Recently, considerable attention has begun to focus on the mediators of hepatic fibrosis, and in particular those factors responsible for enhanced lipocyte ECM synthesis. While it is now evident that a complex interaction of factors is responsible for the development of hepatic fibrosis, cytokines appear to play a primary role in fibrogenesis because of their ability to affect cell phenotype, proliferation, and most importantly, ECM synthesis[9]. Whereas several cytokines appear to be significant in the fibrogenic process, our laboratory has been particularly interested in transforming growth factor-β (TGF-β). This chapter will summarize our *in vitro* studies, as well as those studies of hepatic fibrosis in experimental animals and humans that indicate the importance of TGF-β in liver fibrogenesis.

TRANSFORMING GROWTH FACTOR-β

TGF-β_1 is a homodimer with a molecular weight of 25 kDa; the vast majority of studies have evaluated this isoform and its role as a fibrogenic factor[9]. It has recently been demonstrated that other isoforms of TGF-β exist, and that the physiological roles of these isoforms vary somewhat, as does their regulation[10]. Many cells are known to synthesize TGF-β_1, and Kupffer cells, endothelial cells, and lipocytes are probably the cellular sources of TGF-β_1 in the liver[9]. In addition, essentially all cells have been shown[11] to possess receptors for TGF-β_1. Friedman and Yamasaki[12] have shown that activated hepatic lipocytes possess enhanced binding for TGF-β compared to quiescent lipocytes. They further suggest that enhanced TGF-β receptor expression is associated with lipocyte activation and that this increased receptor expression could augment lipocyte response to this fibrogenic cytokine[12].

Whereas TGF-β_1 is known to have numerous biological effects[11], the activity most germane to our investigations is its ability to enhance extracellular matrix protein synthesis *in vitro* and *in vivo* systems[9]. TGF-β has been shown to enhance the synthesis of collagens, fibronectin, and proteoglycans in a number of systems, including the liver[11]. In addition to TGF-β_1's stimulation of ECM synthesis, it appears to enhance fibrogenesis by inhibiting matrix degradation. It has been shown to decrease the synthesis of proteases and stromelysin and to stimulate the gene expression of tissue inhibitor of metaloproteinase (TIMP)[13]. The stimulation of matrix synthesis, as well as the inhibition of its degradation by TGF-β_1, suggests that this cytokine is an ideal candidate to serve as a modulator of liver fibrosis. Over the past several years we, as well as other investigators, have performed a series of experiments in order to more precisely delineate the role that TGF-β_1 plays in hepatic fibrogenesis.

TRANSFORMING GROWTH FACTOR-β_1 AND HEPATIC FIBROSIS IN ANIMALS

Using two animal models of hepatic fibrosis, we investigated the relationship between the development of hepatic fibrosis and changes in TGF-β_1 expression[14]. Whereas the mechanisms of hepatic injury are different in the models, murine schistosomiasis and CCl_4-induced hepatic fibrosis in rats, the final common pathway is the development of liver fibrosis. The histological development of hepatic fibrosis in both models was associated with an increase in both TGF-β_1 and pro-α_2(I) collagen steady-state mRNA levels, as well as collagen content (Fig. 1). In hepatic schistosomiasis, immunohisto-chemical studies also demonstrated an increase in TGF-β_1 protein in fibrotic livers. The increases in TGF-β_1 and pro-α_2(I) collagen mRNA content in murine schistosomiasis were due to enhanced transcription of their respective

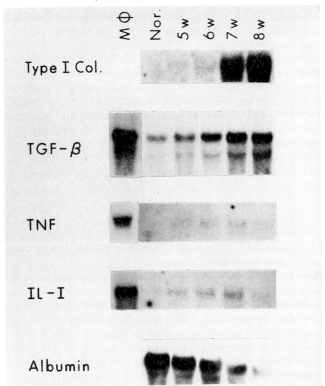

Fig. 1 Autoradiogram of Northern blots with RNA extracted from a macrophage cell line (M①), from livers of control mice (Nor), or from mice infected with *Schistosoma mansoni* and killed after a specified number of weeks of infection (5–8 w). Poly (A$^+$) RNA was prepared from the total RNA samples for use in hybridization studies for TNF and IL-1. The RNA was denatured, electrophoresed, and hybridized with pro-α_2(I) collagen (Type I Col), TGF-β_1, TNF, IL-1, and albumin cDNA probes. (From ref. 14)

genes. The steady-state mRNA levels of two cytokines known to enhance inflammation and to act as mitogens for mesenchymal cells, TNF-α and IL-1 were shown to increase at an early stage of murine schistosomiasis, prior to the increase in TGF-β_1. Other investigators have now confirmed the association of increased TGF-β_1 expression in models of hepatic injury[15–17]. For example, in streptococcal cell wall-induced granulomatous hepatic fibrosis, Manthey and co-workers[15] showed that the development of liver fibrosis was associated with increased TGF-β_1 mRNA content and increased histochemically detectable TGF-β_1 in areas of active fibrogenesis. The streptococcal cell wall-induced granulomas were also demonstrated to release physiologically significant amounts of active TGF-β_1 when they were cultured.

HEPATIC LIPOCYTES AND TRANSFORMING GROWTH FACTOR-β_1

To further elucidate the role of TGF-β_1 in hepatic fibrosis we have examined the effect of TGF-β_1 on hepatic lipocytes. We have shown that TGF-β_1 treatment of cultured lipocytes enhanced their collagen content by 3.5-fold, and that this increase was associated with a similar increase in pro-α_2(I) collagen mRNA content, due to both transcriptional and post-transcriptional mechanisms[18]. TGF-β_1 treatment also increased types III and IV procollagen, fibronectin, and proteoglycan mRNA levels in these cells by a post-transcriptional mechanism. Gressner and Bachem[19] have shown that TGF-β_1 treatment of lipocytes increases their proteoglycan synthesis but that the effect was dependent upon their state of activation; i.e. activated lipocytes demonstrated a greater increase in their proteoglycan synthesis when treated with TGF-β than do quiescent cells[19]. Davis[20] has shown that the effect of TGF-β_1 on Ito cell ECM synthesis is influenced by the matrix on which the cells are cultured, thus suggesting a dynamic interaction between cytokines and the ECM environment.

We, as well as others, have shown that lipocytes are a source of hepatic TGF-β_1 both in normal and fibrotic liver[4,7,19]. Furthermore, TGF-β_1 treatment increased lipocyte TGF-β_1 mRNA content, suggesting an autocrine mechanism for perpetuating the fibrogenic process[7]. It appears that TGF-β_1 may be synthesized by several hepatic cell types during the process of fibrogenesis. We have shown that, in comparison to normal animals, rats with CCl_4-induced hepatic fibrosis have an increase in hepatic TGF-β_1 mRNA content, and that this was associated with a 4-fold increase in hepatic lipocyte TGF-β_1 mRNA content[4] (Fig. 2). A less than 2-fold increase in TGF-β_1 mRNA content was found in the Kupffer/endothelial cell fraction and no increase in hepatocyte TGF-β_1 mRNA content was present[4]. While these findings would suggest hepatic lipocytes are a major source of TGF-β_1 during hepatic fibrogenesis, others would argue[9] that Kupffer cells, or circulating monocytes, or platelets trapped in the damaged liver may be a more important source of TGF-β_1. Another unresolved issue concerning hepatic TGF-β_1 is the mechanism by which it is activated. TGF-β_1 produced by either hepatic lipocytes or Kupffer cells is predominantly in a latent form and must be activated prior to binding to its receptors[11]. Whereas TGF-β_1 can be activated by a low, unphysiological pH, proteases, and glycosidases, the mechanism of its activation in the injured liver remains to be determined. Gressner and Bachen[19] have shown that hepatic lipocytes secrete α_2-macroglobulin which is capable of binding and inactivating TGF-β_1. Moreover, they have shown that TGF-β treatment of myofibroblast-like cells (presumably activated lipocytes) results in their enhanced synthesis of α_2-macroglobulin. These findings suggest the existence of a feedback loop in activated lipocytes for the regulation of TGF-β activity.

Other potential modulators of lipocyte ECM synthesis or hepatic fibrogenesis may exert their effects via their regulation of hepatic lipocyte TGF-β production. For example, a corticosteroid-induced inhibition of lipocyte pro-α_2(I) collagen mRNA content was associated with an inhibition of lipocyte

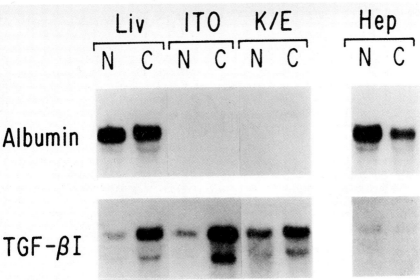

Fig. 2 Northern blot hybridization analysis of total RNA isolated from livers of normal rats (N) and carbon tetrachloride-treated rats (C), and from non-parenchymal and parenchymal cells isolated from these rats. This representative blot demonstrates increased TGF-β_1 mRNA in rat livers from animals treated with CCl$_4$ for 8 weeks. This increase in hepatic TGF-β_1 mRNA was also associated with a 4-fold increase in TGF-β_1 mRNA levels in hepatic lipocytes (Ito) isolated from fibrotic livers, a 2-fold increase in TFG-β_1 mRNA levels in a Kupffer/endothelial cell fraction isolated from similar livers, and no increase in hepatocyte TGF-β_1 mRNA

TGF-β_1 mRNA content (Fig. 3). This suggests that one of the mechanisms whereby steroids may inhibit fibrogenesis is through a suppression of lipocyte TGF-β_1 production[7]. Retinoids have been shown to inhibit lipocyte proliferation, collagen synthesis, and morphological transformation associated with cell culture[21]. We have shown that treatment of cultured lipocytes with retinol caused a decrease in pro-α_2(I) collagen mRNA content as well as decreased levels of TGF-β_1 mRNA[22]. These results suggest that the effects of retinoids on lipocytes may also involve alterations in lipocyte TGF-β_1 production.

HUMAN LIVER DISEASE AND TRANSFORMING GROWTH FACTOR-β_1

We have begun to extend these findings in animal models of hepatic fibrosis and cell culture experiments to determine the role of TGF-β_1 in human liver disease[23]. When compared to patients with normal livers, individuals with active liver disease had a 97% increase in their type I collagen mRNA levels and a 120% increase in their TGF-β_1 mRNA levels (Fig. 4). There was a significant correlation between the steady-state levels of TGF-β_1 and procollagen mRNA. Increase in gene transcription was found to be responsible for the increase in TGF-β_1 mRNA levels in patients with active liver

DEX

− +

Col I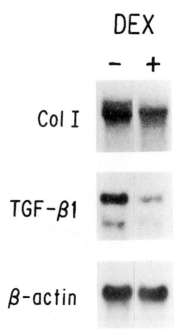

TGF-β1

β-actin

Fig. 3 Northern blot hybridization analysis demonstrating the effects of dexamethasone (DEX) on relative levels of selected mRNA in cultured lipocytes. Total RNA was extracted from (−) untreated lipocytes and (+) lipocytes treated with 100 nmol/l DEX. Col I = pro-α_2(I) collagen. Dexamethasone-treated lipocytes had decreased pro-α_2(I) procollagen and TGF-β_1 mRNA levels compared to untreated cells. (From ref. 7)

disease[23]. These findings have been confirmed by Castillia *et al.*[24], who found that TGF-β_1 mRNA expression correlated closely with type I procollagen mRNA content, serum procollagen type III peptide levels, and with histological activity index in patients with chronic hepatitis and cirrhosis. Collectively these studies provide strong evidence that TGF-β_1 plays a significant role in hepatic fibrogenesis in humans.

TRANSFORMING GROWTH FACTOR-β ISOFORMS

Recently two other members of the TGF-β family, TGF-β_2 and TGF-β_3, have been discovered. Somewhat different physiological roles and regulatory pathways have been demonstrated for these isoforms. We have assessed the role of TGF-β isoforms in CCl_4-induced liver fibrosis in rats[10]. Northern blot hybridization analysis of liver tissue from normal and CCl_4-treated rats revealed significant levels of TGF-β_1 in normal rat livers, increased TGF-β_1 expression after only 2 weeks of CCl_4 administration, and peak levels after 4 weeks of treatment. Levels decreased slightly at later stages of treatment. TGF-β_2 mRNA was also undetectable by Northern blots in normal rats and significant amounts were present only at 4 weeks of

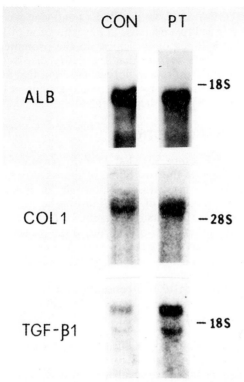

Fig. 4 Autoradiogram of a representative Northern blot hybridization study of total RNA isolated from the liver of a control patient (Con) compared to RNA from a patient with fibrotic liver disease. RNA was obtained from surgical or percutaneous liver biopsy samples. The autoradiogram shows RNA hybridized with either human albumin (ALB), pro-α_1(I) collagen, (COL1) or transforming growth factor-beta1 (TGF-β_1) cDNA probes. The patient with the fibrotic liver had increased TGF-β_1 and pro-α_1(I) collagen mRNA levels compared to an individual with a normal liver. (From ref. 23)

treatment. TGF-β_3 mRNA was undetectable in normal rat liver. Levels peaked at 4 weeks but remained at significant levels at weeks 6 and 8. Thus, there were large increases in the expression of all three isoforms during the period of maximal fibrogenesis. Analysis of the cellular source of these various TGF-β isoforms revealed that only TGF-β_1 mRNA was present in freshly isolated non-parenchymal cells from normal rats. However, activation of lipocytes via cell culture resulted in expression of TGF-β_2 and TGF-β_3 mRNA. As with TGF-β_1, TGF-β_2 and β_3 were capable of stimulating types I and III procollagen mRNA levels in non-parenchymal cells[10].

Because we had shown previously that prostaglandins inhibit hepatic fibrosis in *in vivo* models[25], we attempted to determine the mechanism of the effect of prostaglandins on ECM synthesis by examining the action of PGE$_2$ on non-parenchymal cell TGF-β isoform gene expression. PGE$_2$ treatment of the hepatic cells yielded surprising results. Whereas PGE$_2$ treatment of rat skin fibroblasts led to a 3-fold increase in TFG-β_3 expression (and no change in TGF-β_1 or β_2 levels), PGE_2 treatment of co-cultures of the non-parenchymal cells led to a decrease in the expression of TGF-β_3, despite the presence of a cAMP response element in the promoter region of the TGF-β_3 gene. Our results suggest that the newly discovered isoforms of TGF-β may play a significant role in fibrogenesis, and that an unanticipated inhibition of TGF-β_3 expression by PGE_2 could explain at least in part the antifibrogenic effect of PGE_2 on hepatic fibrosis.

SUMMARY AND NEW DIRECTIONS

The data are now quite compelling that TGF-β_1 plays a significant role in the development of hepatic fibrosis. Some of the issues which still need to be addressed include: the mechanism responsible for induction of TGF-β production; the cellular sources of TGF-β during hepatic fibrogenesis; the mechanism responsible for conversion of latent TGF-β to active TGF-β; and the importance of the other TGF-β isoforms in the process. Whereas most of what we have learned about the role of TGF-β in hepatic fibrogenesis has been accomplished through the study of animal models and cell culture, human studies should be crucial in the future. An understanding of these issues is not only important to our conception of the pathophysiology of hepatic fibrosis but is also crucial for the development of rational therapeutic approaches to its treatment.

A recent focus of our studies has been the attempt to develop new efficacious biological therapies for hepatic fibrosis. One of our initial attempts was the use of neutralizing antibodies to TGF-β_1 and β_2. We employed these antibodies by means of intraperitoneal injections in the murine model of hepatic schistosomiasis with no significant success. This contrasted with the success Ruoslahti and co-workers subsequently had in inhibiting nephro-sclerosis with intravenous administration of neutralizing TGF-β antibodies[26]. Thus it appeared that the targeting of the desirable agents may be crucial in the therapeutic approach to hepatic fibrosis. To accomplish this end we have recently begun to employ liposomes as carriers of therapeutic agents to the liver[27]. The benefit of liposomes is their ability to target the liver selectively with high levels of therapeutic agents that are lipid-soluble or degradable in serum. This approach may be highly successful in targeting cytokine antibodies, antisense, or other agents to the liver in the therapy of hepatic fibrosis.

Whereas this chapter has dealt with the role of TGF-β in the development of liver fibrosis, TGF-β is clearly not the only factor responsible for hepatic fibrogenesis. Other cytokines as well as soluble factors released from Kupffer cells, metabolic products such as acetaldehyde, oxygen free radicals, and other, as yet unidentified factors, may all play roles in the development of hepatic fibrosis. TGF-β appears to be a major component in this cascade of agents responsible for the pathogenesis of chronic liver disease.

Acknowledgement

This work was supported in part by National Institutes of Health grants AA06386 and DK41875 (M.A.Z.).

References

1. Schuppan D. Structure of the extracellular matrix in normal and fibrotic liver: collagens and glycoproteins. Semin Liver Dis. 1990;10:1–10.
2. Schuppan D, Somasundaram R, Just M. The extracellular matrix: A major signal transduction network. In: Clement B, Guillouzo A, editors. Cellular and molecular aspects of cirrhosis. Montrouge, France: John Libbey Eurotext, 1992:115–45.
3. Weiner FR, Czaja MJ, Giambrone M-A et al. Transcriptional and posttranscriptional effects of dexamethasone on albumin and procollagen messenger RNAs in murine schistosomiasis. Biochemistry. 1987;26:1557–62.
4. Weiner FR, Shah A, Biempica L et al. The effects of hepatic fibrosis on Ito cell gene expression. Matrix. 1992;12:36–43.
5. Nehls MC, Rippe RA, Veloz L et al. Analysis of the collagen $\alpha1(I)$ promoter region. Hepatology. 1991;12:919A.
6. Arthur MJP. The metalloproteinases. In: Clement B, Guillouzo A, editors. Cellular and molecular aspects of cirrhosis. Montrouge, France: John Libbey Eurotext, 1992:235–44.
7. Weiner FR, Giambrone M-A, Czaja MJ et al. Ito cell gene regulation and collagen regulation. Hepatology. 1990;11:111–17.
8. Friedman SL. Cellular sources of collagen and regulation of collagen production in liver. Semin Liver Dis. 1990;10:20–29.
9. Weiner FR, Degli Esposti S, Czaja MJ et al. The regulation of hepatic matrix protein synthesis by cytokines. In: Clement B, Guillouzo A, editors. Cellular and molecular aspects of cirrhosis. Montrouge, France, John Libbey Eurotext, 1992:147–56.
10. Degli Esposti S, Frizell E, Abraham A et al. The role of TGF-β isoforms in hepatic fibrosis. Hepatology. 1992;16:130A.
11. Sporn MB, Roberts AB, Wakefield LM et al. Transforming growth factor-beta: biologic functions and chemical structure. Science. 1986;233:532–4.
12. Friedman SL, Yamasaki G. Characterization of TGF-β receptors in cultured rat lipocytes: enhanced expression accompanies cellular activation. Hepatology. 1991;14:113A.
13. Chiang C-P, Nilsen-Hamilton M. Opposite and selective effect of epidermal growth factor and human platelet transforming growth factor-β on production of secreted proteins by murine 3T3 cells and human fibroblasts. J Biol Chem. 1986;261:10478–81.
14. Czaja MJ, Weiner FR, Flander KC et al. In vitro and in vivo association of transforming growth factor-β with hepatic fibrosis. J Cell Biol. 1989;108:2477–82.
15. Manthey CL, Allen JB, Ellingsworth LR et al. In situ expression of transforming growth factor-beta in streptococcal cell wall-induced granulomatous inflammation and hepatic fibrosis. Growth Factors. 1990;4:17–26.
16. Armendariz-Borunda J, Seyer AH, Kang AH et al. Regulation of TGF-beta gene expression in rat liver intoxicated with carbon tetrachloride. FASEB J. 1990;4:215–21.
17. Nakatsukasa H, Nagy P, Evarts RP et al. Cellular distribution of transforming growth factor-beta and procollagen types I, II and IV transcripts in carbon tetrachloride-induced rat liver fibrosis. J Clin Invest. 1990;85:1833–43.
18. Weiner FR, Shah A, Czaja MJ et al. Effect of transforming growth factor-$\beta1$ on Ito cell extracellular matrix gene expression. Hepatology. 1989;10:682A.
19. Gressner AM, Bachen MG. Parasinusoidal lipocytes: their contribution to hepatic connective tissue synthesis and to the mechanisms of matrix amplification in fibrogenesis. In: Clement B, Guillouzo A, editors. Cellular and molecular aspects of cirrhosis. Montrouge, France: John Libbey Eurotext, 1992:157–68.
20. Davis BH. Transforming growth factor-β responsiveness is modulated by the extracellular collagen matrix during hepatic Ito cell culture. J Cell Physiol. 1988;136:547–53.
21. Weiner FR, Blaner WS, Czaja MJ et al. Ito cell expression of a nuclear retinoic acid receptor. Hepatology. 1992;15:336–42.
22. Weiner FR, Shah A. Effects of retinoids on collagen and transforming growth factor-β_1 gene expression in Ito cells. Hepatology. 1989;10:630A.
23. Annoni G, Weiner FR, Zern MA. Increased transforming growth factor-β_1 gene expression in human liver disease. J Hepatol. 1992;14:259–64.
24. Castilla A, Prieto J, Fausto N. Transforming growth factor-β_1 and α in chronic liver disease: Effects of interferon alpha therapy. N Engl J Med. 1991;324:933–40.

25. Degli Esposti S, He Q, Frizell E *et al*. The multifaceted effects of enisprost, a prostaglandin E$_1$ analogue in inhibiting hepatic fibrosis. Hepatology. 1991;14:113A.
26. Border WA, Okuda S, Languanno LR *et al*. Suppression of experimental glomerulonephritis by antiserum against transforming growth factor-β1. Nature. 1990;346:371–4.
27. Yao T, Degli Esposti S, Murphy D *et al*. Vitamin E improves acute hepatic injury: targeted delivery to Kupffer cells by liposomes. Hepatology. 1993;18:323A.

16
Biology and regulation of platelet-derived growth factor

F. MARRA, G. G. CHOUDHURY, B. BHANDARI and H. E. ABBOUD

The observation that bovine serum stimulates the growth of cultured fibroblasts or other mesenchymal cells prompted several laboratories to investigate the molecules responsible for the mitogenic action as potential mechanisms for cell transformation and growth regulation *in vivo*. Since platelets were shown to contain the growth-stimulating activity[1], human platelets were used for purification of a factor that was first accomplished almost simultaneously in several laboratories in 1979[2,3], platelet-derived growth factor (PDGF). Since its discovery, PDGF has represented an area of intense investigation and almost 300 publications dealing with PDGF have appeared in 1992.

DIFFERENT PDGF ISOFORMS

Initial characterization of PDGF showed that it consists of a 30 kDa polypeptide formed by two different chains linked by disulphide bonds[4]. The two chains designated A and B (or 1 and 2) are encoded by two different genes. Comparison of the cDNA clones and of the amino acid sequences reveals a 60% homology between the two chains[5,6]. The homodimer of PDGF-A chains, PDGF AA[7] was first purified from an osteosarcoma cell line. In a similar fashion, a B-chain homodimer, PDGF BB, was found to be present in the material purified from platelets[8]. The major isoform (approximately 70% of the platelet PDGF content) is represented by the heterodimeric form, PDGF AB. The three isoforms interact with different PDGF receptors.

PDGF A- AND B-CHAIN PRODUCTION AND ASSEMBLY

Database comparison of the amino acid sequence of the B-chain revealed a very high homology with p28[sis], the transforming oncogene product of the simian sarcoma virus (v-sis)[9-11]. Transfection into CHO cells showed that part of the recombinant protein is secreted as a 30 kDa form of PDGF BB, whereas a 24 kDa form is retained intracellularly[12]. This is particularly interesting, since p28[sis] is processed as a 24 kDa homodimer that is almost completely retained inside the cell. It has been shown, using chimeric clones of PDGF A- and B-chains, that an 11 amino acid region in the N-terminus of both chains is the signal peptide that determines intracellular retention of the molecule[13]. This peptide is already present in a 56 kDa precursor of the PDGF BB, that is processed in the lysosomes and in the Golgi apparatus to yield the 30 kDa secreted form and the 24 kDa retained form of the molecule[14]. The relative abundance of either form is probably dependent on different activity of intracellular proteases, although the precise mechanism remains to be identified. The A-chain gene consists of seven exons that yield at least two RNA transcripts, originating from alternative splicing. The 'long spliced' A-chain mRNA encodes for a precursor that contains a peptide sequence similar to the one that is associated with intracellular retention of PDGF-BB[15,16]. This mRNA gives rise to an intracellularly bound form of the AA homodimer, whereas the 'short spliced' mRNA encodes for the secreted form[17]. Thus, regulation of the different forms of A- and B-chains occurs at different levels, i.e. alternative splicing or intracellular processing, respectively. Raines and Ross[18] have described the localization of a 40 kDa partially unprocessed form to the plasma membrane and to matrix heparan sulphate proteoglycans. The association with matrix proteoglycans has been reported to occur also with the product of the long spliced form of the A-chain[19]. The different functional significance of these forms is not yet understood. The mechanism of transformation by v-sis is believed to occur in an autocrine manner, and it is possible that interaction with the receptor occurs intracellularly. Although this would suggest a role for intracellularly retained forms of PDGF in transformation, in PDGF-expressing cells a high ability of transformation correlates with receptor activation rather than with the presence of intracellularly retained forms[14,20].

REGULATION OF PDGF A- AND B-CHAIN TRANSCRIPTION

The 5'-flanking sequence of the PDGF A-chain has been reported[15,21]. Transcription starts 845 bp upstream to the translation initiation site. The 5'-flanking region is characterized by the 'TATA box' and a region extremely rich in G and C residues, where three binding sites for SP-1 are located[21] (see Fig. 1). Analysis with S1 nuclease demonstrates that two S1-hypersensitive sites are localized within the G + C rich region, indicating possible regulatory sites for transcription[22]. Moreover, single-stranded oligonucleotides that specifically bind to the C-rich strand of the GC box, inhibit gene transcription, indicating an important role for this region of the promoter[23]. The region including nucleotides from -618 to $+392$ is sufficient to obtain a maximal promoter activity in a CAT reporter construct[24]. Analysis of deletion mutants shows that the most critical regions for promoter activity are located between -558 and -447 bp, and -150 and -33. In this latter region is located the

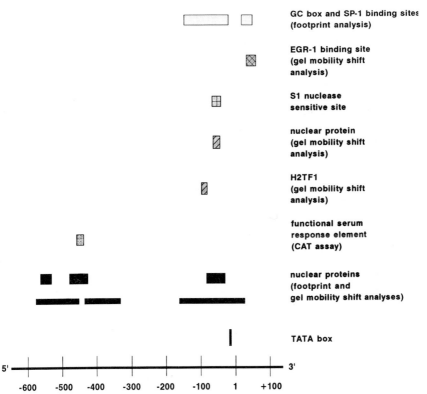

Fig. 1 Summary of the *cis*- and *trans*-acting factors in PDGF-A chain promoter. The figure summarizes location of various *cis*- and *trans*-acting factors identified by gel mobility shift assays, DNA-footprint analysis S1 nuclease analysis and CAT assays. Position of TATA and GC-box is also marked. Numbers represent nucleotide positions relative to the transcription start site. Data are from refs 21–26

GC box. DNA footprint analysis demonstrates that the GC box is protected from DNAse I digestion, and thus is likely a binding site for transcription factors. Therefore, the two S1-hypersensitive regions have been used to construct oligonucleotides to perform gel mobility shift assays. When tested with rhabdomyosarcoma cell nuclear extracts, the region located more upstream binds to a protein that, by comparison with other oligonucleotide sequences, seems to belong to the NF-κB family of transcription factors[24]. Two different proteins interact with the second S1-hypersensitive site, and SP-1 competes for the binding of one of these proteins, consistent with the presence of three SP-1 binding sites[24]. Finally, a serum response element has been localized in the region at bp −558 to −447. Interaction of a serum responsive factor with this element is believed to be responsible for the stimulation of PDGF on A-chain gene transcription and expression[24]. A binding site for EGR-1, a growth factor-inducible transcription factor, has also been demonstrated[25]. On the other hand, the protein encoded by the

Wilms tumour suppressor gene, WT1, acts as a powerful repressor of PDGF A chain transcription[26].

Analysis of the 5′-flanking region of the c-sis gene demonstrated the presence of the TATA box immediately upstream of the first exon[27]. The TATA box is preceded by a potential SP-1 binding site. The transcriptional promoter for normal and transformed cells was found in a region spanning −366 to +37 of the B-chain gene[28]. The same group has also described a region located downstream to the transcription initiation site, in the first intron, encoding untranslated RNA that inhibits translation of the PDGF B-chain mRNA *in vitro*[28,29]. The mechanisms of induction of PDGF B-chain transcription seem to be different in different cell types[30]. Stimulation of PDGF B-chain gene expression by PMA in K562 cells is associated with production of transcription factors that bind to a *cis*-acting element[31], but several, cell-specific, *trans*-acting regulatory regions have also been described[30].

PDGF RECEPTORS

Studies on secretion and structure of PDGF went along with other studies aiming at the purification of the PDGF receptor. In the early 1980s, specific PDGF receptors were demonstrated on mesenchymal and glial cells[32,33], and the receptor was cloned in 1987[34]. It appeared later that different isoforms of PDGF are not equally mitogenic for cultured fibroblasts[35], a finding compatible with the presence of more than one receptor. The existence of a second PDGF receptor was demonstrated in 1988[36,37], and the receptor was eventually cloned[38]. The two receptors share a 44% homology at the amino acid level and show similar structure. The extracellular domain is composed of five immunoglobulin-like domains, linked by a transmembrane segment to an intracellular domain. The cytoplasmic parts of both PDGF receptors constitute two subdomains with very high homology to known tyrosine kinases. These two tyrosine kinase domains are separated by about 100 amino acids called sparex sequences, or kinase insert domain. This structural feature of PDGF-R forms a new family of receptor tyrosine kinases including colony stimulating factor 1 receptor, fibroblast growth factor receptor and c-kit protooncogene product, which is now known as stem cell growth factor receptor. Both PDGF receptors possess a ligand-stimulated tyrosine kinase activity[39,40], that is directed towards the receptor itself (autophosphorylation). This receptor autophosphorylation occurs via inter-molecular transphosphorylation mechanisms. The ligand-activated receptor also phosphorylates other intracellular proteins at tyrosine residues. The two PDGF receptors are termed α and β, and differ in ligand specificity, since the α-receptor binds the A- and B-chains with high affinity, whereas the β-receptor binds only the B-chain of PDGF with high affinity. The mechanism of activation of the PDGF receptor requires dimerization[41]. Thus, PDGF BB will dimerize, and activate, both α- and β-receptors, whereas PDGF AB and AA require the presence of α-receptors to exert their effects (see Fig. 2)[42]. Following ligand binding the receptor is internalized and degraded[43]. Polyubiquitination of the receptor is required for efficient degradation of the

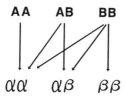

Fig. 2 Schematic representation of the interaction between PDGF dimers and PDGF α- and β-receptors

bound-receptor complex[44]. Very recently a soluble PDGF receptor has been reported in the conditioned medium of human MG-63 cells and in human plasma, thus identifying another possible mechanism relevant to the biological functions of PDGF[45].

SIGNAL TRANSDUCTION

Receptor occupation and dimerization is followed by autophosphorylation on tyrosine residues and acquisition of intrinsic tyrosine kinase activity directed towards other molecules[41]. The receptor tyrosine kinase activity is essential for PDGF-induced mitogenesis and chemotaxis[46,47]. Besides activating the receptor kinase, autophosphorylation on tyrosine provides binding sites for intracellular molecules that are involved in signal transduction. Interaction is mediated by the binding of phosphotyrosine residues of the PDGF receptors to src homology-2 (SH2) domains present in intracellular proteins that determine physical association between the activated receptor and some certain signal transduction proteins[48]. These proteins include phospholipase C-γ1 (PLC-γ1), GTPase activating protein (GAP), phosphatidylinositol-3'-kinase (PI-3-K), and other proteins with SH2 domains[48]. PLC-γ1 catalyses the conversion of phosphatidyl inositol bisphosphate to inositol trisphosphate and diacyl glycerol. The former compound is responsible for the increase in intracellular calcium concentration, whereas diacylglycerol is a known stimulator of protein kinase C, a serine/threonine kinase. The activated PDGF receptor induces phosphorylation on tyrosine of PLC-γ1[49] and probably increases its activity by physical translocation to the plasma membrane, where the availability of substrates for PLC is greater. The consequent activation of protein kinase C (PKC), mediated by diacyl glycerol, contributes to the mitogenic effect of PDGF, since PKC inhibitors inhibit mitogenesis[50]. Following PDGF stimulation, cytosolic PKC is translocated to both the plasma and the nuclear membranes[51]. Translocation to nuclear membranes is associated with increased phosphorylation of the nuclear envelope proteins lamin A and lamin C[51]. Ligand activation of the PDGF receptor is also associated[52] with an increased activation of p21^{ras}. Ras is a family of low molecular weight, GTP-binding proteins that are probably involved in the transduction of mitogenic and transforming signals. Microinjection of Ras antibodies blocks the mitogenic effects of PDGF[53]. RasGAP increases the conversion of the Ras-bound GTP to GDP, and contributes to maintain Ras in an inactive status[54]. PDGF has been shown to induce the association of GAP with the PDGF receptor and to stimulate its phosphorylation[55]. It is possible that sequestration of RasGAP by binding to the PDGF receptor contributes to Ras activation. Recently, however, an alternative pathway has been reported that leads to Ras activation following activation of receptor and non-receptor tyrosine kinases. This pathway involves the binding of Grb2, a protein which contains both SH2 and SH3 domains, to the activated receptor through its SH2 domain. The SH3 domain of Grb2 binds to a protein called Sos, which is the mammalian homologue of *Drosophila* son of sevenless gene. This gene encodes for a guanine nucleotide exchange factor which converts GDP bound Ras to Ras-GTP, resulting in mitogenically active Ras protein. Thus, the Grb2 protein acts as an adaptor molecule between activated PDGF-R and downstream effector molecules functioning in cell growth[56]. Another pathway involved in PDGF receptor signalling is the PI-3-K. PI-3-K is constituted by a heterodimeric complex of an 85 kDa and a 110 kDa protein, and is responsible for the catalytic phosphorylation of the inositol ring in its D-3 position using phosphoinositide as substrate[57]. The 85 kDa regulatory subunit contains SH2 domains and binds to the activated PDGF-R on the phosphorylated tyrosyl residues 740 and 751. The role of PI-3-K in the PDGF mitogenic cascade is not clear, although there is some evidence to indicate that it plays a role in mediating the mitogenic response of PDGF. It has been reported that some products of PI-3-K reaction can stimulate the novel PKC isoform PKC-ζ[58], that is required for mitogenic activation[59]. Valius and Kazlauskas[60] analysed the mitogenic responses mediated by different mutants of the PDGF receptor. A mutant was constructed that lacked the tyrosyl residues needed for binding of different cytosolic molecules, including RasGAP, PLC-γ1 and PI-3-K. Restoration of individual binding sites in 'add-back' mutants allowed the authors to investigate the relative contribution of those molecules in PDGF-dependent mitogenesis. When association of either PLC-γ1 or PI-3-K with the PDGF receptor was restored, DNA synthesis was stimulated, suggesting that PLC-γ1 and PI-3-K are independent downstream mediators of PDGF's mitogenic signalling. Other proteins associate with the PDGF receptor through SH2 domains, like the non-receptor tyrosine kinase p60^{src}, and a 64 kDa protein that corresponds to the recently cloned phosphoprotein phosphatase PTP 1D[61]. The role of this latter molecule is as yet unknown. More distally, the signal transduction pathway that followed PDGF-R activation is only partially known. Similar to other tyrosine kinases, activation of several serine/threonine kinases is likely to occur, with activation of mitogen-activated protein kinase (MAPK), and Raf. Different Raf mutants are able to determine either a block of the mitogenic signal[62] or oncogenic transformation, when a deregulated kinase activity is achieved[63]. Raf kinase activity is increased by PDGF treatment[64], although tyrosine phosphorylation of Raf protein could not be detected in PDGF-treated cells. However, Raf protein is a substrate for PDGF-R *in vitro*[65]. More likely, Raf is controlled by serine/threonine phosphorylation. Although the signal transduction pathways for the α- and β-receptors are considered basically the same, very recently a different pattern of activation of the intracellular transducing molecules has been reported[66], and different signal transduction pathways are activated by different PDGF isoforms in smooth muscle cells[67].

BIOLOGICAL ROLES OF PDGF

The induction of cell proliferation is clearly the most relevant and best-known effect of PDGF. The specificity of this effect is almost exclusively restricted to cells of mesenchymal origin, like fibroblasts or smooth muscle cells, and different types of glial cells. The biological effects of PDGF on cultured cells are, however, much broader. PDGF affects cytoskeletal organization, manifested by the appearance of ruffles on the fibroblast cell surface[68]. This effect is mediated by a rearrangement of actin filaments and requires a functional tyrosine kinase activity[47]. Several groups have also demonstrated that PDGF is chemotactic for fibroblasts, monocytes, smooth muscle cells, and mesangial cells[69-72]. In arterial smooth muscle cells, PDGF up-regulates the production of collagen and extracellular matrix[73,74], and stimulates contraction[75]. PDGF and its β-receptor are markedly expressed in the developing placenta, where they are probably involved in the development of vascular structures[76]. PDGF expression is abundant in the central nervous system, and a role in neural system development and glial regulation has been suggested[77,78]. In an animal model of wound healing, administration of PDGF increased cellular reorganization and wound strength, suggesting a role in the reparative process[79]. Since overexpression of PDGF B- and, to a lesser extent, A-chain confers transforming properties[80,81], several studies were conducted to investigate the role of PDGF in human malignancy. Several tumour cell lines express PDGF A- and B-chain, and autocrine stimulation of cell growth has been reported[82]. In human glioblastoma tissue both PDGF chains are expressed. Whereas the α-receptor is expressed by the neoplastic cells, the β-receptor is expressed by the surrounding stroma[83]. This indicates that PDGF secreted by tumour cells may also contribute to stromal proliferation, thus supporting the growth of neoplastic cells[84]. PDGF release by platelets may trigger smooth muscle cell proliferation and thus contribute to the pathogenesis of atherosclerosis[85]. Support to this view is provided by the observation that PDGF antibodies or platelet depletion inhibit the proliferative response following angioplasty[86]. In the kidney, the expression of PDGF A- and B-chains by glomerular mesangial cells is increased upon stimulation with different growth factors, including PDGF itself, and PDGF is mitogenic for these cells[87,88]. Increased expression of PDGF and PDGF receptor has been described in several animal models of proliferative glomerular disease. Treatment with anti-PDGF antibodies ameliorates cell proliferation[89].

PDGF AND LIVER FAT-STORING CELLS (FSC)

FSC in primary culture are not responsive to the mitogenic effects of PDGF. However, if the cells are pretreated with Kupffer cell-conditioned medium they acquire the ability to proliferate in response to serum, and in particular to PDGF. Anti-PDGF antibodies almost completely inhibit the serum-induced mitogenic effect[90]. This effect was shown to be dependent on the induction of PDGF receptor expression on FSC in response to Kupffer cell-conditioned medium[90]. PDGF is a potent mitogen for rat FSC cultured and passaged on plastic, when transition to a 'myofibroblast-like' phenotype occurs. PDGF stands out as the most potent mitogen among several growth factors tested[91]. The presence of specific PDGF receptor(s) was demonstrated using $[^{125}I]$PDGF-AB isoform. The nature of the PDGF receptor on FSC was addressed in a subsequent study, where the comparative effects of the three different PDGF isoforms on cell proliferation and early signal transduction pathways were investigated in rat FSC[92]. The effects of PDGF AA on DNA synthesis, inositol phosphate accumulation and increase in cytosolic calcium were considerably lower than the ones induced by PDGF-AB or BB. These findings are consistent with the predominance of PDGF β-receptors, with only a minority of α-receptors on FSC. The possible down-regulation of PDGF α-receptors due to endogenous synthesis and release of PDGF AA is unlikely, since pretreatment of FSC with suramin, which inhibits PDGF binding to its receptors, did not modify the response to PDGF-AA[92]. This finding was confirmed by another group of investigators. They reported that another biological effect of PDGF in FSC, the production of hyaluronan, was observed only when PDGF-BB, but not PDGF-AA, was used as an agonist[93]. Several factors have been shown to regulate PDGF-induced mitogenesis in rat liver FSC. Retinoids inhibit PDGF-induced $[^3H]$thymidine incorporation and partially reverse the myofibroblast-like phenotype induced by culturing on plastic[94,95]. The cellular mechanisms by which the modulating effect of retinoids takes place are not known. Retinoic acid does not modify PDGF receptor expression, as assessed by Western blotting[94]. In addition, preliminary data demonstrate that the PDGF signal transduction pathway, including activation of Raf kinase, is not affected by retinoids, suggesting a more distal site of action[96]. IGF-I by itself modestly increases DNA synthesis, but it potentiates the effects of PDGF[97]. Transforming growth factor beta (TGF-β) has been shown to increase[91] or inhibit[94] PDGF-induced mitogenesis. The decrease in mitogenic effect was associated with reduced expression of PDGF receptors. A possible explanation for this discrepancy could be due to the different substrate used for cell culture, i.e. plastic or collagen I. In liver injury, FSC acquire a myofibroblast-like phenotype, which is associated with loss of cellular retinoids. Friedman *et al.*[98] have recently shown that Kupffer cell-conditioned medium and PDGF induce retinol release by FSC in culture. This suggests that PDGF expression may contribute to retinoid loss by activated FSC *in vivo*. The production of several factors that are synthesized by FSC is stimulated by PDGF. Secretion of TGF-β in the conditioned medium is increased by 25% by PDGF-AB[94]. Secretion of insulin-like growth factor I immunoreactivity is stimulated by PDGF-BB, probably through stimulation of IGF-I binding protein(s)[97]. The secretion of macrophage-colony stimulating factor (M-CSF or CSF-1) and its gene expression are stimulated by PDGF in murine FSC. In this respect PDGF appears to be a weaker stimulus than bFGF[99]. On the other hand,

PDGF does not induce production of glycosaminoglycans[100]. We have recently shown that production and gene expression of monocyte chemotactic protein-1 in human FSC is considerably increased by proinflammatory cytokines such as IL-1α and IFN-γ, but only modestly by PDGF[101]. The precise role of PDGF *in vivo* remains to be established. Preliminary data in an acute model of toxic liver injury, show that intense PDGF staining is present 24 h after exposure to the hepatotoxin, and becomes more evident at 48 and 72 h[102]. PDGF B-chain mRNA is expressed at 48 and 72 h, indicating that active synthesis and release of PDGF occurs. It is clear that the diverse biological properties of PDGF make it a strong candidate to mediate or modulate hepatic pathophysiology. The effects of PDGF on growth, development, matrix metabolism and vascular tone are some of the potential mechanisms by which this and other growth factors influence disease processes as diverse as wound healing, hepatic and renal inflammation, atherosclerosis and carcinogenesis.

References

1. Ross R, Glomset J, Kariya B, Harker LA. A platelet-dependent serum factor that stimulates the proliferation of arterial smooth muscle cells in vitro. Proc Natl Acad Sci USA. 1974;71:1207–10.
2. Antoniades HN, Scher CD, Stiles CD. Purification of human platelet-derived growth factor. Proc Natl Acad Sci USA. 1979;76:1809–12.
3. Heldin CH, Westermark B, Wasteson A. Platelet-derived growth factor: purification and partial characterization. Proc Natl Acad Sci USA. 1979;76:3722–6.
4. Johnsson A, Heldin C-H, Westermark B, Wasteson A. Platelet-derived growth factor: identification of constituent polypeptide chains. Biochem Biophys Res Commun. 1982;104:66–74.
5. Betscholtz C, Johnsson A, Heldin C-H et al. cDNA sequence and chromosomal localization of human platelet-derived growth factor A-chain and its expression in tumour cell lines. Nature. 1986;320:694–9.
6. Josephs SF, Guo C, Ratner L, Wong-Staal F. Human proto-oncogene sequences corresponding to the transforming region of simian sarcoma virus. Science. 1984;223:487–90.
7. Heldin C-H, Johnsson A, Wennergren S et al. A human osteosarcoma cell line secretes a growth factor structurally related to a homodimer of PDGF A chains. Nature. 1986;3:19:511–15.
8. Hammacher A, Hellman U, Johnsson A et al. A major part of PDGF purified from human platelets is a heterodimer of one A chain and one B chain. J Biol Chem. 1988;263:16493–8.
9. Devare SG, Reddy EP, Law JP, Robbins KC, Aaronson SA. Nucleotide sequence of the simian sarcoma virus genome: demonstration that its acquired cellular sequences encode the transforming gene product p28sis. Proc Natl Acad Sci USA. 1983;80:731–5.
10. Doolittle RF, Hunkapiller MW, Hood LE et al. Simian sarcoma virus oncogene, v-sis, is derived from the gene (or genes) encoding a platelet-derived growth factor. Science. 1983;221:275–7.
11. Waterfield MD, Scrace T, Whittle N et al. Platelet-derived growth factor is structurally related to the putative transforming protein p28sis of simian sarcoma virus. Nature. 1983;304:35–9.
12. Ostman A, Rall L, Hammacher A et al. Synthesis and assembly of a functionally active recombinant PDGF-AB heterodimer. J Biol Chem. 1988;263:1602–8.
13. Ostman A, Andersson M, Betscholtz C, Westermark B, Heldin C-H. Identification of a cell retention signal in the B-chain of platelet-derived growth factor and in the long splice version of the A-chain. Cell Regul. 1991;2:503–12.
14. Ostman A, Thyberg J, Westermark B, Heldin C-H. PDGF-AA and PDGF-BB biosynthesis:

proprotein processing in the golgi complex and lysosomal degration of PDGF-BB retained intracellularly. J Cell Biol. 1992;118:509–19.

15. Bonthron DT, Morton CC, Orkin SH, Collins T. Platelet-derived growth factor A chain: Gene structure, chromosomal location, and basis for alternative mRNA splicing. Proc Natl Acad Sci USA. 1988;85:1492–6.

16. Rorsman F, Bywater M, Knott TJ, Scott J, Betscholtz C. Structural characterization of the human platelet-derived growth factor A-chain cDNA and gene: alternative exon usage predicts two different precursor proteins. Mol Cell Biol. 1988;8:571–7.

17. Ostman A, Andersson M, Hellman U, Heldin C-H. Identification of three amino acids in the platelet-derived growth factor (PDGF) that are important for binding to the PDGF b-receptor. J Biol Chem. 1991;266:10073–7.

18. Raines EW, Ross R. Compartmentalization of PDGF on extracellular binding sites dependent on exon-6-encoded sequences. J Cell Biol. 1992;116:533–43.

19. Kelly JL, Sanchez A, Brown GS, Chesterman CN, Sleigh MJ. Accumulation of PDGF B and cell-binding forms of PDGF A in the extracellular matrix. J Cell Biol. 1993;121: 1153–63.

20. LaRochelle WJ, Giese N, May-Siroff M, Robbins KC, Aaronson SA. Molecular localization of the transforming and secretory properties of PDGF A and PDGF B. Science. 1990;248:1541–4.

21. Takimoto Y, Wang Z-Y, Kobler K, Deuel TF. Promoter region of the human platelet-derived growth factor A-chain gene. Proc Natl Acad Sci USA. 1991;88:1686–90.

22. Wang Z-Y, Lin X-H, Qui Q-Q, Deuel TF. Modulation of transcription of the platelet-derived growth factor A-chain gene by a promoter region sensitive to S1 nuclease. J Biol Chem. 1992;267:17022–31.

23. Wang Z, Lin X-H, Nobyuoshi M, Qui Q-Q, Deuel TF. Binding of single-stranded oligonucleotides to a non-B-form DNA structure results in loss of promoter activity of the platelet-derived growth factor A-chain gene. J Biol Chem. 1992;267:13669–74.

24. Lin X, Wang Z, Gu L, Deuel TF. Functional analysis of the human platelet-derived growth factor A-chain promoter region. J Biol Chem. 1992;267:25614–19.

25. Wang Z-Y, Deuel TF. An S1 nuclease-sensitive homopurine/homopyrimidine domain in the PDGF A-chain promoter contains a novel binding site for the growth factor-inducible protein EGR-1. Biochem Biophys Res Commun. 1992;188:433–9.

26. Gashler AL, Bonthron DT, Madden SL, Rauscher FJ, Collins T, Sukhatme V. Human platelet-derived growth factor A chain is transcriptionally repressed by the Wilms tumor suppressor WT1. Proc Natl Acad Sci USA. 1992;89:10984–8.

27. van den Ouweland MW, Roebroek AJM, Schalken JA, Claesen CA, Bloemers HPJ, Van de Ven WJM. Structure and nucleotide sequence of the 5′ region of the human and feline c-sis proto-oncogenes. Nucl Acids Res. 1986;14:765–78.

28. Ratner L, Thielan B, Collins T. Sequences of the 5′ portion of the human c-sis gene: characterization of the transcriptional promoter and regulation of expression of the protein product by 5′ untranslated mRNA sequences. Nucl Acids Res. 1987;15:6017–36.

29. Rao CD, Pech M, Robbins KC, Aaronson SA. The 5′ untranslated sequence of the c-sis/platelet-derived growth factor 2 transcript is a potent translational inhibitor. Mol Cell Biol. 1988;8:284–92.

30. Dirks RPH, Jansen HJ, Gerritsma J, Onnekink C, Bloemers HPJ. Localization and functional analysis of DNase-I-hypersensitive sites in the human c-sis/PDGF-β gene transcription unit and its flanking regions. Eur J Biochem. 1993;11:509–19.

31. Pech M, Rao CD, Robbins KC, Aaronson SA. Functional identification of regulatory elements within the promoter region of PDGF2. Mol Cell Biol. 1989;9:396–405.

32. Bowen-Pope DF, Ross R. Platelet-derived growth factor. II. Specific binding on cultured cells. J Biol Chem. 1982;257:5161–71.

33. Heldin CH, Westermark B, Wasteson. Specific receptors for platelet-derived growth factor on cells derived from connective tissue and glia. Proc Natl Acad Sci USA. 1981;78: 3664–8.

34. Yarden Y, Escobedo JA, Kuang W-J et al. Structure of the receptor for platelet-derived growth factor helps define a family of closely related growth factor receptors. Nature. 1986;323:226–32.

35. Nister M, Hammacher A, Mellström K et al. A glioma-derived PDGF A chain homodimer

has different functional activities than a PDGF AB heterodimer purified from human platelets. Cell. 1988;52:791–9.

36. Hart CE, Forstrom JW, Kelly JD *et al.* Two classes of PDGF receptors recognize different isoforms of PDGF. Science. 1988;240:1529–31.

37. Heldin C-H, Backström G, Ostman A *et al.* Binding of different dimeric forms of PDGF to human fibroblasts: evidence for two separate receptor types. EMBO J. 1988;7:1387–94.

38. Claesson-Welsh L, Eriksson A, Westermark B, Heldin C-H. cDNA cloning of the human A type receptor establishes structural similarity to the B type receptor. Proc Natl Acad Sci USA. 1989;86:4917–21.

39. Ek B, Westermark B, Wasteson A, Heldin C-H. Stimulation of tyrosine-specific phosphorylation by platelet-derived growth factor. Nature. 1982;295:419–20.

40. Matsui T, Heidaran M, Miki T *et al.* Isolation of a novel receptor cDNA establishes the existences of two PDGF receptor genes. Science. 1989;243:800–3.

41. Heldin C-H, Ernlund A, Rorsman C, Ronnstrand L. Dimerization of B type receptors occurs after ligand binding and is closely associated with receptor kinase activation. J Biol Chem. 1989;264:8905–12.

42. Hammacher A, Mellstrom K, Heldin C-H, Westermark B. Isoform-specific induction of actin reorganization by platelet-derived growth factor suggests that the functionally active receptor is a dimer. EMBO J. 1989;8:2489–95.

43. Heldin C-H, Wasteson A, Westermark B. Interaction of platelet-derived growth factor with its fibroblast receptor. Demonstration of ligand degradation and receptor modulation. J Biol Chem. 1982;257:4216–21.

44. Mori S, Heldin C-H, Claesson-Welsh L. Ligand-induced ubiquitination of the platelet derived growth factor β-receptor plays a negative regulatory role in its mitogenic signaling. J Biol Chem. 1993;268:577–83.

45. Tiesman J, Hart CE. Identification of a soluble receptor for platelet-derived growth factor in cell-conditioned medium and human plasma. J Biol Chem. 1993;268:9621–8.

46. Escobedo JA, Williams LT. A PDGF receptor domain essential for mitogenesis but not for many other responses to PDGF. Nature. 1988;335:85–7.

47. Westermark B, Siegbahn A, Heldin C-H, Claesson-Welsh L. B-type receptor for platelet-derived growth factor mediates a chemotactic response by means of ligand-induced activation of the receptor protein-tyrosine kinase. Proc Natl Acad Sci USA. 1990;87:128–32.

48. Cantley LC, Auger KR, Carpenter C *et al.* Oncogenes and signal transduction. Cell. 1991;64:281–302.

49. Meisenhelder J, Suh P-G, Rhee SG, Hunter T. Phospholipase C-γ is a substrate for the PDGF and EGF receptor protein tyrosine kinases *in vivo* and *in vitro*. Cell. 1989;57: 1109–22.

50. Ghosh Choudhury G, Biswas P, Grandaliano G, Abboud HE. Involvement of PKC-α in PDGF-mediated mitogenic signaling in human mesangial cells. Am J Physiol. 1993 (In press).

51. Fields AP, Tyler G, Kraft AS, May WS. Role of nuclear protein kinase C in the mitogenic response to platelet-derived growth factor. J Cell Sci. 1990;96:107–14.

52. Satoh T, Endo M, Nakafuku M, Nakamura S, Kaziro Y. Platelet-derived growth factor stimulates formation of active p21^{ras}. GTP complex in Swiss mouse 3T3 cells. Proc Natl Acad Sci USA. 1990;87:5993–7.

53. Mulcahy LS, Smith MP, Stacey DW. Requirement for ras proto-oncogene function during serum stimulated growth of NIH-3T3 cells. Nature. 1985;313:241–3.

54. DeClue JE, Zhang K, Redford P, Vass WC, Lowy DR. Suppression of src transformation by overexpression of full-length GTPase-activating protein (GAP) or of the GAP C terminus. Mol Cell Biol. 1991;11:2819–25.

55. Molloy CJ, Bottaro DP, Fleming RP, Marshall MS, Gibbs JB, Aaronson SA. PDGF induction of tyrosine phosphorylation of GTPase activating protein. Nature. 1989;342: 711–14.

56. Egan SE, Giddings BW, Brooks MW, Buday L, Sizeland AM, Weinberg RA. Association of Sos Ras exchange protein with Grb2 is implicated in tyrosine kinase signal transduction and transformation. Nature. 1993;363:45–92.

57. Auger KR, Cantley LC. Novel phosphoinositides in cell growth and activation. Cancer Cells. 1991;3:263–70.

58. Nakanishi H, Brewer KA, Exton JH. Activation of the ζ isoenzyme of protein kinase C by phosphatidylinositol 3,4,5-trisphosphate. J Biol Chem. 1993;268:13–16.
59. Berra E, Diaz-Meco MT, Dominguez I et al. Protein kinase C ζ isoform is critical for mitogenic signal transduction. Cell. 1993;74:555–63.
60. Valius M, Kazlauskas A. Phospholipase C-γ1 and phosphatidylinositol 3 kinase are the downstream mediators of the PDGF receptor's mitogenic signal. Cell. 1993;73:321–34.
61. Kazlauskas A, Feng G-F, Pawson T, Valius M. The 64 kD protein that associates with the PDGF receptor β subunit via tyrosine 1009 is the SH2-containing phosphotyrosine phosphatase Syp/SH-PTP2/PTP 1D. Proc Natl Acad Sci USA. 1993 (In press).
62. Kolch W, Keidecher G, Lloyd P, Rapp U. Raf-1 protein kinase is required for growth of NIH/3T3 cells induced by serum, TPA, and ras oncogenes. Nature. 1991;349:426–8.
63. Stanton VP, Nichols DW, Laudano AP, Cooper GM. Definition of the human raf amino terminal regulatory region by deletion mutagenesis. Mol Cell Biol. 1989;9:639–47.
64. Morrison DK, Kaplan DR, Escobedo JA, Rapp UR, Roberts TM, Williams LT. Direct activation of the serine/threonine kinase activity of Raf-1 through tyrosine phosphorylation of the PDGFβ-receptor. Cell. 1989;58:649–57.
65. Morrison DK, Kaplan DR, Rapp UR, Roberts TM. Signal transduction from membrane to cytoplasm: growth factors and membrane-bound oncogene products increase raf-1 phosphorylation and associated protein kinase activity. Proc Natl Acad Sci USA. 1988;85:8855–9.
66. Heidaran MA, Beeler JF, Yu J-C et al. Differences in substrate specificities of a and b platelet-derived growth factor (PDGF) receptors. J Biol Chem. 1993;268:9287–95.
67. Kondo T, Konishi F, Inui H, Inagami T. Differing signal transductions elicited by three isoforms of platelet-derived growth factor in vascular smooth muscle cells. J Biol Chem. 1993;268:4458–64.
68. Mellstrom K, Heldin CH, Westermark B. Induction of circular membrane ruffling on human fibroblasts by platelet-derived growth factor. Exp Cell Res. 1988;177:347–59.
69. Williams LT, Antoniades HN, Goetzl EJ. Platelet-derived growth factor stimulates mouse 3T3 cell mitogenesis and leukocyte chemotaxis through different structural determinants. J Clin Invest. 1983;72:1759–63.
70. Seppa H, Grotendorst G, Seppa S et al. Platelet-derived growth factor is chemotactic for fibroblasts. J Cell Biol. 1982;92:584–8.
71. Grotendorst GF, Chang T, Seppa HEJ et al. Platelet-derived growth factor is a chemoattractant for vascular smooth muscle cells. J Cell Physiol. 1982;113:261–6.
72. Barnes JL, Hevey KA. Glomerular mesangial migration in response to platelet-derived growth factor. Lab Invest. 1990;62:379–82.
73. Amento EP, Ehsani N, Plamer H et al. Cytokines and growth factors positively and negatively regulate interstitial collagen gene expression in human vascular smooth muscle cells. Arterioscler Thromb. 1991;11:1223–30.
74. Schonherr E, Jarvelainen HT, Sandell LJ et al. Effects of platelet-derived growth factor and transforming growth factor-beta 1 on the synthesis of a large versican-like chondroitin sulfate proteoglycan by arterial smooth muscle cells. J Biol Chem. 1991;266:17640–7.
75. Berk BC, Alexander RW, Brock TA et al. Vasoconstriction: a new activity for platelet-derived growth factor. Science. 1986;232:87–90.
76. Holmgren L, Glaser A, Pfeifer-Ohlsson S et al. Angiogenesis during human extraembryonic development involves the spatiotemporal control of PDGF ligand and receptor gene expression. Development. 1991;113:749–754.
77. Sasahara M, Fried JW, Raines W et al. PDGF B-chain in neurons of the central nervous system, posterior pituitary, and in a transgenic model. Cell. 1991;64:217–27.
78. Yeh HJ, Ruit KG, Wang YX et al. PDGF A-chain gene is expressed by mammalian neurons during development and maturity. Cell. 1991;64:209–16.
79. Pierce GF, Vande-Berg J, Rudolf R et al. Platelet-derived growth factor-BB and transforming growth factor beta 1 selectively modulate glycosaminoglycans, collagen, and myofibroblasts in excisional wounds. Am J Pathol. 1991;138:639–46.
80. Clarke MF, Westin E, Schmidt D et al. Transformation of NIH 393 cells by a human c-sis cDNA gene. Nature. 1984;308:464–7.
81. Beckmann MP, Betsholtz C, Heldi CH et al. Comparison of biological properties and transforming potential of human PDGF-A and PDGF-B chains. Science. 1988;241:1346–9.

82. Heldin C-H, Westermark B. Growth factors as transforming proteins. Eur J Biochem. 1989;184:487–96.
83. Hermanson M, Funa K, Hartman M et al. Platelet-derived growth factor and its receptors in human glioma tissue: experiments of messenger RNA and protein suggest the presence of autocrine and paracrine loop. Cancer Res. 1992;52:3213–19.
84. Forsberg K, Valyi-Nagi I, Heldin C-H, Herlyn M, Westermark B. Platelet-derived growth factor (PDGF) in oncogenesis: development of a vascular connective tissue stroma in xenotransplanted human melanoma producing PDGF-BB. Proc Natl Acad Sci USA. 1993;90:393–7.
85. Ross R. The pathogenesis of atherosclerosis: a perspective for the 1990s. Nature. 1993;362:801–9.
86. Ferns GAS, Raines EW, Sprugel KH et al. Inhibition of neointimal smooth muscle accumulation after angioplasty by an antibody to PDGF. Science. 1991;253:1129–32.
87. Silver BJ, Jaffer FE, Abboud HE. Platelet-derived growth factor (PDGF) synthesis in mesangial cells: induction by multiple peptide mitogens. Proc Natl Acad Sci USA. 1989;86:1056–60.
88. Schultz PJ, DeCorleto PE, Silver BJ, Abboud HE. Mesangial cells express PDGF mRNAs and proliferate in response to PDGF. Am J Physiol. 1988;255:F674–F684.
89. Abboud HE. Growth factors in glomerulonephritis. Kidney Int. 1993;43:252–7.
90. Friedman SL, Arthur MJP. Activation of cultured rat hepatic lipocytes by Kupffer cell conditioned medium. J Clin Invest. 1989;84:1780–5.
91. Pinzani M, Gesualdo L, Sabbah GM, Abboud HE. Effects of platelet-derived growth factor and other polypeptide mitogens on DNA synthesis and growth of cultured rat liver fat-storing cells. J Clin Invest. 1989;84:1786–93.
92. Pinzani M, Knauss TC, Pierce GF et al. Mitogenic signals for platelet-derived growth factor isoforms in liver fat-storing cells. Am J Physiol. 1991;260:C485–91.
93. Heldin P, Pertoft H, Nordlinder H, Heldin C-H, Laurent T. Differential expression of platelet-derived growth factor α- and β-receptors on fat-storing cells and endothelial cells of rat liver. Exp Cell Res. 1991;193:364–9.
94. Davis BH, Rapp UR, Davidson NO. Retinoic acid and transforming growth factor β differentially inhibit platelet-derived-growth-factor-induced Ito-cell activation. Biochem J. 1991;278:43–7.
95. Pinzani M, Gentilini P, Abboud HE. Phenotypical modulation of liver fat-storing cells by retinoids. Influence on unstimulated and growth factor-induced cell proliferation. J Hepatol. 1992;14:211–20.
96. Davis BH, Coll D, Beno DWA. Retinoic acid suppresses PDGF-induced activation of human Ito cell-like myofibroblasts independent of FOS/EGR expression. Hepatology. 1992;16:96A.
97. Pinzani M, Abboud HE, Aron DC. Secretion of insulin-like growth factor-I and binding proteins by rat liver fat-storing cells: regulatory role of platelet-derived growth factor. Endocrinology. 1990;127:2343–9.
98. Friedman SL, Wei S, Blaner WS. Retinol release by activated rat hepatic lipocytes: regulation by Kupffer cell-conditioned medium and PDGF. Am J Physiol. 1993;264: G947–52.
99. Pinzani M, Abboud HE, Gesualdo L, Abboud SL. Regulation of macrophage colony-stimulating factor in liver fat storing cells by peptide growth factors. Am J Physiol. 1992;262(Cell Physiol 31):C876–81.
100. Bachem MG, Melchior R, Gressner AM. The role of thrombocytes in liver fibrogenesis: effects of platelet lysate and thrombocyte-derived growth factors on the mitogenic activity and glycosaminoglycan synthesis of cultured rat liver fat-storing cells. J Clin Chem Clin Biochem. 1989;27:555–65.
101. Marra F, Valente AJ, Pinzani M, Abboud HE. Cultured human liver fat-storing cells produce monocyte chemotactic protein-1. Regulation by proinflammatory cytokines. J Clin Invest. 1993;92:1674–80.
102. Pinzani M, Weber FL, Gesualdo L, Abboud HE. Expression of platelet-derived growth factor in an in vivo model of acute liver inflammation. Hepatology. 1990;12:920.

17
Inflammatory mediators and fat-storing cell proliferation

M. PINZANI with the collaboration of **F. MARRA, V. CARLONI, A. GENTILINI, R. DE FRANCO, A. CALIGIURI** and **C. SALI**

INTRODUCTION

Studies performed in the past five years have greatly contributed towards clarifying the molecular and cellular events that occur during the progression of liver fibrogenesis. In particular, recent developments in cytokine/polypeptide growth factor research and in the biology of liver non-parenchymal cells have opened new perspectives in this important field of liver pathophysiology. This chapter will outline the biological events that possibly contribute to fat-storing cell (FSC) activation and proliferation and, in particular, will focus on the possible relationships between this cell type, other liver non-parenchymal cells and cells of the inflammatory infiltrate, with particular regard to cytokines, polypeptide growth factors and other soluble mediators.

FAT-STORING CELL ACTIVATION

In conditions of chronic liver damage, FSC undergo a process of activation and phenotypical modulation from the quiescent 'storing' phenotype to the highly proliferative 'myofibroblast-like' phenotype. This transition is gradual and occurs through an intermediate stage defined as 'transitional cell'. A gradual loss of intracellular vitamin A droplets, a significant increase in myofilaments and dense bodies and a general activation of the synthetic properties of the cell are the main features of this transformation. The concept of such a continuum is supported by studies *in vivo* documenting a shift in predominance from FSC to transitional cells following liver injury[1], although it is still unclear whether further activation of transitional cells results in myofibroblast-like cells *in vivo*[2]. Even though *in vitro* studies, utilizing FSC isolated from rat, mouse or human liver, tend to corroborate the concept of a gradual transition to myofibroblast-like cells, the contribution of 'genuine' myofibroblasts or fibroblasts to the fibrogenic process is likely, particularly

Table 1 FSC activation

	Reversible (?)	Irreversible (?)
Cause	Disruption of the normal ECM pattern	Reiterative tissue damage
	Products from hepatocellular damage and necrosis	Loss of retinoids
		TGF-β_1 autocrine loop (?)
	Activation of Kupffer and SEC	PDGF-AA autocrine loop (??)
Effect	Increased expression of PDGF receptors	From 'transitional' to 'myofibroblast-like'
	Proliferation	More proliferative
	Increased production of ECM	Collagen 1 > III > IV
	Contribute to liver regeneration (HGF)	Proinflammatory role (PAF, MCP-1, M-CSF)
	Collagen degradation and remodelling	(Impaired ability to degrade collagen)
		HGF gene down-regulation

in selected areas such as the fibrous septa and around the central vein[3]. It is possible that the same factors determining FSC activation also cause the activation of these other extracellular matrix-producing cell types.

Table 1 summarizes the possible causes and effects of FSC activation. A first important distinction should be made concerning the extent and persistence of liver tissue injury. Indeed, following a single, time-limited liver tissue injury (e.g. single administration of CCl_4 in rats, uncomplicated acute viral hepatitis in humans) the activation of FSC and other liver non-parenchymal cells is likely to play an important role in the tissue repair process. This activation is time-limited and implies proliferation of FSC[4,5] following a rather complex interplay with extracellular matrix (ECM) components, cytokines, growth factors and other soluble factors. At this stage chemotaxis and proliferation of FSC and other ECM-producing cell types towards areas of hepatocyte degeneration and necrosis may represent a key event in the restoration of an ECM network, indispensable for correct tissue repair and, possibly, in providing soluble factors (e.g. hepatocyte growth factor, HGF) necessary for hepatocyte regeneration. Restoration of the normal tissue characteristics is *per se* sufficient to determine the reversibility of this process. On the contrary, in chronic liver diseases, the presence of reiterative tissue damage is likely to represent the major cause leading to a complete phenotypical modulation of FSC towards the myofibroblast-like phenotype. Indeed, the persistence of tissue damage is associated with a chronic inflammatory infiltrate and, consequently, with the presence of high levels of factors modulating the activation and proliferation of mesenchymal cells. In addition, it is possible that these cells acquire the capability of synthesizing and releasing growth factors and cytokines that further contribute to the self-perpetuation of this process through autocrine or paracrine loops. Accordingly, the role of activated FSC and other mesenchymal cells becomes predominant with abundant deposition of fibrillar ECM. In other words, the prolonged activation of tissue repair mechanisms may result in destructive tissue remodelling rather than in effective tissue repair.

CYTOKINES, GROWTH FACTORS AND OTHER MEDIATORS INVOLVED IN FSC ACTIVATION/PROLIFERATION

In conditions of chronic liver damage, and particularly those due to chronic hepatitis virus infection, the inflammatory infiltrate consists of a rather complex association of cells involved in the development of hepatocellular damage (i.e. cells of the immune system) with cells actively participating in the tissue repair process (i.e. platelets, mononuclear cells). This distinction implies that clusters of soluble factors, specifically directed at different cellular targets, are contemporaneously present in the tissue. In addition, resident liver cells, including damaged hepatocytes, may contribute to the release of these factors. Before proceeding further it is important to make a few points. First, it is probable that none of these factors works alone. Second, it is conceivable that a complex network of interactions occurs between these mediators and their targets: the release of one molecule can lead to expression of a second molecule in a target cell that can stimulate either its neighbours in a paracrine way, or itself in an autocrine way.

Growth factors, cytokines and other factors involved in FSC activation/ proliferation are summarized in Fig. 1 together with their potential cellular sources. Studies performed on isolated FSC cultured on plastic, an experimental model that reproduces the activation process *in vitro*, have indicated that all these factors, taken singularly or in combination, have some effect on FSC proliferation, chemotaxis and/or ECM deposition. Cytokines such as interleukin-1 (IL-1), tumour necrosis factor-α (TNF-α), and interferons (IFN), involved in the cross-talk between cells of the immune system, seem to play a negative modulatory role on FSC activation. Both IL-1α and TNF-α, at rather high doses, are weak growth promoters for FSC[6], especially when compared to other mitogens such as platelet-derived growth factor (PDGF) and basic fibroblast growth factor (bFGF)[7]. Moreover, IFN-γ has recently been shown to inhibit FSC proliferation as well as the expression of α-smooth muscle actin, a potential marker for FSC activation[8]. Other possible effects of these inflammatory cytokines could be directed to the modulation of ECM deposition by FSC. Indeed, IL-1α and TNF-α induce a dose-dependent reduction of the synthesis of collagenous and non-collagenous ECM components by FSC[6]. In addition, similar to what was recently reported in human fibroblasts[9], both TNF-α and IFN-γ could be capable of suppressing the activation of type I collagen gene expression induced by transforming growth factor-β_1 (TGF-β).

Several studies performed in the past 5 years have indicated that two polypeptide growth factors, namely PDGF and TGF-β, greatly contribute to the profibrogenic role of FSC. The elements leading to this assumption, and the possible interactions between these two factors, will be outlined in the following sections.

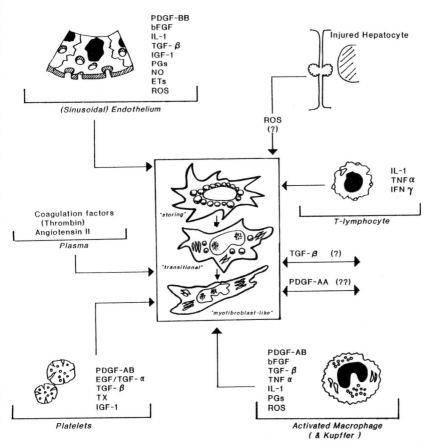

Fig. 1 Growth factors, cytokines and other factors involved in fat-storing cell (FSC) activation/proliferation and their potential sources during acute or chronic liver tissue damage

Platelet-derived growth factor

PDGF, a very potent mitogen for mesenchymal cells, consists of two polypeptide chains, referred to as A- and B-chain, which can form three possible dimeric forms: AA, AB, and BB[10]. The two PDGF receptor subunits (α or type A, and β or type B) differ in their ability to bind different PDGF isoforms[11,12]. Thus, the B-chain of PDGF can bind both α and β subunits, whereas the A-chain can bind only α subunits. Dimerization of the receptor then results in the autophosphorylation and acquisition of the ability to phosphorylate other proteins regulating different intracellular signalling pathways[13]. Although the major determinant in each isoform specificity seems to be the relative number of α and/or β receptors present on the cell surface, recent studies have shown some functional diversities following the activation of the two different receptor subunits[14]. Briefly, the activation of both subunits leads to intracellular signalling pathways stimulating

225

mitogenesis. However, the α receptor seems to have a unique binding site for PDGF-BB to whom PDGF-AA does not bind or binds with very low affinity. Blockade of this site greatly induces the chemotactic response to PDGF-BB. Consequently, the response of cells having both α and β receptors (i.e. fibroblast, smooth muscle cells, and pericytes in general) would be dependent on the isoform of PDGF present: PDGF-AA induces growth, whereas PDGF-AB and -BB induce both growth and chemotaxis. According to a current hypothesis[14], the conclusion of this complex arrangement is the migration of ECM-producing cells into the area of tissue damage due to the action of PDGF-BB or -AB released by platelets and other infiltrating or resident cells. Subsequently, the up-regulation of the α receptor and the PDGF-A chain in the target cells would start an autocrine loop of PDGF-AA, thus maintaining proliferation and reducing chemotaxis.

PDGF, PDGF receptors and FSC growth

Among other polypeptide growth factors potentially involved in chronic tissue inflammation, PDGF is the most potent mitogen for cultured FSC isolated from rat and mouse liver[7,15]. The effects of PDGF, in terms of DNA synthesis and cell proliferation, far exceed those of other polypeptide growth factors in this cell type. The relative mitogenic potential of recombinant PDGF dimeric forms AA, AB and BB on early-passaged rat FSC was evaluated in further studies[16]. All isoforms were able to induce mitogenesis as well as the activation of early signal transduction pathways such as phosphoinositide turnover and intracellular calcium release. However, PDGF-AA was much less potent than PDGF-BB or -AB, indicating a predominant expression of PDGF-receptor β subunits, as also suggested by binding studies[17]. More recently, we have confirmed in cultured human FSC that the expression of the PDGF-β receptor subunit exceeds that of the α subunit (roughly 3:1). Then, similar to what was observed in rat FSC, the mitogenic effect of PDGF-AA is about 30% of that induced by PDGF-BB.

An important element in the process of FSC activation is the expression of growth factor-specific membrane receptors and particularly PDGF receptors (see Table 1). Although PDGF is a key mitogen for FSC in culture, it is likely that *in vivo* the expression of PDGF receptors in this cell type is very low. The still limited experimental evidence suggests that isolated FSC acquire the ability to respond to PDGF by a *de novo* expression of PDGF receptors[18]. In the culture system the enhanced expression of PDGF receptors is probably part of the spontaneous response to the plastic culture substratum[19].

Since other mesenchymal cells potentially related to FSC (i.e. smooth muscle cells, type 1 astrocytes, and glomerular mesangial cells) have been shown to secrete a PDGF-like protein and to stimulate their own growth in an autocrine manner, the possibility that FSC themselves could secrete PDGF isoforms is an additional issue in the relationship between PDGF and FSC. Evidence derived from our studies indicates that cultured rat FSC constitutively express both the PDGF-A and -B chain gene at a very low level of abundance, and do not secrete detectable amounts of PDGF-like activity[16]. However, preliminary results, obtained by Marra and co-workers[20], indicate that cultured human FSC might express the genes encoding for both PDGF-A and -B chain at a higher level of abundance. In particular, Northern blot analysis of poly(A)+ RNA from human FSC hybridized with a cDNA encoding for human PDGF-A chain demonstrated the presence of three transcripts of 2.7, 2.5, and 2.0 kb, respectively. In addition, stimulation of growth-arrested FSC with PMA or PDGF-BB induced a significant increase of PDGF-A chain mRNA levels. Similarly, basal PDGF-B chain mRNA levels, detected by RNase protection assay, were increased by stimulation with PMA and, to a lesser extent, with PDGF-BB. Therefore, the possibility of an autocrine stimulation of FSC growth by PDGF isoforms cannot be excluded.

PDGF and liver fibrosis

A pathogenic role for PDGF has been demonstrated in several fibrogenic disorders, including glomerulosclerosis, pulmonary fibrosis, and athero-sclerosis[21-23]. Evidence from our recent studies indicates that the PDGF-B chain gene expression, absent in normal liver, is markedly upregulated 48 h after a single oral administration of CCl_4, when maximal tissue necrosis and inflammatory infiltration are observed[24]. In addition, the distribution of PDGF protein, closely associated with inflammatory cells surrounding degenerating or necrotic hepatocytes, tends to confirm the role of this growth factor in the tissue repair process. Interestingly, maximal expression of the PDGF-receptor β subunit, localized in mesenchymal cells with perisinusoidal location (most likely FSC), is observed 24 h after CCl_4. At this stage only a certain degree of hepatocellular swelling and a small number of acidophilic bodies are observed. This observation indicates that factors other than tissue necrosis and/or inflammatory infiltration are responsible for the up-regulation of the PDGF-β receptor gene in target cells. It is tempting to speculate that products deriving from damaged hepatocellular membranes or activated Kupffer cells, possibly reactive oxygen species (ROS), may play a certain role in the activation of FSC and, ultimately, in the excessive deposition of ECM as recently reported by Parola and co-workers[25,26]. In addition, the expression of the PDGF-receptor β subunit gene and the correspondent receptor protein in FSC or analogous cell types may represent an early event aimed at preparing an adequate number of 'responsive' cells once the presence of PDGF isoforms in the injured tissue becomes maximal. Along these lines, PDGF seems to play a positive role in the process of tissue repair following acute liver injury by acting as a powerful chemotactic and mitogenic factor for resident or infiltrating mesenchymal cells able to reconstitute an ECM network.

This 'pro-healing' action of PDGF may, however, constitute a major problem in chronic liver diseases, where the presence of reiterative tissue damage associated with a persistent inflammatory state may cause a sustained release of PDGF. In this context the prolonged effects of this growth factor on FSC may contribute to the development of tissue fibrosis rather than to effective tissue repair. Along these lines we have recently evaluated the expression of PDGF and its α and β receptor subunits in surgical specimens obtained from normal liver and from explanted livers of patients undergoing liver transplantation for hepatitis B virus-related liver cirrhosis. In normal human liver, immunoreactivity specific for PDGF-BB is limited to the endothelial layer of blood vessels within the portal tract, whereas no immunoreactivity for PDGF-AA is observed. In cirrhotic liver a marked immunoreactivity for both PDGF isoforms is present along the surface of hepatic sinusoids, around groups or single hepatocytes undergoing acidophilic degeneration and necrosis, and in groups of infiltrating inflammatory cells. These aspects tend to be more pronounced at the edges of fibrous septa. Expression of PDGF α and β receptor subunits was evaluated by *in situ* hybridization and immunohistochemistry. In normal liver, mRNA transcripts, as well as specific immunoreactivity for both subunits, is found over few mesenchymal cells located in portal tract stroma and around large blood vessels. In cirrhotic liver the presence of mRNA transcripts specific for PDGF α and β receptor appears markedly increased and is concentrated in fibrous septa and in perisinusoidal mesenchymal cells adjacent to degenerating or necrotic hepatocytes. The immunoreactivity specific for both subunits is distributed with a similar pattern, although the reaction for the α subunit seems less intense within the fibrous septa. These results, although preliminary, indicate that, in cirrhotic liver, PDGF is co-distributed with mesenchymal cells showing an up-regulation of PDGF-receptor gene expression, and tend to confirm a functional role of this growth factor in the development of liver fibrosis.

Transforming growth factor-β

TGF-β is considered a fundamental regulatory molecule, acting through both autocrine and paracrine mechanisms. As a growth factor, TGF-β is multifunctional since it can either stimulate or inhibit cellular proliferation and/or differentiation. Many different cell types synthesize TGF-β and essentially all have specific high-affinity receptors for this peptide. TGF-β is released in large amounts by platelet and other inflammatory cells. Importantly, TGF-β is produced as an inactive precursor protein which is converted to the mature form by protease cleavage and, *in vitro*, by means of a simple acid treatment. Plasmin has been suggested as one of the proteases that activates TGF-β physiologically. In addition, the activity of TGF-β can be inhibited by the remnant of the precursor protein and by tissue proteoglycans (i.e biglycan and decorin), presumably by competing with the receptor for the binding of TGF-β[27].

One of the most evident effects of TGF-β on fibroblast, myofibroblasts and pericytes in general is the increased synthesis and deposition of collagenous and non-collagenous ECM proteins[28]. In addition, TGF-β is capable of retarding the degradation of such components[29]. Accordingly, TGF-β is considered a key factor in the tissue repair process and in the development of fibrogenic disorders. In the liver, in addition to being a potent inhibitor of hepatocyte growth[30], TGF-β is clearly associated with hepatic fibrosis. Indeed, a positive correlation between TGF-β mRNA expression and mRNAs encoding for one or more procollagens has been reported in different models of liver fibrosis and in patients with chronic liver disease[31–34].

Because of the important role of FSC in the synthesis of ECM components, several studies have evaluated the possible interactions between this cell type and TGF-β. TGF-β does not seem to be, *per se*, a mitogen for FSC but rather a growth inhibitor[6,35]. As expected, TGF-β was found to stimulate procollagen synthesis and release in cultured rat FSC[36–38]. Moreover, cultured FSC have been shown to express TGF-β mRNA and to secrete the corresponding polypeptide[38,39]. Recently, we have confirmed that in FSC isolated from human liver, TGF-β is able to up-regulate its own mRNA and the mRNAs encoding for procollagens I and III, and fibronectin[40]. These observations suggest that TGF-β may act on FSC through an autocrine loop.

TGF-β/PDGF interactions

From the evidence so far presented, it appears that TGF-β exerts direct effects on the excessive deposition of ECM by FSC, whereas PDGF plays an indirect role by promoting FSC proliferation. Interestingly, in our early studies performed in rat FSC, we showed that TGF-β is able to enhance the mitogenic effect of PDGF[7]. Indeed, evidence coming from studies performed in cell types showing morphological and functional similarities with FSC, suggests that TGF-β may affect cell proliferation by modulating the expression of PDGF receptor subunits. We recently tested this hypothesis in cultured human FSC and we observed that TGF-β induces a significant increase of the mitogenic effect of PDGF-BB, whereas the mitogenicity of PDGF-AA and -AB is not affected, thus suggesting a selective effect only on the PDGF-β receptor subunit. This hypothesis was confirmed by regulation experiments showing selective and time-dependent up-regulation of the mRNA encoding for the PDGF-β receptor subunit and the relative protein induced by TGF-β in human FSC. In addition, binding studies demonstrated a parallel increase of PDGF-BB binding sites after incubation with TGF-β. These findings indicate that TGF-β, possibly through an autocrine stimulation of FSC, may contribute to maintain a permanent up-regulation of PDGF-receptor β subunits. Consequently, this effect may contribute to an 'irreversible' transformation towards a progressively more proliferative phenotype.

INTERACTIONS BETWEEN FSC AND INFLAMMATORY CELLS

Infiltration of the portal tract and the hepatic lobule by mononuclear cells is one of the prominent features of chronic, self-perpetuating inflammation of the liver tissue. Recruitment of phagocytes in response to infection or tissue damage occurs through generation of chemotactic gradients that attracts cells to the site of injury. In order to establish the possible role of FSC in this process we have studied whether or not this cell type, once activated, is involved in the production of two important chemotactic mediators, namely monocyte chemotactic peptide-1 (MCP-1) and platelet activating factor (PAF).

MCP-1 is a 76 amino acid monomeric peptide exerting chemoattractant activity for monocytes but not for neutrophils or lymphocytes, which lack MCP-1 receptors[41]. Unstimulated human FSC secrete MCP-1 and express mRNA which encodes for this cytokine. Stimulation with IL-1α, IFN-γ and, to a lesser extent, with TNF-α, induces an increase of MCP-1 mRNA levels as well as of the amount of protein secreted[42]. Importantly, in a parallel study, we observed that MCP-1 mRNA expression is significantly more abundant in liver tissue obtained from patients with chronic active hepatitis than in normal liver tissue.

PAF, a fluid-phase and cell-associated mediator of inflammation, is a potent ether phospholipid implicated in the pathophysiology of several diseases[43]. In the inflammatory process, PAF plays a major role in the adhesion of neutrophils and other inflammatory cells to activated endothelial cells. Upon activation, endothelial cells synthesize PAF, and predominantly its 1-O-acyl analogue, which remains largely cell-associated[44]. Because of their possible role as liver-specific pericytes[45], we have lately evaluated the biosynthesis of PAF by cultured human FSC[46]. Stimulation with the calcium ionophore A23187, as well as with physiological stimuli such as thrombin and lipopolysaccharide (LPS), induced a significant increase of basal PAF synthesis evaluated by measuring [³H]acetate incorporation. Further analysis revealed that over 50% of the newly synthesized PAF species was secreted, whereas the remaining fraction remained cell-associated, with slight differences between the three stimuli. Gas chromatography/mass spectrometry analysis showed that, analogous to what was observed in endothelial cells, a large percentage (74%) of PAF-like lipids synthesized by FSC consisted of 1-O-acyl PAF. As illustrated in Fig. 2, FSC, by releasing PAF species in the subendothelial space, may facilitate the migration of inflammatory cells following their adhesion to sinusoidal endothelial cells. In summary, these findings raise the possibility of an integrated pericyte–endothelium production of PAF species with key functions in the amplification of proinflammatory mechanisms.

Mononuclear cells, once they have completed their migration into the injured tissue through chemotactic gradients, require the continuous availability of highly specific factors that promote their differentiation and long-term survival. Particularly, macrophage-colony stimulating factor (M-CSF, or CSF-1), a glycosylated disulphide-linked dimer with a molecular weight of approximately 70 kDa, is a lineage-specific haematopoietic growth factor that selectively promotes mononuclear phagocyte activities. Interestingly, the expression of M-CSF is markedly increased in experimental liver fibrosis as well as in human liver disease[47,48]. Our studies confirmed that cultured FSC constitutively express M-CSF mRNA, and indicated that PDGF and

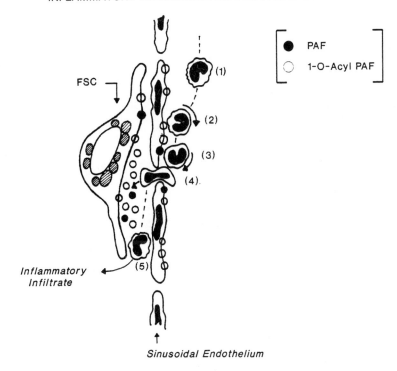

Fig. 2 Integrated pericyte/endothelium production of platelet-activating factor (PAF). Upon stimulation, PAF species produced by endothelial cells remain mainly cell associated, thus acting as adhesion molecules for circulating inflammatory cells (steps 1–4). The production and release of PAF species by FSC, acting as liver-specific pericytes, may create a chemotactic gradient facilitating the migration of inflammatory cell in the subendothelial space (step 5)

bFGF regulate the steady-state expression of M-CSF and the secretion of the encoded protein[15]. Taken into consideration together with our recent findings concerning MCP-1 production by FSC, it is possible to speculate that this cell type, upon stimulation by different subsets of cytokines and growth factors, may provide a complete range of factors facilitating migration and activity of mononuclear cells within the injured tissue (Fig. 3).

CONCLUSIONS

The pathogenesis of liver fibrosis is closely associated with the ubiquitous protective mechanisms involved in inflammation and repair. Once they become excessive and prolonged, the intended protection becomes a disease entity in itself by inducing a chronic fibroproliferative response. The optimization of the inflammatory response may represent, together with the development of antifibrotic drugs, an important approach towards treatment and prevention of this disease.

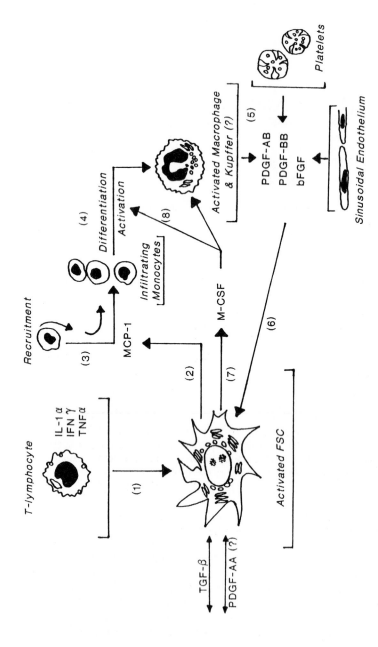

Fig. 3 Cytokines released from cells of the immune system (1) increase the expression and release of MCP-1 by activated FSC (2). MCP-1 contributes to the recruitment of circulating monocytes in the injured tissue (3). Following their activation and differentiation (4), mononuclear cells secrete growth factors involved in the tissue repair process (5). These, in turn, increase the expression and release of M-CSF[6,7]. Then M-CSF induces differentiation of monocytes in macrophages and promotes their long-term survival (8)

Acknowledgements

We would like to thank Professors Paolo Gentilini and Giacomo Laffi for their continuous support and thoughtful advice, and Professor Stefano Milani and Dr Alessandro Casini, together with their co-workers, for sharing with us the everyday delights and sorrows of doing research.

References

1. Mak KM, Lieber CS. Lipocytes and transitional cells in alcoholic liver disease: a morphometric study. Hepatology. 1988;8:1027–33.
2. Maher JJ. Fat-storing cells and myofibroblasts: one cell or two? Hepatology. 1989;6: 903–4.
3. Bhunchet E, Wake K. Role of mesenchymal cell populations in porcine serum-induced rat liver fibrosis. Hepatology. 1992;16:1452–73.
4. Burt AD, Robertson JL, Heir J et al. Desmin-containing stellate cells in rat liver; distribution in normal animals and response to experimental acute liver injury. J Pathol. 1986;150: 29–35.
5. Tanaka Y, Mak KM, Lieber CS. Immunohistochemical detection of proliferating lipocytes in regenerating rat liver. J Pathol. 1990;160:129–34.
6. Matsuoka M, Pham N-T, Tsukamoto H. Differential effects of interleukin-1α, tumor necrosis factor α, and transforming growth factor β1 on cell proliferation and collagen formation by cultured fat-storing cells. Liver. 1989;9:71–8.
7. Pinzani M, Gesualdo L, Sabbah GM et al. Effects of platelet-derived growth factor and other polypeptide mitogens on DNA synthesis and growth in cultured rat liver fat-storing cells. J Clin Invest. 1989;94:1786–93.
8. Rochey DC, Maher JJ, Jarnagin WR et al. Inhibition of rat hepatic lipocytes activation by interferon-gamma. Hepatology. 1992;16:776–84.
9. Kahari V-M, Chen YQ, Su MW et al. Tumor necrosis factor-α and interferon-gamma suppress the activation of human type I collagen gene expression by transforming growth factor-β1. J Clin Invest. 1990;86:1489–95.
10. Ross R. Platelet-derived growth factor. Lancet. 1989;i:1179–82.
11. Claesson-Welsh L, Eriksson A, Westermark B et al. cDNA cloning and expression of the human A-type platelet-derived growth factor (PDGF) establishes structural similarity to the B-type PDGF receptor. Proc Natl Acad Sci USA. 1989;86:4917–21.
12. Hart CE, Forstrom JW, Kelly JD et al. Two classes of PDGF receptor recognize different isoforms of PDGF. Science. 1988;240:1529–31.
13. Cadena DL, Gill GN. Receptor tyrosine kinases. FASEB J. 1992;6:2332–7.
14. Vassbotn FS, Ostman A, Siegbahn A et al. Neomycin is a platelet-derived growth factor (PDGF) antagonist that allows discrimination of PDGF α and β receptor signals in cells expressing both receptor types. J Biol Chem. 1992;268:15635–41.
15. Pinzani M, Abboud H, Gesualdo L et al. Regulation of macrophage colony-stimulating factor in liver fat-storing cells by peptide growth factors. Am J Physiol-Cell Physiol. 1992;262:C876–81.
16. Pinzani M, Knauss TC, Pierce GF et al. Mitogenic signals for platelet-derived growth factor isoforms in liver fat-storing cells. Am J Physiol–Cell Physiol. 1991;29:C485–91.
17. Heldin P, Pertoft H, Nordliner H et al. Differential expression of platelet-derived growth factor α- and β-receptors on fat-storing cells and endothelial cells of rat liver. Exp Cell Res. 1991;193:364–9.
18. Friedman SL, Arthur MJP. Activation of cultured rat hepatic lipocytes by Kupffer cell conditioned medium. Direct enhancement of matrix synthesis and stimulation of cell proliferation via induction of platelet-derived growth factor receptors. J Clin Invest. 1989;84:1780–5.
19. Friedman SL, Roll FJ, Arenson DM et al. Maintenance of differentiated phenotype of cultured rat hepatic lipocytes by basement membrane matrix. J Biol Chem. 1989;264: 10756–62.

20. Marra F, Bhandary B, Pinzani M et al. Regulation of PDGF-A and B-chain gene expression in cultured human liver fat-storing cells (Manuscript in preparation).
21. Gesualdo L, Pinzani M, Floriano JJ et al. Platelet-derived growth factor expression in mesangial proliferative glomerulonephritis. Lab Invest. 1991;65:160–7.
22. Nagaoka I, Trapnell BC, Crystal RG. Upregulation of platelet-derived growth factor-A and -B gene expression in alveolar macrophages of individuals with idiopathic pulmonary fibrosis. J Clin Invest. 1990;85:2023–7.
23. Ross R. The pathogenesis of atheroscerlosis: a perspective for the 1990s. Nature. 1993;362:801–9.
24. Pinzani M, Milani S, Grappone C et al. Expression of platelet-derived growth factor in an in vivo model of acute liver injury. (manuscript submitted).
25. Parola M, Leonarduzzi G, Biasi F et al. Vitamin E dietary supplementation protects against tetrachloride-induced chronic liver damage and cirrhosis. Hepatology. 1992;16:1014–21.
26. Parola M, Muraca R, Dianzani I et al. Vitamin E dietary supplementation inhibits transforming growth factor-β1 gene expression in the rat liver. FEBS Lett. 1992;308:267–70.
27. Border WA, Ruoslahti E. Transforming growth factor-β in disease: the dark side of tissue repair. J Clin Invest. 1992;90:1–7.
28. Raghow R, Postlethwaite AE, Keski-Oja J et al. Transforming growth factor-β increases the steady state levels of type I procollagen and fibronectin mRNAs posttranscriptionally in cultured human dermal fibroblasts. J Clin Invest. 1987;79:1285–8.
29. Edwards DR, Murphy G, Reynolds JJ et al. Transforming growth factor-β modulates the expression of collagenase and metalloproteinase inhibitor. EMBO J. 1987;6:1899–904.
30. Braun L, Mead JE, Panzica M et al. Transforming growth factor-β mRNA increases during liver regeneration: a possible paracrine mechanism of growth regulation. Proc Natl Acad Sci USA. 1988;85:1539–43.
31. Czaja MJ, Weiner FR, Flanders KC et al. In vitro and in vivo association of transforming growth factor-β with hepatic fibrosis. J Cell Biol. 189;108:2477–82.
32. Armendariz-Borunda J, Seyer JM, Kang AH et al. Regulation of transforming growth factor-β expression in rat liver intoxicated with carbon tetrachloride. FASEB J. 1990;4:215–21.
33. Castilla A, Prieto J, Fausto N. Transforming growth factors-β_1 and α on chronic liver disease. N Engl J Med. 1991;324:933–40.
34. Milani S, Herbst H, Shuppan D et al. Transforming growth factors β1 and β2 are differentially expressed in fibrotic liver disease. Am J Pathol. 1991;139:1221–9.
35. Bachem MG, Riess U, Gressner AM. Liver fat-storing cells proliferation is stimulated by epidermal growth factor/transforming growth factor-α and inhibited by transforming growth factor-β. Biochem Biophys Res Commun. 1989;162:708–14.
36. Matsuoka M, Tsukamoto H. Stimulation of hepatic collagen production by Kupffer cell-derived transforming growth factor-β: implication for a pathogenic role in alcoholic liver fibrogenesis. Hepatology. 1990;11:599–605.
37. Maher JJ, McGuire RF. Extracellular matrix expression increases preferentially in rat lipocytes and sinusoidal endothelial cells during hepatic fibrosis in vivo. J Clin Invest. 1990;86:1641–8.
38. Weiner FR, Giambrone M-A, Czaja MJ et al. Ito-cell gene expression and collagen regulation. Hepatology. 1990;11:111–17.
39. Meyer DH, Bachem MG, Gressner AM. Transformed fat-storing cells inhibit the proliferation of hepatocytes by secretion of transforming growth factor-β. J Hepatol. 1990;11:86–91.
40. Casini A, Pinzani M, Milani S et al. Regulation of extracellular matrix synthesis by transforming growth factor-β1 in human fat-storing cells. Gastroenterology. 1993;105:245–53.
41. Yoshimura T, Leonard EJ. Identification of high affinity receptors for human monocyte chemoattractant protein-1 on human monocytes. J Immunol. 1990;145:292–7.
42. Marra F, Valente AJ, Pinzani M et al. Cultured human liver fat-storing cells produce monocyte chemotactic protein-1. Regulation by inflammatory cytokines. J Clin Invest. (In press).
43. Prescott SM, Zimmerman GA, McIntyre TM. Platelet activating factor. J Biol Chem. 1990;265:17381–4.

44. Zimmerman GA, McIntyre TM, Mehra M *et al.* Endothelial cell-associated platelet-activating factor: a novel mechanism for signaling intercellular adhesion. J Cell Biol. 1990;110:529–40.
45. Pinzani M, Failli P, Ruocco C *et al.* Fat-storing cells as liver specific pericytes. Spatial dynamics of agonist-stimulated intracellular calcium transients. J Clin Invest. 1992;90: 642–6.
46. Pinzani M, Carloni V, Marra F *et al.* Biosynthesis of platelet-activating factor and its 1-*O*-acyl analogue by cultured human liver fat-storing cells. (Manuscript submitted).
47. Shu-Ling L, Degli Esposti S, Bartocci A *et al.* Macrophage-colony stimulating factor (CSF-1) is produced by Ito cells in vitro and is elevated in an in vivo model of hepatic fibrosis. Hepatology. 1989;10:632 (abstract).
48. Degli Esposti S, Stanley ER, Zern MA. Macrophage-colony stimulating factor (CSF-1) content is markedly increased in human liver disease. Hepatology. 1990;12:908 (abstract).

18
Gene expression of cytokine receptors during lipocyte activation

S. L. FRIEDMAN, L. WONG and G. YAMASAKI

Activation and accumulation of lipocytes (Ito, stellate, fat-storing cells, vitamin A-storing cells) following liver injury are morphological hallmarks of ongoing hepatic fibrogenesis. Activation is characterized by prominent rough endoplasmic reticulum, reduced intracellular vitamin A content and increased pericellular collagen. A major mode of lipocyte accumulation is the local proliferation of activated cells[1]. Enhanced fibrogenesis has been ascribed to both an increased number of lipocytes, and increased extracellular matrix synthesis per cell.

We have focused on the potential activation of cultured lipocytes by hepatic macrophages (Kupffer cells) because tissue macrophage products in lung and other tissues are potent modulators of mesenchymal proliferation and matrix production.

Previous studies[2,3] suggest that platelet-derived growth factor (PDGF) is an important mitogen for lipocytes. PDGF exerts its effects by binding to specific cellular receptors. The receptor for PDGF is a 160 000–180 000 MW anionic glycosylated protein which can exist as $\alpha\alpha$, $\beta\beta$ or $\alpha\beta$ isoforms. In cultured lipocytes, expression of the β isoform predominates[4].

While PDGF is a major mitogen for lipocytes, transforming growth factor beta (TGF-β) appears to be the primary fibrogenic cytokine. In liver injury TGF-β mRNA expression is markedly increased in situ[5,6] and in extracts of whole liver[7]. Potential cellular sources of TGF-β in liver injury include platelets[8], Kupffer cells[9] and lipocytes[10]. Among the three TGF-β isoforms described to date, TGF-β_1 is most prominent in wound healing, both in liver and other sites[11]. A fibrogenic effect of TGF-β has been confirmed by culture studies in which exogenous TGF-β stimulates extracellular matrix synthesis by lipocytes[12,13].

In most cell types several TGF-β membrane receptor species (types I–V) are expressed. All the receptors characterized to date are proteoglycans, consisting of a core protein to which glycosaminoglycan side-chains are attached; signal transduction only requires the core proteins and not the side-chain[14]. Of the three major receptors only types I and II are signalling

236

molecules[15]. In contrast, the type III receptor, also known as betaglycan, is not signal-transducing and instead may act as a membrane sink for the ligand. Recently, the core proteins for the types I[16], II[17] and III[18,19] receptors have been cloned and sequenced; types I and II receptors contain kinase domains[16,17].

RESULTS

Effects of Kupffer-cell conditioned medium (KCM) on lipocyte morphology

Lipocytes exposed to KCM demonstrated marked nuclear enlargement, cytoplasmic spreading, and apparent loss of retinoid vesicles.

Effects of KCM on lipocyte DNA synthesis

DNA synthesis per cell increased strikingly in KCM-treated lipocytes in the presence of serum, as assessed by incorporation of [^{3}H]thymidine. This incorporation was inhibited 90–95% ($n = 4$, data not shown) by 10 mmol/l hydroxyurea, confirming that DNA synthesis was replicative. Enhanced DNA synthesis was accompanied by a progressive increase in cell number with increasing KCM exposure (not shown).

Mechanism of KCM-induced lipocyte proliferation

We directed our attention to PDGF as a potential mitogen because of evidence that it plays a role in fibrosis of the lung and kidney. Pre-incubation of serum-containing KCM with polyclonal antibody to PDGF blocked DNA synthesis 76–93% (not shown). Responsiveness to PDGF appeared to require activation by Kupffer cells. We examined whether KCM had induced responsiveness to PDGF via induction of receptors for this cytokine. To explore this possibility we performed immunoblot analysis of lipocyte extracts. Receptor for PDGF was not detectable in resting lipocytes in the presence of serum, but was clearly apparent within 24 h after treatment with KCM[2] (with or without serum). The cells displayed both mature and precursor forms of the receptor.

By RNAase protection, induction of receptor protein was preceded and accompanied by increased gene expression for the β isoform of the PDGF receptor.

Effects of KCM on lipocyte collagen and protein synthesis

There was a progressive and parallel increase in both collagen and total protein synthesis by cultured lipocytes exposed to conditioned medium. Unlike proliferation, however, the stimulation of collagen synthesis was not serum-dependent.

Modulation of TGF-β receptors

Previous studies had implicated TGF-β as a major fibrogenic cytokine in Kupffer cell medium[9]. We focused instead on regulation of receptors for TGF-β during the activation response. By affinity labelling, KCM-induced activation was associated with increased expression of types I, II and III receptors. Unlike β-PDGF receptors, however, there was down-regulation of gene expression with culture-induced activation.

DISCUSSION

We have demonstrated that conditioned medium from cultured Kupffer cells of normal rats stimulates hepatic lipocytes in a manner closely parallel to changes observed in hepatic fibrogenesis. Specifically, in addition to morphological activation, KCM induces expression of receptors for PDGF and increased binding activity for TGF-β. The appearance of PDGF receptor is preceded by increased gene expression for the β isoform. The expression of this isoform is consistent with the known bioactivity of the BB PDGF homodimer[2]; β receptors are responsive to either AB or BB isoforms of PDGF. The source of PDGF in liver fibrogenesis is uncertain, however. Since Kupffer cells in this culture model do not secrete bioactive PDGF, an alternative source may be platelets.

The induction of PDGF receptor expression by macrophage-conditioned medium (KCM) is a potentially relevant mode of regulating PDGF responsiveness *in vivo*. Enhanced PDGF receptor expression accompanies vascular inflammation of arteries[20] and synovium[21].

The mechanisms underlying KCM-induced PDGF receptor expression are not yet elucidated. The enhanced expression of PDGF receptors may in part be a spontaneous response to the culture substratum, as well as to specific activating species present in Kupffer cell-conditioned medium.

These data also suggest that lipocyte activation is associated with increased binding activity for TGF-β_1. Interestingly, when binding was low, mRNA levels were high. The results in non-activated cells could be explained by decreased quantity of membrane-associated receptor protein through reduced translation, increased turnover and/or intracellular shunting of receptor protein to degradative pathways in quiescent cells. Alternatively, there may be ample receptor protein, but in a conformation which does not permit ligand binding.

Mechanisms of TGF-β receptor modulation and signalling *in vivo* are not yet completely understood. Concurrent expression of type II receptor may be necessary for type I receptors to bind ligand, although the nature of this interdependence is not certain. A recent study using mutant cell lines has suggested that unmasking of type I receptor binding occurs through 'activation' of latent receptor; this activation may occur through formation of a receptor complex containing the types I and II receptors[22]. In these studies using cell mutants lacking intact type II receptor, previously inapparent type I receptor binding could be uncovered by transfection with

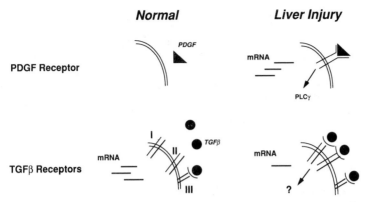

Fig. 1 Contrasting mechanisms of regulation for PDGF and TGF-β receptors during lipocyte activation – a working model. While lipocyte activation is associated with increased binding for both PDGF and TGF-β, gene induction for PDGF receptor is sustained, whereas for TGF-β receptors a divergence develops between levels of binding and mRNA expression. It is possible that TGF-β receptors exist on the cell surface in quiescent cells but lack a conformation which allows binding. Alternatively, there may be decreased translation or increased degradation of the TGF-β receptors

wild-type type II receptor; thus, in this model absence of cell surface binding by TGF-β receptor did not necessarily correlate with absence of receptors, only lack of activation[22]. The findings may be particularly relevant to our lipocyte model, because binding activity for TGF-β_1 was low at a time when gene expression for types II and III receptors was high. This finding raises the possibility that type II receptor is present but not accessible to ligand, because type I receptor was absent, and/or because it lacked the proper conformation (Fig. 1).

In summary, we have presented evidence that Kupffer cell medium stimulates lipocyte proliferation via enhanced gene and protein expression of PDGF receptors, and enhanced fibrogenesis in part through increased binding of TGF-β. Regulation of PDGF receptor gene expression differs from those of TGF-β in that for TGF-β receptors there is a divergent relationship between binding activity and gene expression.

Acknowledgements

This work was supported in part by United States Public Health Service Grants DK 37340, DK 31198, DK 26743 and a grant-in-aid from the American Heart Association, California Chapter (to S.L.F.).

References

1. Geerts A, Lazou JM, Bleser PD *et al.* Tissue distribution, quantitation and proliferation kinetics of fat-storing cells in carbon tetrachloride-injured rat liver. Hepatology. 1990;13:1193–202.

2. Friedman SL, Arthur MJP. Activation of cultured rat hepatic lipocytes by Kupffer cell conditioned medium. J Clin Invest. 1989;84:1780–5.

3. Pinzani M, Gesualdo L, Sabbah GM et al. Effects of platelet-derived growth factor and other polypeptide mitogens on DNA synthesis and growth of cultured rat liver fat-storing cells. J Clin Invest. 1989;84:1786–93.

4. Heldin P, Pertoft H, Nordlinder H et al. Differential expression of platelet-derived growth factor alpha- and beta receptors on fat-storing cells and endothelial cells of rat liver. Exp Cell Res. 1991;193:364–9.

5. Nakatasukasa H, Evarts RP, Hsia C-C, Thorgeirsson SS. Transforming growth factor-beta 1 and type I procollagen transcripts during regeneration and early fibrosis of rat liver. Lab Invest. 1990;63:171–80.

6. Nakatasukasa H, Nagy P, Evarts RP et al. Cellular distribution of transforming growth factor-beta 1 and procollagen types I, III, and IV transcripts in carbon tetrachloride-induced rat liver fibrosis. J Clin Invest. 1990;85:1833–43.

7. Castilla A, Prieto J, Fausto N. Transforming growth factors beta 1 and alpha in chronic liver disease. N Engl J Med. 1991;324:933–40.

8. Assoian RK, Komoriya A, Meyers CA et al. Transforming growth factor β in human platelets; identification of a major storage site, purification and characterization. J Biol Chem. 1983;258:7155–60.

9. Matsuoka M, Tsukamoto H. Stimulation of hepatic lipocyte collagen production by Kupffer cell-derived transforming growth factor beta: implication for a pathogenetic role in alcoholic liver fibrogenesis. Hepatology. 1990;11:599–605.

10. Bachem MG, Meyer D, Melchior R et al. Activation of rat liver perisinusoidal lipocytes by transforming growth factors derived from myofibroblast-like cells. J Clin Invest. 1992;89:19–27.

11. Milani S, Herbst H, Schuppan D et al. Transforming growth factors beta 1 and beta 2 are differentially expressed in fibrotic liver disease. Am J Pathol. 1991;139:1221–9.

12. Ramadori G, Knittel T, Odenthal M et al. Synthesis of cellular fibronectin by rat liver fat-storing (Ito) cells: regulation by cytokines. Gastroenterology. 1992;103:1313–21.

13. Bachem MG, Riess U, Melchior R et al. Transforming growth factors (TGF alpha and TGF beta 1) stimulate chondroitin sulfate and hyaluronate synthesis in cultured rat liver fat storing cells. FEBS Lett. 1989;257:134–7.

14. Massague J. Receptors for the TGF-beta family. Cell. 1992;69:1067–70.

15. Laiho M, Weis FMB, Massague J. Concomitant loss of transforming growth factor (TGF)-beta receptor types I and II in TGF-beta-resistant cell mutants implicates both receptor types in signal transduction. J Biol Chem. 1990;265:18518–24.

16. Ebner R, Chen R, Shum L et al. Cloning of a type I TGFβ receptor and its effect on TGF-β binding to the type II receptor. Science. 1993;260:1344–8.

17. Lin HY, Wang X-F, Ng-Eaton E et al. Expression cloning of the TGF-beta type II receptor, a functional transmembrane serine/threonine kinase. Cell. 1992;68:775–85.

18. Lopez-Casillas F, Cheifetz S, Doody J et al. Structure and expression of the membrane proteoglycan betaglycan, a component of the TGF-beta receptor system. Cell. 1991;67:785–95.

19. Wang X-F, Lin HY, Ng-Eaton E et al. Expression cloning and characterization of the TGF-beta type III receptor. Cell. 1991;67:797–805.

20. Rubin K, Hansson GK, Ronnstrang L et al. Induction of b-type receptors for platelet-derived growth factor in vascular inflammation: possible implications for development of vascular proliferative lesions. Lancet. 1988;1:1353–6.

21. Rubin K, Terracio L, Ronnstrand L et al. Expression of platelet-derived growth factor receptors is induced on connective tissue cells during chronic synovial inflammation. Scand J Immunol. 1989;27:285–94.

22. Wrana JL, Attisano L, Carcamo J et al. TGFbeta signals through a heteromeric protein kinase receptor complex. Cell. 1992;71:1003–14.

Section V
Selected oral presentations

19
Hepatocyte growth factor/scatter factor expression is a marker for the quiescent state of rat fat-storing cells

M. ODENTHAL, A. GEERTS, W. JUNG, B. GILBERG, H. P. DIENES and P. SCHIRMACHER

INTRODUCTION

Hepatocyte growth factor/scatter factor (HGF/SF) is a pleiotropic cytokine effecting cell motility and cell proliferation of various endothelial and epithelial cell types (for review see ref. 1). The growth factor was first detected as a highly potent mitogen for hepatocytes in primary culture in the sera of hepatectomized rats[2,3]. Since acute hepatic injury in rat and fulminant hepatic failure in humans lead to a dramatic increase of HGF/SF serum level, its mitogenic activity on hepatocytes suggests an important function in liver regeneration processes. The genes of human and rat HGF have been cloned and sequenced[4], revealing identity with the morphogenic and motogenic acting, fibroblast-derived scatter factor[5,6]. HGF/SF cDNA encodes for a 90 kDa heterodimer related in sequence and in overall structure to proteins involved in coagulation processes such as plasminogen, prothrombin and others[4,7]. Therefore HGF/SF represents a new type of cytokine. The high-affinity receptor of HGF/SF was found to be identical with the protooncogene, c-met, a membrane anchored receptor protein with intrinsic tyrosine kinase activity[8].

METHODS

Induction of acute and chronic liver damage

Acute liver damage was induced by a single, intraperitoneal administration of 200 μl CCl_4 per 100 g body weight mixed with silicon oil in a ratio 1:1. At 24, 48, and 72 h after the treatment rats were sacrificed and livers were excised. For induction of liver fibrosis rats received an intraperitoneal administration of 100 μl CCl_4 per 100 g body weight twice a week. After 6 weeks of treatment followed by 7 days of recovery, fibrotic livers were removed for analysis of HGF/SF expression.

Isolation of parenchymal and mesenchymal liver cells

Hepatocytes were isolated by the collagenase-perfusion procedure according to the method of Seglen[9]. After perfusion of untreated and fibrotic rat livers with pronase and collagenase, mesenchymal cell types were separated from parenchymal cell debris by Nycodenz density gradient centrifugation and Kupffer and endothelial cells were further purified by centrifugal elutriation as described earlier[10]. FSC were plated in DMEM supplemented with 5% FCS and maintained in culture for 30 days. Composition of the cell preparations was determined by transmission electron microscopy.

In situ hybridization

Cryostat sections of normal, acutely and chronically damaged livers were hybridized with ^{35}S-labelled sense and antisense riboprobes, representing the β-chain of HGF/SF[10] or with a riboprobe recognizing *c-met* transcripts[11]. The specimens were coated with Kodak NTB-2 emulsion, exposed for 10 days, counterstained and analysed by light and dark field microscopy.

Northern blot hybridization

Total RNA of the different cell populations from control and fibrotic rat liver was extracted, separated by agarose gel electrophoresis and immobilized onto nylon membranes. Hybridization was performed with HGF/SF cDNA of the pRBC-1 plasmid[10]. Isolated total RNA from rat liver was also hybridized with a cDNA probe spanning the intracellular kinase domain of human *c-met*[11]. Total RNA subjected to HGF/SF-cDNA hybridization was estimated by rehybridization of filters with a GAPDH-cDNA probe[12].

RESULTS AND DISCUSSION

In the normal rat liver, transcripts for both HGF/SF and its receptor *c-met* are present (Fig. 1). *In situ* hybridization demonstrates that HGF/SF is synthesized by a subpopulation of sinusoidal liver cells, while *c-met* transcripts are evenly distributed over the parenchyma (Fig. 3A,C). In order to identify the HGF/SF expressing cell type we analysed RNA from isolated liver cells. Among the different cell populations, FSC strongly express HGF/SF, whereas parenchymal and Kupffer cells do not take part in HGF/SF synthesis (Fig. 2)[10]. HGF/SF transcripts detectable in the endothelial cell isolates could be attributed to contaminating FSC[10].

In response to a CCl_4-induced acute liver injury pericentral proliferation of FSC takes place, leading to a significant accumulation of FSC in the

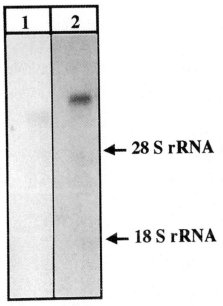

Fig. 1 HGF/SF- (1) and *c-met*-gene expression (2) in normal rat liver; Northern blot hybridization of 20 µg total RNA with HGF/SF cDNA (1) or with *c-met* cDNA (2)

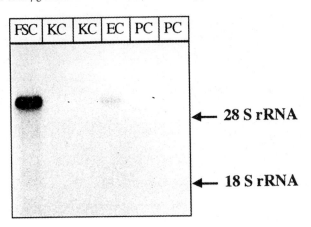

Fig. 2 HGF/SF expression in fat-storing cells (FSC), Kupffer cells (KC), endothelial cells (EC), and hepatocytes (PC) isolated from normal rat livers; Northern blot hybridization of total RNA with HGF/SF cDNA

necrotic parenchyma[13,14]. By *in situ* hybridization we could also show a moderate increase in the number of HGF/SF-expressing cells in comparison to control liver (Fig. 3C,E). Seventy-two hours after a single CCl_4 administration additional HGF/SF synthesis was detected in cells infiltrating perivenular necroses (Fig. 3F). Therefore infiltrating immune cells may also contribute to HGF/SF synthesis after acute inflammation.

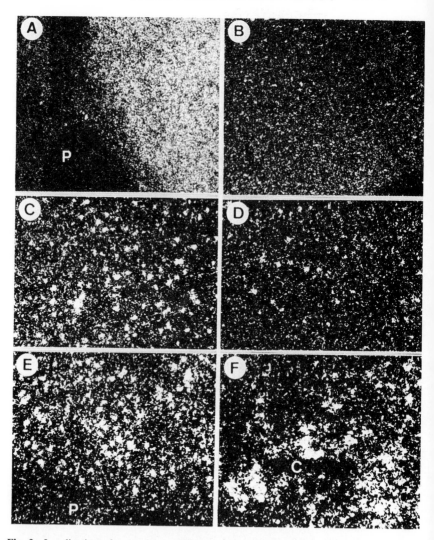

Fig. 3 Localization of *c-met* (**A**) or HGF/SF transcripts (**B–F**) by *in situ* hybridization in normal rat liver (**A, B, C**), in chronically diseased rat liver (**D**), and in rat liver at 24 h (**E**) or 72 h (**F**) after a single dose of CCl_4; representative dark-field illuminations of liver tissue hybridized with the respective ^{35}S-labelled riboprobes; hybridization with the sense HGF/SF-riboprobe was performed as a control (**B**)

In contrast to the elevated number of HGF/SF expressing cells in the acutely injured rat liver, in the fibrotic liver the number of cells bearing transcripts for HGF/SF is reduced in comparison to normal liver (Fig. 3C,D). We reasoned that this loss of HGF/SF expressing cells can be due to down-regulated HGF/SF synthesis in activated FSC. During primary culture FSC undergo a transformation into myofibroblast-like cells that mimics the

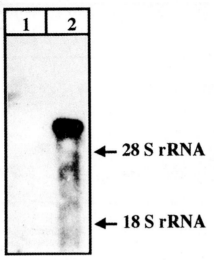

Fig. 4 HGF/SF-gene expression in myofibroblast-like cells derived from FSC after long-term primary culture (1) and in freshly isolated FSC (2); Northern blot hybridization of the respective total RNA with HGF/SF cDNA

altered phenotype observed after activation upon liver injury or intoxication. Prolonged primary culture leads to a down-regulation of HGF/SF-transcript level[10,15], and after 30 days of cultivation no HGF/SF-mRNA is detectable (Fig. 4). In order to investigate whether activated FSC also lose their ability to express HGF/SF *in vivo*, we isolated different mesenchymal cell types from fibrotic liver. In agreement with suppressed HGF/SF gene expression after activation of FSC during primary culture, in activated FSC isolated from fibrotic liver the HGF/SF mRNA level is decreased (Fig. 5). However, in the endothelial cell isolates from the fibrotic liver, HGF/SF transcripts were detectable to an extent that is not explained by contaminating FSC (Fig. 5, Table 1).

Our results demonstrate that HGF/SF is produced by quiescent FSC. Via HGF/SF FSC may be involved in paracrine regulation of parenchymal cell growth during regenerating processes. The synthesis of other cytokines such as TGF-β or TGF-α produced by FSC is induced upon their transition into myofibroblast-like cells[16,17]. In contrast HGF/SF is expressed in quiescent FSC but completely abolished after their transition into myofibroblast-like cells during primary culture[10,15] and greatly reduced in isolated FSC from chronically injured rat liver, most likely corresponding to the extent of myofibroblast-like transition. Therefore HGF/SF expression is a marker for the quiescent state of FSC *in vitro* and *in vivo*. Analysis of regulatory genetic elements may give new insights in factors controlling HGF/SF-gene expression in dependence of the state of FSC differentiation.

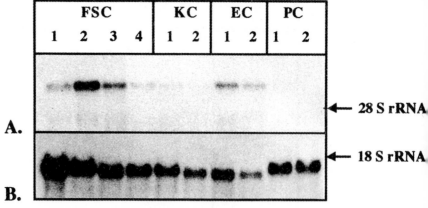

Fig. 5 HGF/SF expression in different isolates of fat-storing cells (FSC), Kupffer cells (KC), endothelial cells (EC) and parenchymal cells (PC) from the fibrotic liver. Northern blot hybridization of 10 μg total RNA with the HGF/SF cDNA (**A**); rehybridization of the blot with GAPDH cDNA probe (**B**)

Table 1 Composition of the different cell isolates from fibrotic rat liver determined by transmission electron microscopy (see Fig. 5); parenchymal cells (PC), endothelial cells (EC), Kupffer cells (KC), fat-storing cells (FSC), lymphocytes (LY)

	PC	EC	KC	FSC	LY	Others
PC1	85.5	12.2	0.5	1.6	0	0.5
PC2	81.9	8.7	0	3.9	0	5.5
EC1	0	78.8	0.8	1.35	9.3	9.7
EC2	0	77.4	0.6	1.3	10.2	10.5
KC1	0	1.1	91.5	0	0.7	6.6
KC2	0	25.4	63.9	1.0	6.5	3.1
FSC1	0	34.7	4	52.5	3.3	5.4
FSC2	—	—	—	—	—	—
FSC3	0	21.3	6.5	64	3.3	5.0
FSC4	0	7.26	8.3	78.8	1.7	3.9

Acknowledgement

This work was supported by the grant Schi 273/3-1 from the Deutsche Forschungsgemeinschaft.

References

1. Michalopoulos GK, Zarnegar R. Hepatocyte growth factor. Hepatology. 1992;15:149–55.
2. Nakamura T, Nawa K, Ishihara A. Partial purification and characterization of a hepatocyte growth factor from serum of hepatectomized rats. Biochem Biophys Res Commun. 1984; 122:1450–9.
3. Zarnegar R, Michalopoulos G. Purification and biological characterization of human hepatopoietin A, a polypeptide growth factor for hepatocytes. Cancer Res. 1989;49: 3314–20.

4. Nakamura T, Nishizawa T, Hagiya M *et al.* Molecular cloning and expression of human hepatocyte growth factor. Nature. 1989;342:440–3.
5. Stoker M, Gherardi E, Perryman M *et al.* Scatter factor is a fibroblast-derived modulator of epithelial cell mobility. Nature. 1987;327:239–42.
6. Weidner KM, Arakaki N, Hartmann G *et al.* Evidence for the identity of human scatter factor and human hepatocyte growth factor. Proc Natl Acad Sci USA. 1991;8:7001–5.
7. Seki T, Hagiya N, Shimonishi M *et al.* Organization of the human hepatocyte growth factor-encoding gene. Gene. 1991;213:213–19.
8. Naldini L, Vigna E, Narsimhan RP *et al.* Hepatocyte growth factor (HGF) stimulates the tyrosine kinase activity of the receptor encoded by the proto-oncogene c-met. Oncogene. 1991;6:501–4.
9. Seglen PO. Preparation of isolated liver cells. In: Prescott D, editor. Methods in cell biology, Vol. XIII. New York/London: Academic Press; 1976:29–83.
10. Schirmacher P, Geerts A, Pietrangelo A *et al.* Hepatocyte growth factor/hepatopoietin A is expressed in fat-storing cells from rat liver but not myofibroblast-like cells derived from fat-storing cells. Hepatology. 1992;15(1):5–11.
11. Park M, Dean M, Cooper C *et al.* Mechanism of *met* oncogene activation. Cell. 1986;45:895–904.
12. Tso JY, Sun XH, Kao T *et al.* Isolation and characterization of rat and human glyceraldehyde-3-phosphate dehydrogenase cDNAs: genomic complexity and molecular evolution of the gene. Nucl Acids Res. 1985;13(7):2485–92.
13. Geerts A, Lazou JM, De Bleser P *et al.* Tissue distribution, quantitation and proliferation kinetics of fat-storing cells in carbon tetrachloride-injured rat liver. Hepatology. 1991;13(6):1193–202.
14. Burt AD, Robertson JL, Heir J *et al.* Desmin containing stellate cells in rat liver, distribution in normal animals and in response to experimental acute liver injury. J Pathol. 1986;150:29–35.
15. Ramadori G, Neubauer K, Odenthal M *et al.* Hepatocyte growth factor (hepatopoietin A, Scatrin)-gene expression in quiescent fat-storing cells of rat liver: downregulation by transforming growth factor-β. Biochem Biophys Res Commun. 1992;183(2):739–42.
16. Weiner FR, Shah A, Biempica L *et al.* Cellular sources of increased collagen and transforming growth factor β_1 gene expression in fibrotic rat liver. Hepatology. 1989;10:629–35.
17. Bachem MG, Meyer D, Melchior R *et al.* Activation of rat liver perisinusoidal lipocytes by transforming growth factors derived from myofibroblast-like cells. J Clin Invest. 1992;89:19–27.

20
Iron overload in rodents leads to hepatic cirrhosis through enhancement of collagen gene expression into non-parenchymal cells

A. PIETRANGELO, R. GUALDI, G. CASALGRANDI, G. MONTOSI and E. VENTURA

In iron storage diseases (e.g. idiopathic haemochromatosis (IH), thalassaemic syndromes, transfusional iron overload, alcoholic cirrhosis, porphyria cutanea tarda), the liver is a major target organ of injury, and hepatic fibrosis and cirrhosis are the major pathological hallmarks of the disease[1,2]. In general, hepatic fibrosis is viewed as a secondary effect following cell injury and death. However, in metabolic diseases, such as IH or Wilson's disease, hepatic fibrosis may be seen without accompanying necroinflammatory events. Indeed, in individuals with IH, early periportal fibrosis may occur with heavy parenchymal iron deposition, but in the absence of obvious cell necrosis and inflammation[3,4], suggesting that excess tissue iron may provide a direct stimulus to collagen synthesis. Our finding of an early activation of hepatic pro-α_2(I) collagen gene expression in rats chronically fed with carbonyl iron in the absence of histological signs of liver damage or alteration in differentiated functions[5], gave support to the notion that iron *per se* may act as a profibrogenic agent.

Type I collagen is the most abundant extracellular matrix protein found in liver cirrhosis[6]. In recent years, understanding of the molecular mechanisms controlling collagen I gene expression and, particularly, identifying the hepatic cell type responsible for collagen synthesis in normal and fibrotic liver have been the subject of active investigation[7-13]. Most of these observations have been collected by using experimental models of postnecrotic and/or inflammatory fibrosis.

In human iron overload (i.o.) disorders iron can preferentially accumulate into parenchymal or non-parenchymal cells of the liver[3]. In fact, in conditions in which i.o. is caused by increased influx from the portal blood (e.g. idiopathic haemochromatosis), the metal accumulates into parenchymal cells, whereas during secondary i.o. due to blood transfusions, hepatic iron is mainly localized into reticuloendothelial cells. The possibility that the accumulation of the metal in a particular liver cell type might differently influence the pathobiology of the i.o. disease, and specifically the fibrogenic process, has not been addressed so far.

The present study was designed: (a) to determine whether accumulation of excess iron into different hepatic cells *in vivo* would differently affect collagen gene expression and ultimately lead to hepatic cirrhosis; (b) to investigate the role of hepatocytes during hepatic fibrogenesis under these circumstances.

We induced in animals (A) parenchymal cell i.o. (2.5% carbonyl iron diet for 6 months), (B) Kupffer and endothelial cell i.o. (i.m. weekly injections of 1 mg/g body weight iron–dextran in rats for 4 months), or (C) 'focal' i.o. (s.c. injections of 1 mg/g body weight iron–dextran in gerbils). Control animals were fed a normal diet (group A) or treated with i.m. injections of dextran alone (groups B and C).

Histochemical evaluation of iron deposition demonstrated, as expected, a preferential accumulation of iron into hepatocytes in zone 1 and 2 (group A) or into non-parenchymal cells (mainly Kupffer cells) (group B), and into microscopic haemorrhagic lesions[14] throughout the hepatic lobule (group C). All iron-intoxication protocols achieved a comparable amount of hepatic iron content, as assessed by atomic absorption spectroscopy (20–30-fold increase as compared to control animals). As far as the accumulation of collagen is concerned, histological evaluation with a trichrome staining was performed. Tissue specimens from animals of group A showed signs of periportal fibrosis, those from rats of group B were essentially negative, the gerbils showed collagen deposition around iron foci at 6 weeks and developed micronodular cirrhosis after 4 months.

To investigate whether excess iron accumulation into different hepatic cells differently affects the expression of collagen gene, we used an *in situ* hybridization assay which would be highly sensitive and most suitable to detect different cellular and lobular patterns of gene expression. To this purpose an EcoR I-Hind III 1300 bp fragment of rat pro-α_1(I) collagen cDNA[15] was subcloned in pGEM1 plasmid. To generate run-off transcripts of the antisense or sense strands, respectively, 1 μg of plasmid linearized with either Hind III or EcoRI restriction endonucleases and 10 units of T7 or SP6 RNA polymerases were added to a 10 μl reaction mixture containing 100 μCi of [^{35}S]uridine-5′-thiotriphosphate (1250 Ci/mmol, Amersham, UK); 1 mmol/l each of adenosine, cytidine and guanosine-5′-triphosphate; 10 mmol/l DTT; 25 units of human placental RNAase inhibitor; 6 mmol/l MgCl$_2$; 40 mmol/l Tris-HCl, pH 7.5; 2 mmol/l spermidine; 10 mmol/l NaCl; and incubated 1 h at 37°C for T7 or 40°C for SP6 RNA polymerase. Plasmid DNA was removed by digestion with 2 units of RNAase free-DNAase I at 37°C for 15 min, followed by phenol–chloroform extraction and ethanol precipitation. To increase the penetration into tissue, the size of the ^{35}S riboprobe was adjusted to 50–200 bases length by controlled alkaline hydrolysis in 80 mmol/l $NaHCO_3$; 120 mmol/l Na_2CO_3, pH 10.2; 10 mmol/l DTT at 60°C. After neutralization in 0.2 mol/l sodium acetate, pH 6.0; 1% acetic acid; 120 mmol/l Na_2CO_3, pH 10.2 and 10 mmol/l DTT and ethanol precipitation, RNA probes were stored at −80°C.

Frozen tissue sections (5 μm thick) were collected onto 3-aminopropyl-triethoxysilane (TES) coated slides, air-dried, fixed in a 4% solution of paraformaldehyde in 0.1 mol/l PBS (pH 7.4) containing 5 mmol/l $MgCl_2$ for 15 min. After serial washes in PBS, dehydration in graded ethanols and short air-drying, sections were acetylated with 0.1 mol/l triethanolamine, pH 8.0, containing 0.25% acetic anhydride (vol/vol) for 10 min and washed twice in 0.2 × standard saline citrate (20 × SSC is 3 mol/l NaCl, 0.3 mol/l sodium citrate) for 10 min at room temperature. Sections were air-dried and prehybridized in 50% formamide; 2.5% Denhardt's solution (100 × Denhardt's solution is: 2% bovine serum albumin, 2% polyvinylpyrrolidone, MW 360 000, 2% ficoll, MW 400 000); 150 μg/ml salmon sperm DNA; 0.6 mol/l NaCl; 10 mmol/l Tris HCl, pH 7.5; 1 mmol/l EDTA, pH 8.0; 0.1% SDS and 0.05 mg/ml yeast tRNA, at 45°C for 2 h. Hybridization was performed in the same solution with the addition of 10% dextran sulphate, 10 mmol/l DTT and 1 × 10^6 cpm/slide of [^{35}S]UTP-labelled rat pro-α_1(I) collagen probes for an additional 16 h at 45°C. Probe excess was removed by washing the slides twice in 4 × SSC/50% formamide/10 mmol/l DTT at 50°C for 15 min and in 2 × SSC at room temperature. This was followed by RNAase treatment for 30 min at 37°C with 20 μg/ml RNAase A in 0.5 mol/l NaCl, 10 mmol/l Tris, 1 mmol/l EDTA. After dehydration in graded ethanols containing 0.3 mol/l ammonium acetate and air-drying, slides were exposed to Kodak X-OMAT-AR films (Eastman Kodak, Rochester, NY) at −70°C for 2–4 days. Subsequently, the slides were coated with Kodak NTB-2 emulsion and exposed at 4°C for several weeks, typically 4–6 weeks. After development in Kodak D19 developer and fixation in Kodak fixer, the slides were counterstained with H&E, mounted, and viewed under the light microscope in dark or bright field.

In iron-fed animals a higher hybridization signal for α_1(I) collagen mRNA was detected in non-parenchymal cells adjacent to heavily iron-laden hepatocytes. The higher signal for collagen mRNA was mainly detected in non-parenchymal cells zones 1 and 2. Over iron-laden parenchymal cells, no grains with a typical 'cluster' distribution detected on non-parenchymal cells were found. Negative results for hybridization signal over hepatocytes were also collected when serial sections of the liver tissue were hybridized with the ^{35}S-collagen cRNA. On the other hand, in the rats treated with parenteral injections of iron–dextran (group B) no specific hybridization signal was detected in iron-laden reticuloendothelial cells (mainly Kupffer cells) or in nearby parenchymal or non-parenchymal cells. In the gerbils a strong activation of collagen gene expression was detected in non-parenchymal cells surrounding iron-laden lesions. No signal of collagen gene activation was detected in nearby hepatocytes. As mentioned above, only in this group was it possible to achieve a micronodular cirrhosis.

In human iron overload states, different or changeable patterns of iron distribution into cells of the hepatic lobule may be encountered, with preferential parenchymal or non-parenchymal cell iron accumulation. Each cell type of the hepatic lobule (hepatocyte, Kupffer cell, endothelial cell, fat-storing cell) may be involved in hepatic fibrogenesis, being directly responsible for collagen biosynthesis or contributing to the production of diffusible factors mediating the fibrogenic process[16,17]. In the present study we used different experimental models of hepatic iron overload (enteral or parenteral iron administration in the rat and in the gerbil), which allowed us to target the hepatotoxin (i.e. iron) selectively to a specific liver cell type, to test whether the cell localization of excess iron might affect collagen gene expression differently. Although in both enterally and parenterally iron-treated rats a comparable amount of hepatic iron burden was reached, a significant activation of collagen gene expression into non-parenchymal cells surrounding iron-laden hepatocytes was detected only in livers of enterally intoxicated rats. It has been reported that iron-induced lipid peroxidation may enhance collagen gene transcription in cultured fibroblasts[18]. Since iron-catalysed lipid peroxidation has been documented in both experimental models of iron overload[19], one would expect to find signs of collagen gene activation in both enterally and parenterally iron-treated rats. This was not the case in our study. Thus, if lipid peroxidation by-products mediate enhancement of collagen gene expression during experimental siderosis, the cell context in which the oxidative damage occurs must dictate the differential response of the collagen gene.

The basis for the stimulatory effect of parenchymal iron on collagen gene activation in fat-storing cells remains to be determined. Lipid peroxidation by-products released from iron-laden hepatocytes may elicit their stimulatory effect on the collagen gene in neighbouring fat-storing cells, directly, or through activated Kupffer cells. The latter might respond by increasing the generation of oxygen radical species and/or releasing fibrogenic factors. Selective loading of Kupffer and endothelial cells with iron does not appear to elicit any activation of collagen gene activity. On the other hand, the fact that, in the gerbil (upon accumulation of iron into microscopic lesions containing non-parenchymal cells and necrotic hepatocytes) a strong activation of collagen gene expression and micronodular cirrhosis were achieved, may suggest that hepatic reticuloendothelial iron overload may be pathogenetically linked to the fibrogenic process when iron accumulation in these cells is secondary to hepatocellular necrosis (sideronecrosis) and mainly due to the phagocytic activity of necrotic iron-laden hepatocytes. In this case the activated reticuloendothelial cell would strongly activate collagen biosynthesis into nearby non-parenchymal cells, most likely Ito cells. Future studies will attempt to identify the molecular basis for the stimulatory effect of iron overload on collagen gene activity into non-parenchymal liver cells.

References

1. Bonkovsky HL. Iron and the liver. Am J Med Sci. 1991;301:32–43.
2. Deugnier YM, Loréal O, Turlin B et al. Liver pathology in genetic hemochromatosis: a review of 135 homozygous cases and their bioclinical correlations. Gastroenterology. 1992;102:2050–9.

3. Tavill AS, Sharma BK, Bacon BR. Iron and the liver: genetic hemochromatosis and other hepatic iron overload disorders. Prog Liver Dis. 1990;9:281–305.
4. Weintraub LR, Goral A, Grasso J *et al.* Collagen biosynthesis in iron overload. Ann NY Acad Sci. 1988;526:179–84.
5. Pietrangelo A, Rocchi E, Schiaffonati L *et al.* Liver gene expression during chronic dietary iron overload in rats. Hepatology. 1990;11:798–804.
6. Rojkind M. From regeneration to scar formation: the collagen way. Lab Invest. 1992;64: 131–4.
7. Tseng SCG, Lee PC, Ells PF *et al.* Collagen production by rat hepatocytes and sinusoidal cells in monolayer culture. Hepatology. 1982;2:13–18.
8. Diegelmann RF, Guzelian PS, Gay R *et al.* Collagen formation by the hepatocyte in primary monolayer culture and *in vivo*. Science. 1983;219:1343–5.
9. Chojkier M, Lyche KD, Filip M. Increased production of collagen *in vivo* by hepatocytes and nonparenchymal cells in rats with carbon tetrachloride-induced hepatic fibrosis. Hepatology. 1988;8:808–14.
10. Milani S, Herbst H, Schuppan D *et al.* In situ hybridization for procollagen types I, III and IV mRNA in normal and fibrotic rat liver: evidence for predominant expression in nonparenchymal liver cells. Hepatology. 1989;10:84–92.
11. Milani S, Herbst H, Schuppan D *et al.* Procollagen expression by nonparenchymal rat liver cells in experimental biliary fibrosis. Gastroenterology. 1990;98:175–84.
12. Nakatsukasa H, Nagy P, Evarts RP *et al.* Cellular distribution of transforming growth factor-beta 1 and procollagen types I, III and IV transcripts in carbon tetrachloride-induced rat liver fibrosis. J Clin Invest. 1990;85:1833–43.
13. Maher JJ, McGuire RF. Extracelluar matrix gene expression increases preferentially in rat lipocytes and sinusoidal endothelial cells during hepatic fibrosis in vivo. J. Clin Invest. 1990;86:1746–51.
14. Carthew P, Edwards RE, Smith AG *et al.* Rapid induction of hepatic fibrosis in the gerbil after the parenteral administration of iron-dextran complex. Hepatology. 1991;13:534–9.
15. Genovese C, Rowe D, Kream B. Construction of DNA sequences complementary to rat alpha-1 and alpha-2 collagen mRNA and their use in studying the regulation of type I collagen synthesis by 1,25-dihydroxyvitamin D. Biochemistry. 1984;23:6210–16.
16. Bissell DM. Lipocyte activation and hepatic fibrosis. Gastroenterology. 1992;102:1803–5.
17. Friedman SL. The cellular basis of hepatic fibrosis. Mechanisms and treatment strategies. N Engl J Med. 1993;328:1828–34.
18. Chojkier M, Houglum K, Solis-Herruzo J *et al.* Stimulation of collagen gene expression by ascorbic acid in cultured human fibroblasts. J Biol Chem. 1989;264:16957–62.
19. Bacon BR, Britton RS. The pathology of hepatic iron overload: a free radical-mediated process? Hepatology. 1990;11:127–37.

Section VI
New perspective in the clinical management of chronic liver disease and liver fibrosis

21
Fibrosis of the liver: a pathologist's view

V. J. DESMET

INTRODUCTION

Fibrosis of the liver is part of the liver alterations in most chronic liver diseases.

In the past, fibrosis was usually considered as an excess of collagen (fibre) deposition in the organ, mostly thought of as a stable and irreversible increase in collagen. Research over the past two decades, however, has revealed an extraordinary complexity of the extracellular matrix in general, and new insights into its composition in the liver. In addition, evidence was brought forward for the dynamic aspects of fibrosis, including synthesis, deposition and degradation of matrix components, rendering the fossil 'stability' of fibrosis obsolete[1]. Furthermore, recent investigations have focused on the cells of origin, and their mechanisms of matrix formation and degradation, revealing a remarkably complex network of cellular interactions and cytokines.

Hence, fibrosis has come to be considered as a disturbance in the delicate equilibrium of a hepatic bioecological system[2] resulting in the deposition of excess quantities of numerous extracellular matrix components, including glycoproteins and proteoglycans[3,4].

Fibrosis occurs in different patterns. The pattern of fibrosis appears to be related to some extent to the pathogenetic mechanism of disease, explaining the relative diagnostic usefulness of various patterns of fibrosis for the liver histopathologist.

However, patterns of fibrosis are also related to the structural organization of the liver organ, since the spatial juxtaposition of epithelial cells, mesenchymal cells, matrix components and blood vessels are the fundamental determinants of normal hepatic structure and function, and the starting point from which fibrosis develops in its various patterns.

The uniqueness of the structure of the normal liver, including its integrated extracellular matrix, and the organ-specificity of numerous hepatic functions, explain why hepatic fibrosis differs from interstitial fibrosis in the lung or any other organ, although the basic mechanisms for the deposition of excess quantities of extracellular matrix components may be largely the same[5].

THE NORMAL LIVER: EXTRACELLULAR MATRIX AND ANGIOARCHITECTURE

Extracellular matrix

The extracellular matrix of the liver comprises extralobular and intralobular components. Extralobular components are represented by the liver capsule (capsule of Glisson), the portal tracts and a small amount of matrix surrounding the efferent veins. The intralobular component corresponds to the extracellular matrix in the space of Disse.

The portal tracts correspond to a sheet of connective tissue surrounding the afferent vessels (hepatic artery, portal vein) and the intrahepatic bile ducts. The portal tracts with their enclosed vascular and biliary channels represent a three-dimensional, tree-like arborizing system, which alternates, in an interdigitating way, with a branching tree of efferent vessels (hepatic veins). The space between the portal tracts and efferent veins is occupied by the liver parenchyma and its sinusoids. Hepatic arterial and portal venous blood perfuses, in an unidirectional way, the sinusoids from the terminal ramifications of the portal tracts to the finest radicles of the efferent veins (so-called centrolobular veins or terminal hepatic venules)[6].

The portal tracts in normal liver are sharply delineated from the surrounding lobular parenchyma by the limiting plate (a parenchymal cell muralium modelled around the portal tract).

The portal mesenchyme comprises all classical components of connective tissue. The constituent mesenchymal cells are fibroblasts, which may show slight phenotypic heterogeneity even in normal rat liver, since a few of these cells express α-smooth muscle-actin[7,8], in line with the heterogeneity of fibroblasts demonstrated in other locations and pathological states[9].

The extracellular matrix comprises collagens type I, type III, type V, type VI, fibronectin and undulin, whereas the basement membranes surrounding bile ducts contain collagen type IV, and laminin[10-13] and perlecan[14].

The mesenchyme surrounding the terminal hepatic veins is composed of 'second layer cells' – a mesenchymal cell type different from endothelial cells and myofibroblasts[15] – and the stromal components: collagen type I, type III, type V, type VI, fibronectin, undulin, and as subendothelial basement membrane components: collagen type IV and laminin[10,13].

The perisinusoidal space of Disse, located between the sinusoidal endothelial lining and the liver cell plates, contains a unique type of matrix, with perisinusoidal cells (Ito cells, fat-storing cells) and collagen type I, type III, type IV, type VI[16], fibronectin, undulin[17], small amounts of collagen type V and laminin[10,13], tenascin[18-20], thrombospondin[21] and heparan sulphate proteoglycan[14].

In spite of the presence of several basement membrane components, no continuous subendothelial basement membrane can be demonstrated by transmission electron microscopy[22,23].

A remarkable feature of the hepatic structural and functional organization is the heterogeneity of parenchymal cells, sinusoidal lining cells and matrix components in the space of Disse along the portal–hepatic axis.

Heterogeneity of parenchymal cells has been demonstrated for several structural aspects and functional characteristics of hepatocytes[24], best established for glucose metabolism[25] and ammonia metabolism[26].

Sinusoidal endothelial cells show phenotypic heterogeneity between periportal and centrolobular zones, and are distinctly different from endothelial cells in portal vessels and hepatic veins[27]. Kupffer cells are more numerous in periportal zones, whereas perisinusoidal cells predominate in centrolobular areas[23].

The matrix components in the space of Disse comprise more basement membrane constituents and hyposulphated proteoglycans in periportal zones, whereas fibrillar collagens and sulphated proteoglycans are more strongly represented in centrolobular areas[28–30].

Lobular parenchymal heterogeneity has been explained by portal–hepatic gradients in oxygen, metabolites and hormones. 'Compartmental' expression of particular functions without clear-cut gradient, as may be the case for pericentral expression of glutamine synthetase, has been explained by phenotypic determination by stromal components[31,32].

The question remains what determines the stromal and sinusoidal cell heterogeneity along the portal–central axis, be it as gradient or as compartment. Presumably, this relates to the different levels of regulation of the biological ecosystem of cells and matrix in the liver[2]. A first level of regulation is determined by the immediate microenvironment. A second level operates between different microenvironments, and may include reciprocal metabolic pathways between periportal and pericentral hepatocytes or complex networks of cytokines and intercellular reactions resulting in secondary and focally effective signals. A third level of regulation is at the inter-organ level, between the liver and other organs of the body[2].

A further explanation for parenchymal and stromal heterogeneity is provided by the 'streaming liver' concept[33] and dependence of hepatocellular and mesenchymal differentiation on lineage-position[28–30]. The 'master' regulator, which represents the basic level on which primary, secondary and further loops and networks of intercellular interactions are based – and which could explain gradients, compartments and lineage-position dependence – is the basic angioarchitecture of the liver with its interdigitating systems of afferent and efferent vessels.

Angioarchitecture

In early embryonic development of the liver the left umbilical vein is the major component of the afferent blood supply to the liver, since the placenta is the sole source of nutrients[34]. Hepatic segmentation[35] appears to be initiated and maintained by the direction and force of blood flow through the left umbilical vein[36]. At birth the ductus venosus Arantii is closed, blood flow ceases in the umbilical vein, and afferent supply is taken over by the portal vein.

In early stages of embryonic development, therefore, the primitive intrahepatic branches of the nutrient 'portal' veins comprise the umbilical vein ramifications as well as the portal vein branches (derived from the omphalomesenteric or vitelline veins)[37]. In contrast to the efferent veins of the liver, which remain thin-walled, the afferent 'portal' vessels are surrounded by a cuff of mesenchyme[38]. This observation suggests that in these early stages of development the (future) portal vein wall or its content (placental blood) induces the development of a layer of mesenchyme, a property not shared by the efferent (hepatic) veins. This periportal sleeve of mesenchyme appears to be crucial for the development of the intrahepatic bile ducts through induction of the 'ductal plate' which represents the most primitive appearance of intrahepatic bile ducts[37,39]. It thus appears that the early branching of the (future) portal vein initiates, maintains and directs the further development and structural organization of the liver.

In the adult liver the vectorial transit of portal blood from the finest ramifications of the afferent portal veins to the finest radicles of the efferent hepatic veins, along the liver sinusoids, presumably remains the key determinant of normal liver structure and function.

The heterogeneity of parenchymal cells, sinusoidal lining cells and matrix components along the portal–hepatic sinusoidal axis is usually described in terms of liver 'units'. Continuing controversy exists about the definition of the structural and functional unit of the human liver, resulting in numerous proposals: the hepatic lobule[40], the portal lobule[41], the liver acinus[42], the primary hepatic lobule[43] and the metabolic lobulus[44]. These liver 'units' can be viewed as so many aspects of structural and functional organization of the liver, perceived from different viewpoints: anatomical[40,41], angioarchitectural[43], angioarchitectural and pathological[42] or metabolic[44]. The fact remains that the human liver has no clearly defined, structurally delineated anatomical units, but rather represents a large 'continuum' of hepatic parenchyma and sinusoids[45].

The flow of blood in the sinusoids throughout this huge continuum is locally determined by the interdigitating ramification patterns of afferent and efferent vessels. In this sense the hepatic angioarchitecture is the key determinant of structural and functional organization of the liver, including the topography and heterogeneity of its mesenchymal and extracellular matrix components. Without recognition of this underlying angioarchitectural determinant it is hard to conceive why the liver looks and functions as it does, with structural landmarks such as portal tracts, central veins and lobular (or acinar) gradients and compartments. Disturbance of this normal angioarchitectural pattern is a key determinant for the irreversibility of fibrosis in case of end-stage liver fibrosis (see further: cirrhosis).

FIBROSIS OF THE LIVER

Morphological study of fibrosis

As mentioned above, the term 'fibrosis' refers to an increase in extracellular matrix components, not necessarily maintaining the normal relative proportions[1]. Three periods can be distinguished in hepatic fibrosis research[46]. The first was a descriptive period, dealing with morphological and biochemical observations, during which the increase in connective tissue in the liver was considered stable and inert. The second period, starting in the mid-1960s, could be designated as the physiological period, during which basic research on connective tissue indicated that hepatic fibrosis is a dynamic process of formation and degradation of matrix components. The third period followed since the 1980s, with quantitation of cellular and molecular events in fibrosis, characterizing it as the kinetic period[46].

Histological studies on liver fibrosis have mainly been performed with classical 'connective tissue stains'. Silver impregnation techniques for the demonstration of 'reticulin fibres' are extremely helpful in histopathological diagnostic work. It should be realized, however, that 'reticulin' does not refer to a well-defined molecule. Reticulin fibres demonstrated by empirical (and sometimes capricious) silver impregnation correspond to collagen type III with attached fibronectin and glycoprotein[47,49] and forming hybrid fibrils with collagen type I[50].

Collagen and presumably other matrix components are demonstrated with classical but non-specific 'connective tissue stains', such as Masson's trichrome, Von Gieson and Goldner stains[49].

A specific stain for collagen is Sirius red[51]. Sirius red staining for collagen allows for quantitative assessment of collagen deposition by photometric determination of eluted dye[52,53] or by quantitative histophotometry and spectrophotometry of tissue sections[54]. 'Dense connective matrix organization'[55] is recognized under the microscope by its birefringence when using polarized light[56]. Elastin is demonstrated by classical elastica stains such as orcein and victoria blue, which are useful to demonstrate areas of older collapse fibrosis[57,58].

More recent application of immunohistochemical techniques (immunofluorescence, immunoperoxidase) allows for demonstration of individual matrix components by use of appropriate monoclonal or polyclonal antibodies[14,16,18,48,49,59-62], whereas in-situ hybridization techniques confirm the synthesis of matrix molecules in particular cells by demonstration of their mRNA[63-65].

Quantitation of hepatic fibrosis by morphology-based techniques is attempted by histophotometry[54], morphometry and by the application of semi-quantitative scoring systems[66-68].

Patterns of liver fibrosis

The disadvantage of morphological techniques as compared to the biochemical approach is their qualitative rather than quantitative result. However, the advantage of morphological study lies in the possibility of recognizing different patterns of fibrosis, which allow some insight into pathogenesis of disease. Furthermore, refinements of morphological investigation by immunohistochemistry allow investigation of the change in phenotype of Ito cells involved in fibrogenesis[7,8,69-75].

Classically recognized patterns of fibrosis include the following[76].

1. *Portal fibrosis* describes increased density and fibrous enlargement of portal tracts.
2. *Pipe-stem fibrosis* (Symmer's fibrosis) is typically seen in hepatic schisto-somiasis[77].
3. *Hepatoportal sclerosis* corresponds to phlebosclerosis of portal vein branches as a result of organized mural thrombi or of portal hypertension, usually associated with some degree of portal and periportal fibrosis[78-80].
4. *Periportal fibrosis* refers to fibrous extensions irradiating from portal tracts. It may be rich in inflammatory cells (piecemeal necrosis in chronic hepatitis[81]) or paucicellular (as in alcoholic liver disease).
5. *Concentric periductal fibrosis* occurs in several 'vanishing bile duct disorders' typically in primary sclerosing cholangitis, and is a synonym of fibro-obliterating cholangitis[82]. A sequence of changes appears to occur during development of periductal fibrosis, with transient deposition of tenascin during earlier stages, followed by collagens type III and I in later stages[83].
6. *Periductular fibrosis* accompanies 'ductular reaction' in chronic cholestatic liver diseases. Ductular reaction with its accompanying periductular fibrosis is the pacemaker for progression to advanced biliary fibrosis and cirrhosis in chronic cholestatic liver disease[84,85]. Also in periductular fibrosis, tenascin expression precedes the subsequent deposition of collagens[18].
7. *Perivenular fibrosis* refers to a fibrous thickening of the wall of the terminal hepatic venule of at least 4 μm in thickness over at least two-thirds of the venular perimeter[86]. Whether this lesion indicates the alcoholic patient at risk of developing liver cirrhosis remains a matter of debate[87].
8. *Centrolobular (acinar zone 3) fibrosis* describes fibrous scarring around the terminal hepatic venules. It may be conspicuous in some forms of alcoholic liver disease, corresponding to 'sclerosing hyaline necrosis'[88].
9. *Pericellular or perisinusoidal fibrosis* refers to collagen and matrix deposition around single liver parenchymal cells or small groups of hepatocytes, predominantly in acinar zone 3. In alcoholic liver disease this pattern was described as 'chicken-wire fibrosis'[78-80].
10. *Septal fibrosis* indicates fibrosis in the form of fibrous sheets. It occurs in various topographical patterns (portal–portal septa; central–central septa; portal–central septa) according to the type of vascular canals linked by connective tissue membranes[89,90]. The mesenchymal cells in fibrous septa include Ito cells[91,92] and fibroblasts[15].
11. *Portal–portal septa* link adjacent portal tracts. They result from extending ductular reaction in chronic cholestasis, or from progressive piecemeal necrosis in chronic active hepatitis.
12. *Central–central septa* extend between adjacent terminal hepatic venules (or central veins), representing the scarring stage of central–central bridging necrosis (confluent necrosis in the microcirculatory periphery

of the complex acinus according to Rappaport)[89].

13. *Portal–central septa* connect portal tracts and central veins, usually resulting from portal–central bridging necrosis (confluent necrosis in the microcirculatory periphery of the simple acinus according to Rappaport)[89].

14. *Active septa* represent connective tissue sheets which are infiltrated by mononuclear inflammatory cells with imprecise delineation from the adjacent parenchyma. They can be conceived of as representing extensive degrees of piecemeal necrosis[89]. Immunologically competent cells in active septa may stimulate progressive fibrosis by production of fibrogenic cytokines[93].

15. *Passive septa* are connective tissue membranes which are rich in fibres and poor in cells, sharply delineated from the adjacent parenchyma. They derive from postnecrotic collapse and fibrous healing after extensive confluent lytic necrosis[78,89]. Older passive septa (more than 6 months) contain elastic fibres[57].

16. *Primary collapse* indicates postnecrotic collapse and fibrous scarring after confluent necrosis in a previously normal parenchyma. The topographical spacing of the approximated portal tracts and terminal hepatic venules is more or less preserved[79].

17. *Secondary collapse* corresponds to postnecrotic collapse and fibrous scarring following extensive necrosis in abnormal parenchymal territories (e.g. in cirrhosis), resulting in loss of the reciprocal spacing of afferent and efferent vessels[79].

18. *Biliary fibrosis* is characterized by periportal and portal–portal septa, encircling garland-shaped parenchymal nodules. It represents an advanced but potentially reversible state of chronic bile-duct disease[94,95], often confused with true biliary cirrhosis. It differs from cirrhosis in that the basic lobular architecture and vascular relationships are preserved[79,82,84,96].

19. *Cirrhosis* is a special form of fibrosis, discussed under a separate section below.

CIRRHOSIS OF THE LIVER

Definition

Cirrhosis of the liver is defined as 'a diffuse process characterized by fibrosis and a conversion of normal architecture into structurally abnormal nodules'[97,98]. Implicit in this definition is the association of important vascular changes: the development of intrahepatic porto-hepatic vascular shunts[99]. The diffuse nature of liver cirrhosis excludes from its definition focal lesions such as focal nodular hyperplasia, which – like cirrhosis – are characterized by fibrous septa and parenchymal nodules. The septal fibrosis distinguishes cirrhosis from non-fibrotic lesions such as nodular regenerative hyperplasia which – like cirrhosis – are diffuse and nodular. The nodularity of cirrhosis (with the associated abnormality in intrahepatic blood flow) distinguishes cirrhosis from other forms of diffuse fibrosis, e.g. pipe-stem fibrosis in chronic schistosomiasis.

Pathogenesis

Virtually all chronic progressive liver diseases may lead to the end stage of liver cirrhosis. Different main pathogenetic pathways for cirrhosis development can be recognized, some of them combined in a single liver disease[100].

1. *The hepatitic pathway* is typically involved in chronic active hepatitis, whatever its aetiology. The main mechanisms involved are piecemeal necrosis and confluent lytic necrosis (portal–central bridging necrosis and multilobular necrosis).
2. *The steatohepatitis pathway* involves mechanisms of acinar zone 3 damage and pericellular fibrosis, progressively extending to the portal tracts. It operates in alcoholic liver disease, and in non-alcoholic liver disease resembling alcoholic hepatitis, which may be observed in obese patients with non-insulin-dependent diabetes and in amiodarone toxicity[100].
3. *The portal–periportal fibrosis* pathway is mostly seen in chronic biliary disease and in genetic haemochromatosis[100].
4. *The acinar zone 3 fibrosis* (centrolobular scarring pathway) is typically seen in prolonged venous outflow block at any level from the smaller draining veins (veno-occlusive disease) to the pericardium (constrictive pericarditis)[100].

The last two pathways do not lead by themselves to true cirrhosis, since the development of fibrotic septa in both instances leads to connections between vessels of the same type: afferent vessels in the portal–periportal fibrosis pathway and efferent vessels in the centrolobular scarring pathway.

This explains why normal lobular metabolic zonation is preserved in the parenchymal nodules in both conditions[101–103], but with opposite directions of blood flow; the efferent vessels are at the nodular periphery in 'toxic' (centrolobular scarring pathway) 'cirrhosis', whereas afferent vessels occupy the nodular periphery in experimental biliary 'cirrhosis'.

However, in both pathways the key disturbance of intrahepatic microcirculation typical for true cirrhosis is lacking, since neither pathway by itself leads to the development of direct portal–central connections associated with extraparenchymal shunting of blood. This event occurs only in later complicated stages of these conditions, explaining the slow development of true cirrhosis in only a small percentage of such cases[84,96,100].

Disturbance of intrahepatic circulation

These observations indicate that the quintessence of a 'cirrhotic' pattern of fibrosis implies a disturbance in intrahepatic angioarchitecture with development of intrahepatic portal–hepatic shunts[99,104]. The portal–hepatic shunts have classically been interpreted as being derived from sinusoids which remained open and perfused in the collapsing stroma[105,106]. However, new formation of vessels (neoangiogenesis) is apparently also involved[104].

In a true cirrhotic pattern of fibrosis the parenchymal nodules lack normal metabolic gradients[104]; the corollary is a great diversity in sinusoidal abnormalities[107].

Reduction or lack of portal blood flow in the sinusoids (arterialization) causes alterations in sinusoidal lining cells and in matrix components of the space of Disse, as demonstrated after portacaval shunt in experimental animals[108].

In true cirrhosis of the liver, vascular networks develop in the fibrous septa surrounding the nodules. These networks include portal–hepatic anastomoses[105,106] and feeding vessels which vascularize the parenchymal nodules from their periphery[99]. The feeding vessels are predominantly arterial, leading to 'arterialization' of cirrhotic nodules[109-111]. Consequently, the development of intrahepatic portal–hepatic shunts has profound effects on liver structure and function. First, it leads to loss of normal gradients of hepatocellular function and of sinusoidal phenotype, as mentioned above. Second, it is the key event which determines the irreversibility of the cirrhotic pattern of fibrosis.

Fibrosis by itself is potentially reversible, due to the existence of numerous mechanisms and enzymes involved in degradation of extracellular matrix components[112,113]. However, fibrosis associated with an altered intrahepatic angioarchitecture has evolved beyond a point of no return, and becomes irreversible. Published reports on reversibility of cirrhosis are subject to criticism, since most reported cases correspond to advanced biliary fibrosis rather than true cirrhosis[96], and because liver biopsy studies may suffer from sampling errors[114]. These considerations do not deny that some forms of fibrosis may become less degradable due to inter- and intra-crosslinking of matrix molecules[115,116].

It appears that hepatic angioarchitecture is a master regulator not only of liver development, structure and function (see above), but also a basic determinant of the irreversibility of the cirrhotic pattern of fibrosis.

Liver dysfunction in cirrhosis

Disturbance of liver parenchymal function in cirrhosis results from an interplay of numerous contributing factors. The development of extrahepatic portosystemic shunts and intrahepatic portal–hepatic anastomoses deprives the liver parenchyma from a variable part of the afferent blood supply, which may have repercussions on functional reserve capacity of the liver. In cirrhotic nodules the sinusoidal lining is changed, corresponding to 'capillarization of sinusoids'[117]. Although this change may not be universal throughout each nodule[107], it hampers the normal metabolic exchange between blood and hepatocytes[118-120].

The regenerating parenchyma in cirrhotic nodules appears hyperplastic, with liver cell plates more than one cell thick (muralium multiplex)[45], thus lowering the accessibility of numerous hepatocytes for nutrients supplied by sinusoidal blood[121]. Furthermore, regenerating parenchyma may be variably immature, and deficient in more or less highly specialized functions characteristic of fully differentiated parenchyma.

Loss of normal metabolic gradients and/or compartments may have repercussion on metabolic pathways based on reciprocal gene expression in opposite acinar locations, as is the case for glucose[25] and ammonia metabolism[26], and result in less altruistic and more autistic behaviour of cirrhotic nodules[25,122].

Parenchymal cell disturbance and even necrosis may result from anoxia precipitated by variceal haemorrhage due to portal hypertension[123]. In addition, parenchymal function may be reduced by hepatocellular lesions intrinsic to the primary hepatic disease which caused the progressive fibrosis and eventually cirrhosis: perpetuation of necro-inflammatory lesions in chronic viral hepatitis B, D and C, and in autoimmune and drug-induced chronic hepatitis; continuing bile acid overload and retention of cholephiles in prolonged cholestatic and biliary disease; progressive iron or copper overload in idiopathic haemochromatosis or Wilson's disease; persistence of hepatocellular lesions in chronic alcoholism, and increasing overload of metabolites due to genetic enzyme defects in several storage diseases.

All these variables may differ between individual patients, and may even fluctuate during the evolution of the cirrhogenic disease in individual patients. A typical example is provided by the exacerbations of disease activity in chronic viral hepatitis B and C. It follows that no single experimental model of cirrhosis is equal to the pathological condition in humans[124,125].

Experimental cirrhosis

Experimental models of liver cirrhosis produced in laboratory animals are nonetheless of great value, and continue to provide new insights in cellular and molecular mechanisms of fibrogenesis and physiopathological consequences of chronic fibrosing liver disease, provided that extrapolation from experimental results to the human disease is applied with due caution.

Experimental cirrhosis in animals has been produced by various procedures[125]. Toxic agents used include carbon tetrachloride, dimethylnitrosamine and thioacetamide. Nutritional manipulations comprise diets rich in fat and low in choline and protein, or low protein–low methionine diets supplemented with ethionine. Immunological induction of experimental cirrhosis is achieved by injection of heterologous serum, bacterial cell walls, endotoxin or infestation with *Schistosoma mansoni*.

Biliary cirrhosis is readily induced by ligation of the common bile duct, whereas alcohol-induced cirrhosis is obtained in baboons by an ethanol-containing liquid diet and in rats by intragastric infusion of ethanol and a high-fat diet[125].

Classification of cirrhosis

Numerous attempts at classification of cirrhosis during the past century may have created more confusion than insight[126,127]. At present a morphological classification of cirrhosis distinguishes between micronodular, macronodular and combined micro-macronodular cirrhosis[97,98]. A somewhat special variant of the macronodular variety is so-called incomplete septal cirrhosis[128,129].

More important than the morphological subgroups is an aetiological classification of cirrhosis, which includes virtually all types of chronic liver disease: toxic and drug-induced liver disease, infections (hepatitis viruses B, C, D and *Schistosoma japonicum*), autoimmune liver disease (chronic active hepatitis and primary biliary cirrhosis), metabolic liver diseases, biliary obstruction, vascular lesions and a miscellaneous group of conditions including so-called neonatal hepatitis and sarcoidosis.

Actual aetiological classifications of cirrhosis are tabulated and extensively described in recent textbooks[113,130,131]. Even today, each aetiological classification of cirrhosis includes the category of 'cryptogenic' cirrhosis, awaiting the new discoveries still to be made.

Differential diagnosis of cirrhosis

During the second half of this century a number of conditions have been identified which clinically or morphologically may be confused with cirrhosis of the liver[126,132].

1. *Idiopathic portal hypertension* (or hepatoportal sclerosis) refers to patients with portal hypertension, in whom all other causes of portal hypertension, including cirrhosis, have been excluded[133]. The incomplete septal type of macronodular cirrhosis appears to be on the borderline between cirrhosis and non-cirrhotic portal hypertension[129,134].
2. *Nodular regenerative hyperplasia* is characterized by diffuse, regular nodularity of the liver without real septal fibrosis. It appears to be related to obliterative lesions of intrahepatic portal vein branches[135,136]. The same applies to *partial nodular transformation*[135,136].
3. *Focal nodular hyperplasia* resembles a biliary type of cirrhosis microscopically[137] but is a focal lesion, also associated with portal vascular lesions[135,136].
4. *Congenital hepatic fibrosis* can be conceived of as a biliary type of fibrosis, with intrahepatic bile ducts in immature, embryological shapes[138,139].

Use of liver biopsy in cirrhosis

Liver biopsy is essential for confirmation of the diagnosis of cirrhosis, although sampling errors should always be kept in mind, especially in the case of macronodular cirrhosis[80,113,132,140].

Microscopic examination of the liver biopsy allows for[114,132]:

1. confirmation of the presence of cirrhosis;

2. evaluation of the stage of progression of cirrhosis (early, fully developed, advanced);
3. evaluation of the activity of the disease;
4. contribution to the aetiological diagnosis of cirrhosis;
5. identification of complications of cirrhosis, including hepatocellular carcinoma.

References

1. Gressner AM. Major topics of fibrosis research: 1990 update. In: Wisse E, Knook DL, McCuskey RS, editors. Cells of the hepatic sinusoids, Vol. 3. Leiden: Kupffer Cell Foundation; 1991:136–44.
2. Rojkind M, Greenwel P. Pathophysiology of liver fibrosis. In: McIntyre N, Benhamou J-P, Bircher J et al., editors. Oxford textbook of clinical hepatology, Vol. I. Oxford: Oxford University Press; 1991:375–80.
3. Gressner AM, Mayer D. The role of proteoglycans in liver fibrogenesis. In: Gressner AM, Ramadori G, editors. Molecular and cell biology of liver fibrogenesis. Dordrecht: Kluwer; 1992:115–36.
4. Trelstad RL. Glycosaminoglycans: mortar, matrix, mentor. Lab Invest. 1985;53:1–4.
5. Bruggeman LA, Kopp JB, Klotman PE. Progressive renal failure: role of extracellular matrix protein deposition in the renal mesangium. In: Clément B, Guillouzo A, editors. Cellular and molecular aspects of cirrhosis, Vol. 216. London: Colloque INSERM/John Libbey Eurotext; 1992:199–209.
6. Takahashi T. Lobular structure of the human liver from the viewpoint of hepatic vascular architecture. Tohoku J Exp Med. 1970;101:119–40.
7. Miyazaki H, Van Eyken P, Roskams T et al. Transient expression of tenascin in experimentally induced cholestatic fibrosis in rat liver: an immunohistochemical study. In: Gressner AM, Ramadori G, editors. Molecular and cell biology of liver fibrogenesis. Dordrecht: Kluwer; 1992:176–80.
8. Miyazaki H, Van Eyken P, Roskams T et al. Transient expression of tenascin in experimentally induced cholestatic fibrosis in rat liver. An immunohistochemical study. J Hepatol. 1993 (In press).
9. Sappino AP, Schürch W, Gabbiani G. Differentiation repertoire of fibroblastic cells: expression of cytoskeletal proteins as marker of phenotypic modulations. Lab Invest. 1990;63:144–61.
10. Schuppan D. Structure of the extracellular matrix in normal and fibrotic liver: collagens and glycoproteins. Semin Liver Dis. 1990;10:1–10.
11. Schuppan D, Somasundaram R, Just M. The extracellular matrix: a major signal transduction network. In: Clément B, Guillouzo A, editors. Cellular and molecular aspects of cirrhosis. London: Colloque INSERM/John Libbey Eurotext; 1992:115–34.
12. Schuppan D, Milani S. The extracellular matrix in cellular communication. In: Gressner AM, Ramadori G, editors. Molecular and cell biology of liver fibrogenesis. Dordrecht: Kluwer; 1992:52–71.
13. Martinez-Hernandez A, Amenta PS. Morphology, localization, and origin of the hepatic extracellular matrix. In: Zern MA, Reid LM, editors. Extracellular matrix: chemistry, biology and pathobiology with emphasis on the liver. New York: Marcel Dekker; 1993:255–327.
14. Rescan P-Y, Loréal O, Hassell JR et al. Distribution and origin of the basement membrane component perlecan in rat liver and primary hepatocyte culture. Am J Pathol. 1993;142:199–208.
15. Bhunchet E, Wake K. Role of mesenchymal cell populations in porcine-serum-induced rat liver fibrosis. Hepatology. 1992;16:1452–73.
16. Griffiths MR, Shepherd M, Ferrier R et al. Light microscopic and ultrastructural distribution of type VI collagen in human liver: alterations in chronic biliary disease. Histopathology. 1992;21:335–44.

17. Knittel T, Armbrust T, Schwögler S et al. Distribution and cellular origin of undulin in rat liver. Lab Invest. 1992;67:779–87.
18. Van Eyken P, Sciot R, Desmet VJ. Expression of the novel extracellular matrix component tenascin in normal and diseased human liver. An immunohistochemical study. J Hepatol. 1990;11:43–52.
19. Van Eyken P, Geerts A, De Bleser P et al. Localization and cellular source of the extracellular matrix protein tenascin in normal and fibrotic rat liver. Hepatology. 1992;15:909–16.
20. Ramadori G. The stellate cell (Ito cell, fat storing cell, lipocyte, perisinusoidal cell) of the liver. New insights into an intriguing cell. Virchows Arch B. 1991;61:147–58.
21. Rieder H, Ramadori G, Schwögler S et al. Thrombospondin, a matrix protein of the Disse space, is mainly produced by sinusoidal endothelial liver cells. In: Gressner AM, Ramadori G, editors. Molecular and cell biology of liver fibrogenesis. Dordrecht: Kluwer; 1992: 172–5.
22. Bioulac-Sage P, Lafon ME, Le Bail B et al. Ultrastructure of sinusoids in liver disease. In: Bioulac-Sage P, Balabaud C, editors. Sinusoids in human liver: health and disease. Rijswijk: Kupffer Cell Foundation; 19988:223–78.
23. Desmet VJ. Organizational principles. In: Arias I, Boyer J, Fausto N et al., editors. The liver: biology and pathobiology, 3rd edn. New York: Raven Press (In press).
24. Gumucio JJ, Chianale J. Liver cell heterogeneity and liver function. In: Arias IM, Jakoby WB, Popper H et al., editors. The liver: biology and pathobiology, 2nd edn. New York: Raven Press; 1988:931–47.
25. Jungermann K, Katz N. Functional hepatocellular heterogeneity. Hepatology. 1982;2: 385–95.
26. Häussinger D. Nitrogen metabolism in liver: structural and functional organization and physiological relevance. Biochem J. 1990;267:281–90.
27. Scoazec J-Y, Racine L, Couvelard A et al. Endothelial cell heterogeneity in the normal human liver acinus: in situ immunohistochemical demonstration. Liver (In press).
28. Reid LM, Fiorino AS, Sigal SH et al. Extracellular matrix gradients in the space of Disse: relevance to liver biology. Hepatology. 1992;15:1198–203.
29. Sigal SH, Brill S, Fiorino AS et al. The liver as a stem cell and lineage system. Am J Physiol. 1992;263:G139–48.
30. Sigal SH, Brill S, Fiorino AS et al. The liver as a stem cell and lineage system. In: Zern MA, Reid LM, editors. Extracellular matrix: chemistry, biology and pathobiology with emphasis on the liver. New York: Marcel Dekker; 1993:507–38.
31. Lamers WH, Moorman AFM, Charles R. The metabolic lobulus, a key to the architecture of the liver. In: Gumucio JJ, editor. Revisiones sobre biologia cellular. Cell biology reviews, Vol. 19. Berlin: Springer; 1989:5–26.
32. Gebhardt R, Ebert A, Bauer G. Heterogeneous expression of glutamine synthetase mRNA in rat liver parenchyma revealed by in situ hybridization and northern blot analysis of RNA from periportal and perivenous hepatocytes. FEBS Lett. 1988;241:89–93.
33. Arber N, Zajicek G, Ariel I. The streaming liver. II. Hepatocyte life history. Liver. 1988;8:80–7.
34. MacSween RNM, Scothorne RJ. Developmental anatomy and normal structure. In: MacSween RNM, Anthony PP, Scheuer PJ, editors. Pathology of the liver, 2nd edn. Edinburgh: Churchill Livingstone; 1987:1–45.
35. Couinaud C. Le foie. Etudes Anatomiques et Chirurgicales. Paris: Masson; 1957.
36. Lassau JP, Bastian D. Organogenesis of the venous structures of the human liver: a hemodynamic theory. Anat Clin. 1983;5:97–102.
37. Desmet VJ. Embryology of the liver and intrahepatic biliary tract, and an overview of malformations of the bile duct. In: McIntyre N, Benhamou J-P, Bircher J et al. The Oxford textbook of clinical hepatology, Vol. 1. Oxford: Oxford University Press; 1991:497–519.
38. Mollier S. Die Entwicklung des periportalen Gallengangnetzes und der Gefäsze in der embryonalen Leber des Menschen. Gegenbaurs Morphol Jahrb. 1939;83:569–600.
39. Van Eyken P, Sciot R, Callea F et al. The development of the intrahepatic bile ducts in man: a keratin-immunohistochemical study. Hepatology. 1988;8:1586–95.
40. Kiernan F. The anatomy and physiology of the liver. Phil Trans R Soc Lond. 1833;123: 711–70.

41. Mall FP. A study of the structural unit of the liver. Am J Anat. 1906;5:227–308.
42. Rappaport AM. The microcirculatory acinar concept of normal and pathological hepatic structure. Beitr Pathol. 1976;157:215–43.
43. Matsumoto R, Kawakami M. The unit-concept of hepatic parenchyma – a re-examination based on angioarchitectural studies. Acta Pathol Jpn. 1982;32:285–314.
44. Lamers WH, Hilberts A, Furt E et al. Hepatic enzymic zonation: a reevaluation of the concept of the liver acinus. Hepatology. 1989;10:72–6.
45. Elias H, Sherrick JC. Morphology of the liver. New York: Academic Press; 1969.
46. Popper H. Summary of the conference. In: Gerlach U, Pott G, Rauterberg J et al., editors. Connective tissue of the normal and fibrotic human liver. Stuttgart: Georg Thieme Verlag; 1982:246–58.
47. Unsworth DJ, Scott DL, Almond TJ et al. Studies on reticulin. Stereological and immunohistological investigation of the occurrence of collagen type III, fibronectin and the non-collagenous glycoprotein of Pras and Glynn in reticulin. Br J Exp Pathol. 1982;63:154–66.
48. Martinez-Hernandez A. The hepatic extracellular matrix. I. Electron immunohistochemical studies in normal rat liver. Lab Invest. 1984;51:57–74.
49. Martinez-Hernandez A. The hepatic extracellular matrix. II. Electron immunohistochemical studies in rats with CCl$_4$-induced cirrhosis. Lab Invest. 1985;53:166–86.
50. Geerts A, Schuppan D, Lazeroms S et al. Collagen type I and III occur together in hybrid fibrils in the space of Disse of normal rat liver. Hepatology. 1990;12:233–41.
51. Junqueira LCA, Bignolas G, Brentani RR. A simple and sensitive method for the quantitative estimation of collagen. Anal Biochem. 1979;94:96–9.
52. Lopez de Leon A, Rojkind M. A simple micromethod for collagen and total protein determination in formalin-fixed paraffin-embedded sections. J Histochem Cytochem. 1985;33:737–43.
53. Jimenez W, Pares A, Caballeria J et al. Measurement of fibrosis in needle liver biopsies: evaluation of a colorimetric method. Hepatology. 1985;5:815–18.
54. James J, Bosck KS, Aronson DC et al. Sirius Red histophotometry and spectrophotometry of sections in the assessment of the collagen content of liver tissue and its application in growing rat liver. Liver. 1990;10:1–5.
55. Grimaud J-A, Druguet M, Peyrol S et al. Collagen immunotyping in human liver: light and electron microscope study. J Histochem Cytochem. 1980;28:1145–56.
56. Popper H, Udenfriend S. Hepatic fibrosis. Am J Med. 1970;49:707–21.
57. Scheuer PJ, Maggi G. Hepatic fibrosis and collapse: histological distinction by orcein staining. Histopathology. 1980;4:487–90.
58. Bedossa P, Lemaigre G, Paraf F, Martin E. Deposition and remodelling of elastic fibres in chronic hepatitis. Virchows Arch A. 1990;417:159–62.
59. Clément B, Grimaud JA, Campion JP et al. Cell types involved in collagen and fibronectin production in normal and fibrotic human liver. Hepatology. 1986;6:225–34.
60. Clement B, Loreal O, Rescan P-Y et al. Cellular origin of the hepatic extracellular matrix. In: Gressner AM, Ramadori G, editors. Molecular and cell biology of liver fibrogenesis. Dordrecht: Kluwer; 1992:85–98.
61. Porto LC, Chevallier M, Guerret S et al. Elastin in alcoholic liver disease. An immunohistochemical and immunoelectron microscopic study. Pathol Res Pract. 1990;186:668–79.
62. Peyrol S, Grimaud JA. Perisinusoidal connective matrix. Immunohistochemical mapping of the major matricial components. In: Bioulac-Sage P, Balabaud C, editors. Sinusoids in human liver: health and disease. Rijswijk: Kupffer Cell Foundation; 1988:323–40.
63. Milani S, Herbst H, Schuppan D et al. Procollagen expression by nonparenchymal rat liver cells in experimental biliary fibrosis. Gastroenterology. 1990;98:175–84.
64. Milani S, Herbst H, Schuppan D et al. Transforming growth factors β1 and β2 are differentially expressed in fibrotic liver disease. Am J Pathol. 1991;139:1221–9.
65. Herbst H, Milani S, Heinrichs O et al. Pathomorphologie akuter und chronischer Stadien der CCl$_4$-induzierten Leberfibrose: immunohistochemische und in situ Hybridisierungsuntersuchungen. Z Gastroenterol. 1992;30(Suppl 1):21–8.
66. Knodell RG, Ishak KG, Black WC et al. Formulation and application of a numerical scoring system for assessing histological activity in asymptomatic chronic active hepatitis. Hepatology. 1981;1:431–5.

67. Scheuer PJ. Classification of chronic viral hepatitis: a need for reassessment. J Hepatol. 1991;13:372–4.
68. Chevallier M, Chossegros P, Guerret S et al. Validation of a histological scoring system for hepatic fibrosis: comparison with morphometric data. Hepatology. 1992;16:181A.
69. Ballardini G, Fallani M, Biagini G et al. Desmin and actin in the identification of Ito cells and in monitoring their evolution to myofibroblasts in experimental liver fibrosis. Virchows Arch B Cell Pathol. 1988;56:45–9.
70. Ballardini G, Giostra F, Groff P et al. Co-distribution in normal and diseased liver of iso-alpha-actin-positive cells and collagen type III. In: Gressner AM, Ramadori G, editors. Molecular and cell biology of liver fibrogenesis. Dordrecht: Kluwer; 1992:75–7.
71. Schmitt-Gräff A, Krüger S, Bochard F et al. Modulation of alpha smooth muscle actin and desmin expression in perisinusoidal cells of normal and diseased human livers. Am J Pathol. 1991;138:1233–42.
72. Johnson SJ, Hines JE, Burt AD. Phenotypic modulation of perisinusoidal cells following acute liver injury: a quantitative analysis. Int J Exp Pathol. 1992;73:765–72.
73. Nouchi T, Tanaka Y, Tsukada T et al. Appearance of alpha smooth-muscle-actin positive cells in hepatic fibrosis. Liver. 1991;11:100–5.
74. Rockey DC, Boyles JK, Gabbiani G et al. Smooth muscle specific actin in an experimental model of hepatic fibrosis. In: Wisse E, Knook DL, McCuskey RS, editors. Cells of the hepatic sinusoid, Vol. 3. Leiden: Kupffer Cell Foundation; 1991:177–9.
75. Tanaka Y, Nouchi T, Yamane M et al. Phenotypic modulation in lipocytes in experimental liver fibrosis. J Pathol. 1991;164:273–8.
76. Desmet VJ. General pathology. In: McIntyre N, Benhamou J-P, Bircher J et al., editors. Oxford textbook of clinical hepatology, Vol. 1. Oxford: Oxford University Press; 1991:263–9.
77. Grimaud JA, Borojevic R. Chronic human Schistosomiasis mansoni. Pathology of the Disse's space. Lab Invest. 1977;36:268–73.
78. Bianchi L. Liver biopsy interpretation in hepatitis. Part I. Presentation of critical morphologic features used in diagnosis (Glossary). Pathol Res Pract. 1983;178:2–19.
79. Popper H. General pathology of the liver: light microscopic aspects serving diagnosis and interpretation. Semin Liver Dis. 1986;6:175–84.
80. Scheuer PJ. Liver biopsy interpretation, 4th edn. London: Baillière Tindall; 1988.
81. Takahara T, Nakayama Y, Itoh H et al. Extracellular matrix formation in piecemeal necrosis: immunoelectron microscopic study. Liver. 1992;12:368–80.
82. Ludwig J. New concepts in biliary cirrhosis. Semin Liver Dis. 1987;7:293–301.
83. Van Eyken P, Desmet V. Immunohistology of primary sclerosing cholangitis. In: Meyer zum Büschenfelde KH, Hoofnagle J, Manns M, editors. Immunology and liver. Dordrecht: Kluwer; 1993:307–17.
84. Desmet VJ. Cirrhosis: aetiology and pathogenesis: cholestasis. In: Boyer JL, Bianchi L, editors. Liver cirrhosis. Falk Symposium 44. Lancaster: MTP Press; 1987:101–18.
85. Desmet VJ. Cholestasis: extrahepatic obstruction and secondary biliary cirrhosis. In: MacSween RNM, Anthony PP, Scheuer PJ, editors. Pathology of the liver, 2nd edn. Edinburgh: Churchill Livingstone; 1987:364–423.
86. Van Waes L, Lieber CS. Early perivenular sclerosis in alcoholic fatty liver: an index of progressive liver injury. Gastroenterology. 1977;73:646–50.
87. Maher JJ. Hepatic fibrosis caused by alcohol. Semin Liver Dis. 1990;10:66–74.
88. Edmondson HA, Peters RL, Reynolds TB et al. Sclerosing hyaline necrosis in the liver of the chronic alcoholic. A recognizable syndrome. Ann Intern Med. 1963;59:646–73.
89. International Group. Acute and chronic hepatitis revisited. Lancet. 1977;2:914–19.
90. Desmet VJ. Acute viral hepatitis: hepatitis B. In: Gitnick G, editor. Modern concepts of acute and chronic hepatitis. New York: Plenum; 1989:87–111.
91. Ballardini G, Degli Esposti S, Bianchi FB et al. Correlation between Ito cells and fibrogenesis in an experimental model of hepatic fibrosis. A sequential stereological study. Liver. 1983;3:58–63.
92. Takahara T, Kojima T, Miayabayashi C et al. Collagen production in fat-storing cells after carbon tetrachloride intoxication in the rat. Immunoelectron microscopic observation of type I, type III collagens, and prolyl hydroxylase. Lab Invest. 1988;59:509–21.
93. Kovacs EJ. Fibrogenic cytokines: the role of immune mediators in the development of scar tissue. Immunol Today. 1991;12:17–22.

271

94. Aronson DC, Chamuleau RAFM, Frederiks WM et al. Reversibility of cholestatic changes following experimental common bile duct obstruction: fact or fantasy? J Hepatol. 1993;18:85–95.
95. Abdel-Aziz G, Lebeau G, Rescan PY et al. Reversibility of hepatic fibrosis in experimentally induced cholestasis in rat. Am J Pathol. 1990;137:1333–42.
96. Weinbren K, Hadjis NS, Blumgart LH. Structural aspects of the liver in patients with biliary disease and portal hypertension. J Clin Pathol. 1985;38:1013–20.
97. Anthony PP, Ishak KG, Nayak NC et al. The morphology of cirrhosis: definition, nomenclature and classification. Bull WHO. 1977;55:521–40.
98. Anthony PP, Ishak KG, Nayak NC et al. The morphology of cirrhosis. J Clin Pathol. 1978;31:395–414.
99. Rappaport AM, McPhee PJ, Fisher MM et al. The scarring of the liver acini (cirrhosis). Tridimensional and microcirculatory considerations. Virchows Arch [A]. 1983;402: 107–37.
100. Scheuer PJ. Cirrhosis: pathology. In: McIntyre N, Benhamou J-P, Bircher J et al., editors. Oxford textbook of clinical hepatology, Vol. 1. Oxford: Oxford University Press; 1991: 371–5.
101. Sokal EM, Collette E, Buts JP. Persistence of a liver metabolic zonation in extra-hepatic biliary atresia cirrhotic livers. Pediatr Res. 1991;30:286–9.
102. Sokal EM, Trivedi P, Portmann B et al. Adaptive changes of metabolic zonation during the development of cirrhosis in growing rats. Gastroenterology. 1990;99:785–92.
103. Sokal EM, Mostin J, Buts J-P. Liver metabolic zonation in rat biliary cirrhosis: distribution is reverse of that in toxic cirrhosis. Hepatology. 1992;15:904–8.
104. Gaudio E, Pannarale L, Onori P et al. A scanning electron microscopic study of liver microcirculation disarrangement in experimental rat cirrhosis. Hepatology. 1993;17: 477–85.
105. Popper H, Elias H, Petty DE. Vascular patterns of the cirrhotic liver. Am J Clin Pathol. 1952;22:717–29.
106. Popper H. Pathologic aspects of cirrhosis. Am J Pathol. 1977;87:228–64.
107. Bioulac-Sage P, LeBail B, Carles J et al. and the PATH group. Ultrastructure of sinusoids in human cirrhotic nodules. In: Clément B, Guillouzo A, editors. Cellular and molecular aspects of cirrhosis. London: Colloque INSERM/John Libbey Eurotext; 1992:91–101.
108. Dubuisson L, Bedin C, Boussarie L et al. Liver sinusoids and hemodynamic disturbance. In: Bioulac-Sage P, Balabaud C, editors. Sinusoids in human liver: health and disease. Rijswijk: Kupffer Cell Foundation; 1988:279–98.
109. Yamamoto T, Kobayashi T, Phillips MJ. Perinodular arteriolar plexus in liver cirrhosis. Scanning electron microscopy of microvascular casts. Liver. 1984;4:50–4.
110. Haratake J, Hisaoka M, Yamamoto Y et al. Morphological changes of hepatic microcirculation in experimental rat cirrhosis: a scanning electron microscopic study. Hepatology. 1991;13:952–6.
111. Hirooka N, Iwasaki I, Horie H et al. Hepatic microcirculation of the liver cirrhosis studied by corrosion cast/scanning electron microscope examination. Acta Pathol Jpn. 1986;36: 375–87.
112. Arthur MJP. The role of matrix degradation in liver fibrosis. In: Gressner AM, Ramadori G, editors. Molecular and cell biology of liver fibrogenesis. Dordrecht: Kluwer; 1992: 213–27.
113. Friedman SL, Millward-Sadler GH, Arthur MJP. Liver fibrosis and cirrhosis. In: Millward-Sadler GH, Wright R, Arthur MJP, editors. Wright's liver and biliary disease. Pathophysiology, diagnosis and management, Vol. 2, 3rd edn. London: WB Saunders; 1992:821–81.
114. Scheuer PJ. Liver biopsy in the diagnosis of cirrhosis. Gut. 1970;11:275–8.
115. Ricard-Blum S, Bresson-Hadni S, Vuitton DA et al. Hydroxypyridinium collagen cross-links in human liver fibrosis: study of alveolar echinococcosis. Hepatology. 1992;15: 599–602.
116. Clément B, Loréal O, Levavasseur F et al. New challenges in hepatic fibrosis. J Hepatol. 1993;18:1–4.
117. Schaffner F, Popper H. Capillarization of hepatic sinusoids in man. Gastroenterology. 1963;44:239–42.

118. Martinez-Hernandez A, Martinez J. The role of capillarization in hepatic failure: studies in carbon tetrachloride-induced cirrhosis. Hepatology. 1991;14:864–74.

119. Couvelard A, Scoazec JY, Feldmann G. Expression of laminin receptors and intercellular adhesion molecules by sinusoidal endothelial cells is correlated with laminin deposition in the perisinusoidal matrix of human cirrhotic nodules. Hepatology. 1992;16:101A.

120. Mori T, Okanoue T, Sawa Y et al. Defenestration of the sinusoidal endothelial cell in a rat model of cirrhosis. Hepatology. 1993;17:891–7.

121. Martinez-Hernandez A, Martinez Delgado F, Amenta PS. The extracellular matrix in hepatic regeneration. Localization of collagen types I, III, IV, laminin and fibronectin. Lab Invest. 1991;64:157–66.

122. Nuber T, Teutsch HF, Sasse D. Metabolic zonation in thioacetamide-induced liver cirrhosis. Histochemistry. 1980;69:277–88.

123. Popper H, Schaffner F. Liver: structure and function. The Blakiston Division. New York: McGraw-Hill; 1957.

124. Perez Tamayo R. Is cirrhosis of the liver experimentally produced by CCl_4 an adequate model of human cirrhosis? Hepatology. 1983;3:112–20.

125. Tsukamoto H, Matsuoka M, French SW. Experimental models of hepatic fibrosis: a review. Semin Liver Dis. 1990;10:56–65.

126. Desmet V. Liver cirrhosis: evolving aspects of an old problem. In: Clément B, Guillouzo A, editors. Cellular and molecular aspects of cirrhosis. Montrouge: Colloque INSERM/John Libbey Eurotext; 1992:1–9.

127. Schaffner F, Sieratzki JS. The early history of cirrhosis. In: Boyer JL, Bianchi L, editors. Liver cirrhosis. Lancaster: MTP Press; 1987:57–72.

128. Popper H. What are the major types of hepatic cirrhosis? In: Ingelfinger F, Relman A, Finland M, editors. Controversy in internal medicine. Philadelphia: Saunders; 1966: 233–43.

129. Sciot R, Staessen D, Van Damme B et al. Incomplete septal cirrhosis: histopathological aspects. Histopathology. 1988;13:593–603.

130. Sherlock S, Dooley J. Diseases of the liver and biliary system, 9th edn. Oxford: Blackwell Scientific Publications; 1993:360–1.

131. Erlinger S, Benhamou J-P. Cirrhosis: clinical aspects. In: McIntyre N, Benhamou J-P, Bircher J et al., editors. Oxford textbook of clinical hepatology, Vol. 1. Oxford: Oxford University Press; 1991:380–90.

132. Desmet VJ, Sciot R, Van Eyken P. Differential diagnosis and prognosis of cirrhosis: role of liver biopsy. Acta Gastroenterol Belg. 1990;53:198–208.

133. Okuda K, Benhamou JP (editors). Portal hypertension: clinical and physiological aspects. Tokyo: Springer Verlag; 1991.

134. Sciot R, Van Damme B, Desmet VJ. Does incomplete septal cirrhosis link non-cirrhotic nodulations with cirrhosis? Histopathology. 1989;15:318–20.

135. Wanless IR. The pathophysiology of non-cirrhotic portal hypertension: a pathologist's perspective. In: Boyer JL, Bianchi L, editors. Liver cirrhosis. Lancaster: MTP Press; 1987:293–311.

136. Wanless IR. Micronodular transformation (nodular regenerative hyperplasia) of the liver: a report of 64 cases among 2500 autopsies and a new classification of benign hepatocellular nodules. Hepatology. 1990;11:787–97.

137. Butron Vila MM, Haot J, Desmet VJ. Cholestatic features in focal nodular hyperplasia of the liver. Liver. 1984;4:387–95.

138. Desmet VJ. What is congenital hepatic fibrosis? Histopathology. 1992;20:465–77.

139. Desmet VJ. Congenital diseases of intrahepatic bile ducts: variations on the theme 'ductal plate malformation'. Hepatology. 1992;16:1069–83.

140. Thaler H. Leberkrankheiten. Klinisch-morphologische Diagnostik und ihre Grundlagen, 2nd edn. Berlin: Springer-Verlag; 1987.

22
Laboratory diagnosis and treatment of liver fibrosis

D. STROBEL and E. G. HAHN

In the clinical management of liver fibrosis diagnosis is based on clinical symptoms, laboratory tests, liver biopsy, histological and imaging techniques including ultrasound, CT scanning and NMR.

Liver fibrosis develops slowly over a period of time depending upon constant stimulation by the aetiological factor. Clinical features of liver fibrosis such as jaundice, ascites, gastrointestinal bleeding, and hepatic encephalopathy are seen in a later stage of disease, when hepatocellular failure and portal hypertension have occurred.

It is particularly important to recognize patients in the clinical latent phase of disease, or even before cirrhosis has developed. Therefore we need tests which are valid to detect fibrosis, to direct the diagnostic work-up, to estimate the severity of disease, to assess prognosis, and to evaluate therapy.

Conventional blood tests cannot diagnose or predict liver fibrosis; therefore histopathology is and will be the golden standard to diagnose liver fibrosis and cirrhosis. In the clinical management of liver fibrosis, however, conventional serum markers are commonly used to assess liver function. Conventional blood tests such as serum enzymes and bilirubin indicate the degree of cell damage and cholestasis. Standard tests for the synthetic function are plasma proteins such as albumin and prothrombin time. Detailed information about the cytosolic, microsomal and excretory function of the liver in fibrotic diseases can be obtained by more sophisticated tests such as galactose elimination and indocyanine green clearance. These techniques, however, are more complex and therefore not widely accepted.

In the clinical management of fibrotic liver diseases the pattern of conventional liver parameters such as bilirubin and enzymes leads to more specific diagnostic tests with regard to the aetiology of fibrotic liver diseases including viral hepatitis markers.

In Europe and the United States alcoholic liver disease and fibrosis due to chronic hepatitis B and C account for the majority of liver fibrosis. In addition plasma proteins in metabolic disorders, e.g. haemochromatosis and Wilson's disease, and autoimmune markers such as smooth muscle, mitochondrial, and nuclear antibodies should be assessed. Biliary obstruction, as in sclerosing cholangitis or atresia, or vascular causes of fibrosis such as the Budd–Chiari syndrome, can be suspected by clinical appearance and conventional liver laboratory tests. However, diagnosis in these conditions is based on imaging techniques such as ultrasound, CT scanning, NMR, endoscopy or angiography.

To assess fibrogenic activity in fibrotic liver diseases, and to control potential antifibrogenic therapy, a non-invasive diagnostic tool is needed. Based on the growing knowledge of structure, function, and metabolism of extracellular matrix we estimate fibrosis by several tests measuring various circulating connective tissue-related compounds. The composition, structure, and localization of the hepatic connective tissue components have been studied intensively to find a non-invasive serum parameter for liver fibrosis. Enzymes and metabolic products of collagen and extracellular glycoproteins have been widely used for some time to quantitate changes in connective tissue metabolism. During the past 10 years or so several tests have been developed to measure circulating connective tissue-related components. Some of them are commercially available, and the number of published methods is increasing rapidly.

In this context it is important to clearly define what we are talking about. Histomorphological fibrosis is an excess of connective tissue at a certain point in time. Based on the studies about biology of hepatic extracellular matrix components today we also understand fibrosis as a dynamic process which is contributed by matrix synthesis, degradation, and remodelling. In this dynamic process hepatic fibrogenesis can be correlated with an increase of the aminoterminal propeptide of type III procollagen (PIIINP). Serum assays for type IV procollagen propeptides (PIVNP, PIVCP) and laminin (Lam P1) reflect the turnover of basement membranes. Collagen type VI and undulin are located in the interstitium where they are associated with the large collagen fibrils. Serum assays for collagen type VI (CVI) and undulin (Un) may therefore be helpful markers for matrix degradation and fibrolysis. Serum levels of one or a combination of these extracellular matrix components can indicate activity of fibrogenesis or fibrolysis in patient follow-up.

Persistent elevation of PIIINP correlates with the activity of hepatic fibrogenesis and predicts the development of chronic active fibrogenic liver disease. It is possible to differentiate alcoholic fatty liver from alcoholic hepatitis, chronic active from persistent viral hepatitis and to predict outcome in primary biliary cirrhosis. PIIINP is not a useful marker of fibrogenesis in childhood because of growth-related procollagen turnover. Collagen type IV peptides and laminin can be used as markers in small children; they further help to distinguish between chronic persistent and active hepatitis. As markers for basement membrane turnover and sinusoidal capillarization they show a good correlation to portal hypertension in cirrhosis, which is of practical clinical value. More recently collagen VI and undulin may serve as markers for matrix degradation and need to be evaluated in clinical studies. In clinical terms the correlations of these serum parameters may be more valuable than strict measurement of matrix content, because they offer prognostic information for some forms of liver disease. It remains to be determined whether measurement of these circulating polypeptides mirrors hepatic matrix synthesis, degradation and remodelling, and whether these tests are broadly applicable in all types of liver injury. Thus the high expectations of finding a reliable non-invasive tool to diagnose liver fibrosis/ cirrhosis which could substitute for morphological assessment have not yet been fulfilled, but in clinical management of liver fibrosis serum levels of one or a combination of these extracellular matrix components may indicate activity of fibrosis in patient follow-up, and may be helpful to monitor patients under antifibrinogenic therapy.

Current therapies for liver fibrosis naturally include withdrawal of the disease stimulus, reduction of hepatic inflammation, and cell injury. Severe cases may demand surgical procedures such as liver transplantation. Removal of the aetiological agents such as alcohol and hepatotoxic drugs prevents progression of fibrosis. In viral hepatitis, progression to chronic infection always precedes fibrosis, implying that viral clearance will remove the stimulus of fibrogenesis. There is some success to clear hepatitis B and C viruses with interferon-alpha (IFN-α); but it is not yet known whether reduction in inflammation by IFN-α without viral clearance will reduce liver fibrosis. Metabolic disorders such as haemochromatosis and Wilson's disease are controlled by phlebotomy and chelation therapy when diagnosed early. In α_1-antitrypsin deficiency the future development of somatic gene therapy might have beneficial effects on these forms of hepatic fibrosis. In primary biliary cirrhosis there is no evidence that pharmacological intervention will reduce long-term fibrogenesis, but clinical trials using ursodeoxycholic acid and immunosuppressive drugs are still ongoing. In autoimmune hepatitis immunosuppressive drugs such as prednisolone and azathioprine can reduce inflammation and cell injury, and thus prevent fibrosis. In advanced stages of fibrotic liver diseases liver transplantation must be considered.

New therapeutic perspectives in treatment of hepatic fibrosis will arise from growing knowledge of the biology of matrix modulation in hepatic fibrosis. Again potential pharmaceutical intervention is based on the understanding of the molecular basis of matrix synthesis and degradation, and more recently on the understanding of cytokines involved in hepatic fibrogenesis.

Most attempts to interfere with matrix synthesis have focused on collagen biosynthesis. A number of agents inhibit collagen biosynthesis on a transcriptional level. These include corticosteroids, interferon-gamma (IFN-γ) and retinoids. Clinical trials of these agents are limited so far; IFN-γ can reduce matrix deposition in murine schistosomiasis but has not been examined in humans. Use of retinoids shown to prevent fibrosis in animal experiments is limited because of potential toxicity. Transcriptional feedback inhibition by collagen propeptides has been reported in cultured fibroblasts but has not been used *in vivo*. Currently drugs such as prolyl 4-hydroxylase inhibitors are promising. These drugs lead to destabilization of the triple helical structure in procollagen without affecting mRNA levels of collagen I, III, or prolyl 4-hydroxylase. Unstable procollagen then undergoes intracellular degradation or incomplete extracellular processing. Clinical studies using these inhibitors have been started; data concerning efficiency are expected shortly. Collagen synthesis may also be inhibited at the stage of fibril crosslinking by inhibitors of lysyl oxidase. Penicillamine blocks aldehyde formation during collagen crosslinking, but has so far failed to demonstrate significant antifibrotic activity in clinical studies in Wilson's disease.

Other therapeutic strategies for the future include the augmentation of extracellular proteases for degrading connective tissue. This would be helpful in advanced fibrotic liver diseases, when excess connective tissue deposition has already taken place. Very few agents with potential effect on matrix degradation have been tested *in vivo*. Colchicine has been studied in cell culture and animal models. In cultured cells colchicine can stimulate collagenase activity, but this effect remains to be shown in clinical studies. Matrix metalloproteinases in culture models may be stimulated by cytokines such as interleukin-1, tumour necrosis factor alpha (TNF-α) and platelet derived growth factor (PDGF), and may be inhibited by transforming growth factor beta (TGF-β). However, regulation of metalloproteinase activity *in vivo* is complex and not yet well understood. Efforts to enhance endogenous activity of metalloproteinases require better understanding of the cellular localization and regulation by metalloproteinase inhibitors, which may interfere with potential therapeutic drugs.

Increased matrix synthesis in liver fibrogenesis is mainly located in activated lipocytes. Initiation and perpetuation of lipocyte activation in hepatic fibrosis therefore offer interesting routes for potential antifibrotic therapy. Since fat-storing cell activation is accompanied by cell proliferation and enhanced matrix synthesis neutralizing antibodies of cytokines such as PDGF and TGF-β might inhibit fibrogenesis. In cell cultures neutralizing antibodies against TGF-β have been shown to suppress matrix suppression. Whether hepatic matrix suppression *in vivo* can be also reduced has not been shown yet. We have learned a lot about the prominent role of lipocyte activation and subsequent matrix production in liver fibrogenesis; but regulation of hepatic matrix synthesis by cytokines is increasingly complex and requires more studies *in vivo* to identify potential sites for therapeutic intervention.

Therapeutic strategies for the future include the possibility of somatic gene therapy. This approach seems to be successful for metabolic disorders, e.g. α_1-antitrypsin deficiency or cystic fibrosis where the molecular defect is characterized.

Blocking the synthesis of connective tissue proteins by somatic gene therapy is an interesting futuristic approach and more understanding of the regulatory elements in matrix gene expression *in vivo* is required. In addition a very important requirement for all future therapies is to target potential pharmaceutical agents or gene products to the liver *in vivo* specifically to prevent alterations in collagen metabolism or unwanted side-effects in other organs.

In summary, based on the growing understanding of connective tissue metabolism we approach new perspectives for a specific antifibrotic therapy in liver fibrosis. Closest to practical application so far are inhibitors of collagen synthesis as prolyl 4-hydroxylase inhibitors, which are currently evaluated in clinical studies. New potential sites for therapeutic intervention in liver fibrosis are arising from the new insights into matrix synthesis inhibition, augmentation of matrix degradation, interference with cytokines by neutralizing antibodies, and somatic gene therapy. There are still many open questions; liver-specific targeting is only one – but intensive research in this field may solve some of these questions in future. Diagnosis for liver fibrosis is still lacking a specific non-invasive serum test which can substitute histomorphological evaluation. Histology is the golden standard of the diagnostic work-up. Clinical symptoms and conventional bloods test rather indicate hepatocellular function in liver fibrosis, and often become evident only in advanced stages of fibrotic liver disease. We have learned that measurement of connective tissue polypeptides cannot diagnose liver fibrosis, but conclusions may indicate activity of fibrosis and prognosis; thus they may be a helpful serum parameter to control antifibrotic therapy, which now for the first time becomes feasible.

References

1. Schuppan D. Structure of the extracellular matrix in normal and fibrotic liver: collagens and glycoproteins. Semin Liver Dis. 1990;10:1–10.
2. Schuppan D. Connective tissue polypeptides in serum as parameters to monitor antifibrotic treatment in hepatic fibrogenesis. J Hepatol. 1991;13(Suppl 3):17–25.
3. Friedman SL. The cellular basis of hepatic fibrosis. N Engl J Med. 1993;328:1828–35.
4. Liver selective fibrosuppression: a new approach in therapy of liver fibrosis. J Hepatol. 1991;13(Suppl.3).
5. Clement B, Loreal O, Levavasseur F et al. New challenges in hepatic fibrosis. J Hepatol. 1993;18:1–4.

23
Pathogenetic mechanisms of intrahepatic cholestasis

P. GENTILINI, R. G. ROMANELLI, M. FOSCHI and R. MAZZANTI

GENERAL ELEMENTS

The term 'cholestasis' indicates a clinical and biochemical syndrome generally characterized by jaundice, itching and increased serum levels of bile acids and of cholephilic enzymes, such as alkaline phosphatase and gamma-glutamyl-transpeptidase (γ-GT). It is based on an impairment of bile secretion, with specific organic anion secretory defects[1-5]. Though the presence of jaundice due to increased conjugated bilirubin is often observed in this condition, the essential feature of the syndrome is represented by the abnormal retention of bile acids in serum; this phenomenon has eventually been linked to itching[6-11]. Due to the fact that jaundice is not an invariable feature of cholestasis, and can follow the onset of symptoms such as pruritus and biochemical alterations such as raised serum alkaline phosphatase by weeks or even years, familial cholemic syndromes (i.e. Dubin-Johnson and rotor syndromes, characterized by increased serum level of bilirubin), are excluded from the definition. On the contrary, anicteric forms, such as intrahepatic cholestasis of pregnancy or the first stage of primary biliary cirrhosis, characterized only by pruritus, with concomitant increased total bile acid levels in serum, must be included[1,2,12].

Experimental studies have confirmed the elevation of serum levels of bile acids as the pivotal element of intrahepatic cholestasis. Administration of ethinyloestradiol, a hormone that is a component of the contraceptive pill and a molecule known to induce a decrease in bile flow, has been demonstrated capable of inducing an increase in serum levels of bile acids. This is due to an impaired uptake of bile acids on the sinusoidal domain of the hepatocyte during enterohepatic circulation, which normally occurs up to 10 times a day in humans and leads to a total of more than 30 g of bile acid entering the intestinal lumen[2,10,11].

In a second phase, other cholestatic signs are present, such as increased levels of alkaline phosphatase and γ-GT, followed by an increment in conjugated bilirubin, serum levels of cholesterol, phospholipids, β-globulins and other cholephilic molecules.

Considering intrahepatic cholestasis as a clinical–biochemical syndrome, one or more alterations in physiological cellular mechanisms of bile flow generation may be responsible. Modifications of membrane structures (ionic pumps, membrane carriers, ionic channels, etc.), an altered membrane lipid composition (with a decrease in phospholipid amount with absolute increase in cholesterol content), functional impairment of one or more intracytoplasmatic organelles involved in the establishment and maintenance of cellular polarity, have been demonstrated[9,10]. According to the sequence it is possible to draw up a list of disorders potentially involved in the occurrence of cholestatic syndromes, which can play a prevalent or secondary role in determining the manifestation of the syndrome itself (Table 1). However, a simple list of these disorders does not always permit individuation of precise pathogenetic mechanisms of intrahepatic cholestasis, even though recent years have seen great improvements in our understanding of specific steps in bile acid metabolism and bile formation. Thus, even in considering recent papers or reviews in this field[10–12], other factors could be considered, and further research is necessary.

Considering these different steps, other factors should be taken into consideration: (1) Some pathogenetic mechanisms are based on experimental data not sufficiently proven with research in humans; (2) pathogenetic mechanisms involved in the development of cholestatic syndrome can be multiple, for even the same molecule. Typical examples are represented by ethinyloestradiol and chlorpromazine: the first compound, administered to animals – in addition to an impairment of bile acid uptake on the sinusoidal domain of the hepatocytes, without significant alterations of the excretion of bile acids through the canalicular pole, at least in the initial period[13] – also acts through other mechanisms. This is due to an altered ratio between cholesterol and phospholipids of the membrane, with a consequent alteration in membrane fluidity, a dissipated sodium gradient and a decrease in sinusoidal Na,K-ATPase activity, which is only in part responsible for the impaired bile acid uptake[14–16]. Furthermore, prolonged administration of ethinyloestradiol determines altered ATP-dependent bile acid secretion on the canalicular domain and/or altered transcytotic vesicular transport of bile acids through the bile canaliculus[17–20]. Chlorpromazine, a drug with well-known cholestatic potential, also decreases membrane fluidity and inhibits Na,K-ATPase and Mg-ATPase activities. Previous data showed an association between chlorpromazine and cholangiolytic syndrome through a sensitization mechanism (for which the term 'allergic cholangiolitis' was proposed)[21–24]. In fact, at normal dosage of the drug it is possible to have an autoimmune process with cholestatic syndrome, with ultrastructural hepatocellular and ductular alterations. This syndrome is progressive, almost insensitive to pharmacological treatment and often evolves towards real biliary cirrhosis[12,25]. Later, two other mechanisms were recognized. Chlorpromazine may cause cholestasis through one or more metabolites, and also in cases where increased dosages of the drug were used, the cholestatic syndrome (perhaps on the basis of different mechanisms) could be elicited in about 2% of patients treated[1,2,12].

Table 1 Pathogenetic mechanisms of intrahepatic cholestasis with some experimental and clinical examples

I Mechanism (increased permeability) Total parenteral nutrition (TPN) Ethinyloestradiol Lithocholic acid Phalloidin Manganese–bilirubin complexes	*VII Mechanism (Golgi apparatus impairment)* Alagille's syndrome (arteriohepatic dysplasia) *VIII Mechanism (cytoskeleton hyperplasia)* Byler's disease Cytochalasin B Phalloidin
II Mechanism (decreased membrane fluidity) Ethinyloestradiol Jaundice in pregnancy Spironolactone Chlorpromazine Lithocholic acid	*IX Mechanism (cytoskeleton disruption)* North American Indian children, severe cholestasis Phalloidin Colchicine Norethandrolone Chlorpromazine
III Mechanism (impaired Na,K-ATPase activity) Hypopituitarism Protoporphyria (?) Endotoxins Chlorpromazine Cardiac glycosides	*X Mechanism (tight junction alterations)* Phalloidin Ethinyloestradiol α-Naphthylisothiocyanate (ANIT)
IV Mechanism (decreased bile acid membrane carrier activity) Phalloidin and phallotoxins Taurolithocholic acid Load of amino adic (TPN) Mechanical obstacle (bile duct ligation) Rifampin	*XI mechanism (intracanalicular precipitation)* Lithocholic acid Protoporphyria (?) Chlorpromazine
V Mechanism (mitochondrial and endoplasmic reticulum alterations) Trihydroxycoprostanic acidaemia (THCA-demia) α₁-Antitrypsin deficiency Alcoholic hepatitis Cirrhosis (?) Metabolic and energetic defects	*XII Mechanism (intrahepatic mechanical cholestasis)* (a) Ductular infiltration and disruption primary biliary cirrhosis cholangitis primary sclerosing cholangitis biliary atresia vanishing bile duct syndrome cholestatic–cholangiolytic hepatitis (b) Portal tract invasion sarcoidosis Hodgkin's disease multinodular carcinoma
VI Mechanism (peroxisomal paucity) Zellweger's syndrome (cerebrohepatorenal syndrome)	(c) Lymph vessel hypoplasia Aagenaes's syndrome (hereditary cholestasis with lymphoedema)

This drug can cause cholestasis by affecting different structures of liver cells, particularly by altering membrane lipid composition, membrane Na,K-ATPase activity, microfilament function and intracytoplasmic vesicular transport, and by determining insoluble complexes that precipitate in bile canaliculi and ductules[24].

The inhibition of bile flow may be related to the local increased release of prostanoids (arachidonic acid metabolites), since chlorpromazine-induced cholestasis can be prevented by the administration of indomethacin and other cyclooxygenase inhibitors[26,27].

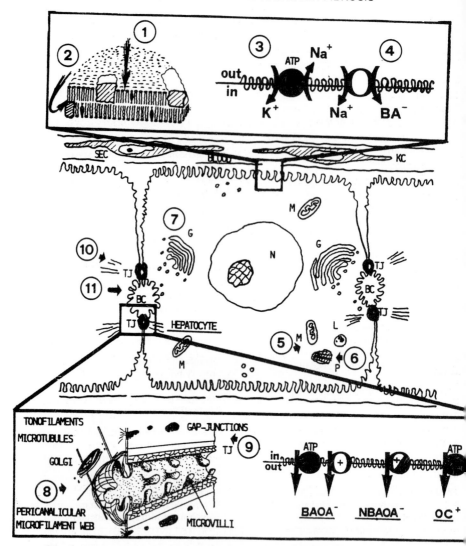

Fig. 1 Diagrammatic representation of localization of morphological and functional defects of the hepatocyte during cholestasis (the twelfth defect is not shown, due to the mechanical nature of this type of non-hepatocellular cholestasis)

SPECIFIC ALTERATIONS IN BILE SECRETION

Liver injuries may lead to cholestasis through different pathogenetic mechanisms with consequent osmotic driving force decrease. As shown in Table 1, it is possible to identify at least 12 different mechanisms leading to cholestasis (Fig. 1). Early impairment of ultrastructural and biochemical energy-dependent processes, involved in the generation of bile flow, leads to impaired bile salt uptake and the establishment of a reflux of biliary molecules from the bile canaliculus to the sinusoidal space and the systemic circulation[10]. However, when the first and prevalent phenomenon is represented by an alteration of the liver cell's sinusoidal membrane, there is at first only an increase in the circulating levels of bile salts. On the other hand, when the prevalent defect is localized at or around the bile canaliculus, there are first morphological alterations of the liver cell with possible regurgitation of bile salts, followed by altered uptake. Moreover, it is possible to have apparently primitive alterations of the ductular cells, i.e. during primary biliary cirrhosis, during which the most important phenomenon is represented by bile stagnation and cholephilic material regurgitation, followed by a defect in bile acid uptake.

However, whatever the specific site of the altered mechanism may be, the end stage of cholestasis is represented by bile salt accumulation both in the liver and in systemic circulation. In these cases, light microscopic examination of liver biopsies only occasionally suggests a definite aetiology; other parameters are thus necessary for differential diagnosis, such as circulating antibodies, increased serum levels of immunoglobulins, lipids, cholephilic enzymes, i.e. serum alkaline phosphatase and γ-GT. Sometimes, in differential diagnosis with extrahepatic biliary obstruction, liver biopsy evaluation and biliary imaging techniques, including ultrasound scan, CT scan, radionuclide imaging and cholangiographic techniques are necessary.

Considering the *increase in membrane permeability* as the first pathogenetic step, one of the most frequent clinical conditions is represented by total parenteral nutrition (TPN), during which a slight increase in serum level of lithocholic acid (and other monohydroxy bile acids) has been found[28,29]. Monohydroxy bile acids, such as lithocholic acid and its conjugates 3-hydroxy-5β-cholenoate and the allo derivative 3-hydroxy-5α-cholenoate, have been shown to be toxic for the liver and other tissues, and increased during progressive childhood cholestasis and primary biliary cirrhosis[2,6,30].

Whatever the primary mechanism of cholestasis, retention of monohydroxy and other bile acids induces hepatocellular damage, with consequent altered membrane permeability, which may initiate a vicious cycle of cell injury[31-36]. These compounds have been proven to be potent cholestatic agents in experimental conditions; this toxicity is due to their detergent activity and hydrophobicity[35,37], with increased intracellular concentration of calcium ions. This increment determines haemolysis in red blood cells and affects several other functions[38,39]. Increase in calcium ions seems to be secondary to a specific release from intracellular stores, in particular endoplasmic reticulum[40]. In addition, lithocholic acid induces a change in lipid composition of plasma membranes, characterized by an increased cholesterol/phospholipid ratio[35,37]. These bile acids can determine an increase in membrane permeability of tight junctions (junctional permeability)[41,42], possibly secondary to the high calcium-binding capacity of these molecules[43,44]. This leads to reflux of bile acids and organic anions from bile to the paracellular space and sinusoidal domain; more specifically there is an inverse process in respect of the physiological vesicular transcytosis from the sinusoidal to the canalicular plasma membrane, the so-called 'diacytosis', or back-diffusion of biliary content into intracytoplasmatic vesicles[45]. However, it is possible that

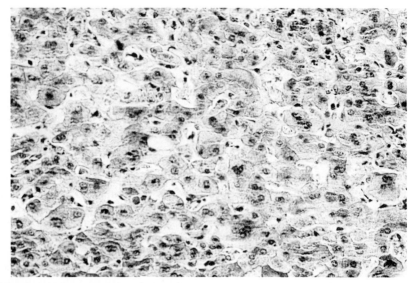

Fig. 2 Post-partum cholestatic jaundice (II mechanism). Presence of mesenchymal cell activation, mild necrosis and diffuse small intracellular deposits of bile pigment. H&E x 234

the increased membrane permeability could be secondary to the intracellular bile salt accumulation after cholestasis is initiated by other events, the so-called *cholate stasis*, which first occurs in acinar zone 1 of Rappaport acinus[2–5,12,46].

A second mechanism to affect in bile secretion and bile acid metabolism is based on *decrease in membrane fluidity*, which can be altered secondarily to increased accumulation of cholesterol into membranes, with a consequent altered ratio between cholesterol and phospholipids and modification of activity of many membrane-bound enzymes[47,48]. Examples of this condition are represented by reversible cholestatic syndromes, such as cholestasis in pregnancy (Figs 2 and 3), ethinyloestradiol-induced and lithocholate- and conjugate-induced cholestasis. Altered fluidity may impair bile acid carrier function of isolated membrane vesicles from the sinusoidal domain, with tightly associated inhibition of Na,K-ATPase activity[49,50]. Ethinyloestradiol administration in experimental conditions leads to decreased bile salt uptake (inhibition of sodium/bile acid symport), in particular with taurocholate and glycocholate and other trihydroxy bile acids[14,15]. Spironolactone, like ethinyloestradiol, has been found to decrease membrane fluidity and Na,K-ATPase activity in experimental conditions[51,52], with a consequent alteration in bile acid transport; the same phenomenon has been observed in chlorpromazine-induced cholestasis[27,53,54].

Monohydroxy bile acids can lead to membrane fluidity and lipid composition alterations, so that modified fluidity and membrane permeability can be linked to each other in this particular form of intrahepatic cholestasis[35–37,41].

Another mechanism which leads to decreased bile acid uptake and a

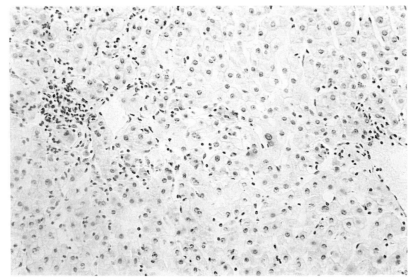

Fig. 3 Chlorpromazine-induced cholestasis (II and XI mechanism). A large number of intracellular biliary deposits, together with mild intralobular flogistic reaction, are shown. × 93

consequent bile secretory failure is represented by the *decrease in Na,K-ATPase activity*. Even if this defect is often associated with changes in membrane fluidity, specific inhibition can be induced by administration of ouabain and other cardiac glycosides, or ethacrynic acid; however, these compounds, even if capable of inducing a sodium pump function impairment, do not induce cholestasis: after secretion into bile canaliculus these molecules provide an osmotic driving force which maintains bile flow[32,55].

The fourth mechanism of cholestasis is represented by an extension of the *sodium-dependent bile acid uptake* on the sinusoidal domain of the plasma membrane which can be specifically altered during intrahepatic cholestasis. Bile acid uptake defect can be determined by rifampin, even if morphological alterations are represented by biliary deposits in the cytoplasm and in the bile canaliculi, suggesting a possible intracellular transport impairment with consequent precipitation of metabolites into the bile canaliculi (Fig. 4).

Inhibition of bile acid transport, which can be elicited after administration of phalloidin or other phallotoxins, can lead to the reduction of the so-called *bile acid-dependent flow (BADF)*. This inhibition is competitive, so it is conceivable that these compounds enter hepatocytes through the bile acid carrier[55-57]. Other bile salts, such as taurolithocholate and its 3-β-OH isomer, are non-competitive inhibitors of bile acid uptake[58,59]. TPN, with competition between amino acids and bile salts and consequent dissipation of sodium gradient, is a clinical cholestatogen condition[60,61].

During mechanical biliary obstruction, induced by bile duct ligation, there are two different phenomena: a disruption of tight junctions and a contemporary loss of functional polarity of the hepatocyte, so that there is dissipation of the osmotic driving forces for bile secretion[62,63]. Canalicular

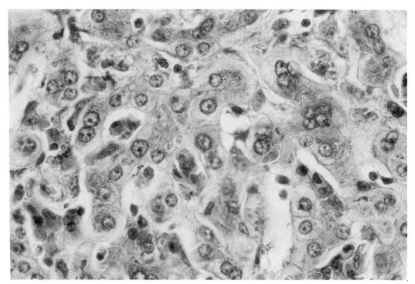

Fig. 4 Severe cholestatic jaundice due to rifampin (IV mechanism). It is possible to observe intracellular and extracellular biliary deposits, associated with slight necrosis in the absence of inflammatory reaction ($\times 300$)

bile acid carriers migrate from the canalicular domain and relocalize themselves on the sinusoidal membrane, possibly to prevent bile acid and cholephilic compounds (such as IgA) accumulation in hepatocytes[2,62,63].

A further pathogenetic mechanism in intrahepatic cholestasis is represented by an *alteration in bile acid synthesis*, which can occur in situations leading to morphological alterations of mitochondria and endoplasmic reticulum; one particular form is represented by THCA-demia, a syndrome characterized by an abnormal increased synthesis of trihydroxycoprostanoic acid (THCA-demia). Such a defect leads to an accumulation of this bile acid in bile, urine and serum; this syndrome is due to an enzymatic defect in the conversion of this acid to varanic acid (cholic acid precursor), or a decrease in 3β-hydroxydehydrogenase/isomerase, another bile acid synthetic enzyme[64].

α_1-Antitrypsin deficiency, a congenital autosomic recessive disease, is more frequent than THCA-demia and is histologically characterized by PAS-positive diastasis-resistant globular deposits in the liver cell, due to the precipitation of α_1-antitrypsin (Fig. 5). These deposits are visible in rough endoplasmic reticulum, which appears swollen and altered under electron microscopic observation[12]. In this case, some other alterations of cytoskeleton and other organelles can be detected and interpreted as a consequence of intracellular bile acid accumulation[65-67]. Because of these complex phenomena, this cholestatic syndrome becomes irreversible, progressing towards liver cirrhosis, which frequently occurs in young adults.

The intracellular alterations of mitochondria and other organelles may explain the cholestatic syndrome occurring in some cases of alcoholic hepatitis or liver cirrhosis[66].

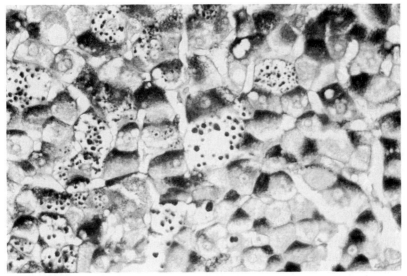

Fig. 5 Cholestatic hepatitis due to α_1-antitrypsin deficiency (V mechanism). The specific PAS staining shows a large number of intracellular globular deposits, due to precipitation of α_1-antitrypsin ($\times$ 375)

Progressive cholestasis – with growth and mental retardation, hepatomegaly, renal cysts and a characteristic facies – is represented by Zellweger's syndrome; in this condition the primary defect (the eighth pathogenetic mechanism) lies in an ultrastructural *alteration of peroxisomes*, unable to oxidize fatty acids and side-chain shortening of bile acid precursors[68–71]. These bile acid precursors increase in the bile, serum and urine of these patients. Liver biopsy shows bile duct paucity, mild hepatocellular damage and the absence of peroxisomes.

Another pathogenetic mechanism of intrahepatic cholestasis is represented by *Golgi apparatus impairment*, with hypoplasia and loss of interlobular bile ducts, ultrastructural accumulation of pigment in the intercellular space and in the hepatocyte (vesicles, lysosomes and Golgi regions on the basolateral site of the cell)[72,73]. The clinical syndrome is known as Alagille's syndrome, or arteriohepatic dysplasia, and is characterized by extrahepatic clinical and radiological abnormalities such as distinct facies, cardiac and pulmonary defects, growth and mental retardation with hypogonadism. The ultrastructural defect seems to be a bile secretory failure on the apical or canalicular domain of the hepatocyte. This entity, typical of childhood, progresses to cirrhosis and portal hypertension with hepatic encephalopathy in 10% of cases[74].

Morphological changes occur in experimental and clinical forms of intrahepatic cholestasis, particularly regarding cytoskeleton and tight junctions.

Disruption of cytoskeleton of the hepatocyte can be provoked by phalloidin or cytochalasin B exposure; the first compound inhibits F-actin depolymeriz-

287

ation with pericanalicular web condensation, consequent accumulation of microfilaments in the liver and, decreased bile flow, with contemporary increase in paracellular permeability[75,76]. In addition, ATP depletion, generally secondary to a variety of causes, such as hypoxic injuries, substrate depletion or mitochondrial damage, can induce actin depolymerization, due to the energy-dependent mechanism of polymerization of G (globular) to F (filamentous) actin[55]. Phalloidin, in experimental conditions, is able to induce a cholestatic syndrome similar to that occurring in familial cholestasis of North American Indian children[77] and extrahepatic cholestasis[75,78]. Cytochalasin B is a fungus alkaloid, known as an inhibitor of microfilament function; it detaches actin microfilaments from the plasma membrane and, on electron microscopic examination, induces granular deposit in the pericanalicular region of the hepatocyte. Other phenomena are represented by a decrease in number and tonicity of bile canaliculus microvilli, hypertrophy of vesicles budding from the Golgi apparatus and a 50% decrease in bile flow[79,80].

These agents are able to reduce the rhythmic canalicular contractions that propel bile fluid in the canalicular area, which furthermore can prove the pivotal role played by cytoskeleton in the physiology of bile secretion[81,82].

Colchicine, a microtubular system inhibitor through its action on micro-tubular protein tubulin, seems to inhibit intracytoplasmic microtubule-dependent vesicle transport of bile acids (*transcytotic vesicular pathway for bile acids*[83]), particularly in advanced forms of cholestasis after administration of supraphysiological levels of bile acids and when bile acid flux is increased[2,84,85]. Colchicine-induced cholestasis can be experimentally counteracted by β-murocholic acid (or taurine conjugated β-murocholic acid) administration in the rat liver perfusion system[86].

Chlorpromazine has been demonstrated as being able to inhibit transcellular horseradish peroxidase transport, a well-known marker of fluid phase endocytosis[2-4].

In some familial cholestatic syndromes, the so-called *cytoskeleton hyperplasia*, with microfilament disorder and secondary accumulation of intracellular organelles in the bile canaliculus, can be observed[87]. This disorder has been described in Byler's disease, a progressive childhood cholestasis, which is characterized by ultrastructural features resembling those reported in experimental phalloidin-induced cholestasis[75]. Serum levels of monohydroxy bile acids and other toxic molecules, such as lithocholic acid, can be found increased in this condition, as can other serum bile acids[88,89].

As mentioned above, phalloidin, cytochalasin B and colchicine, impair (in different ways) the cytoskeletal apparatus of the hepatocyte (microtubules, microfilaments and intermediate filaments) and, at the same time, may induce an *alteration of tight junction structure and function*. These structures contribute to maintaining the physiological polarity of the cell, which is the basis for bile secretion through the generation of osmotic forces from the sinusoidal membrane and bile canaliculus. Tight junction alterations, quite often encountered after experimental bile duct ligation and in spontaneous bile mechanical obstruction, can lead to an increase in number and density of interconnecting 'strands' which separate canalicular lumen from the intercellular space[2-5]. This can also occur during experimental mechanical obstruction of bile ducts[90,91].

Some potent cholestatic drugs such as cyclosporine, an immunodepressive drug used in transplanted patients, have been shown able to reduce the concentration and biliary secretion of bile acids, cholesterol and phospholipid output in experimental animals, together with a decreased secretion in alkaline phosphatase and γ-GT in a dose-dependent manner[92,93]. Furthermore, this drug has been shown to be capable of uncoupling biliary lipid secretion from bile acid secretion, suggesting that it may be able to induce a fall in bile acid output, perhaps acting through the transcytotic vesicular pathway, even if some other mechanisms are involved, such as intracellular transport impairment of vesicles derived from Golgi apparatus and directed towards canalicular membranes, decrease in canalicular membrane fluidity and/or other intracanalicular events[94]. The cholestatic effect of cyclosporine has also been shown in humans, in which the chronically administered drug has been shown capable of inducing a decrease in hepatic excretory function, leading to cholestasis, without signs of hepatotoxicity[95]. The cholestatic potency of this drug could be related to the high hydrophobicity of the molecule, which seems to be responsible for the aspecific interaction of this drug with membrane carriers of the bile canaliculus domain[96]. This particular form of cholestasis seems to be counteracted by intravenous taurocholate and per os UDCA (ursodeoxycholic acid) administration[97]. Cyclosporine-induced cholestasis, with morphological changes in bile canaliculi with loss of microvilli, should be considered to be based on a complex mechanism possibly involving contractile as well as membrane transport systems. However, more data in humans are still necessary to confirm hypothetical mechanisms for drug-induced cholestasis in transplanted patients[98-100].

More recently, the ATP-dependent export carriers for bile acids and cysteinyl leukotrienes in the hepatocyte canalicular membrane have been found to be targets for inhibitory side-effects of cyclosporine. Thus, inhibition of bile acid transport in the presence of physiological concentrations of cyclosporine (such as those used in transplanted patients) may induce cholestasis[101]. Another transporter has been identified recently in canalicular membrane vesicles, the ATP-dependent transport system for bile acids, which is distinct from the P-glycoprotein and the organic anion transporter[102]. This has been successively characterized in mutant rats[103]. Further research is necessary to establish if the ATP-dependent transport system for bile acids is distinct from the membrane potential-dependent transport activity previously discovered[104]. Regarding leukotrienes, an ATP-dependent transport system responsible for the hepatobiliary export of LTC4 and its metabolites has been identified in liver canalicular membranes[105]. This system has also been identified in mastocytoma vesicles[106]. This system is responsible for the transport of DNP-glutathione and glutathione S-conjugates through the canalicular membrane[107,108]. Successively, another ATP-dependent transport of bilirubin mono- and diglucuronides in canalicular membrane vesicles was demonstrated[109]. Another transporter not yet purified is the non-bile acid organic anion transporter, or the multispecific organic anion transporter (MOAT) responsible for transport of sulphobromophthalein (BSP) and its conjugates, such as BSP-GSH (glutathione)[110,111]. More recently some particular physiological findings have been made regarding another ATP-dependent carrier of the canalicular domain of the hepatocyte: the multidrug resistance (mdr1) gene product, p-glycoprotein (gp-170)[112]. This carrier, resembling the ATP/ADP exchanger of mitochondria, is a 170-kDa membrane phosphoglycoprotein which binds ATP and drug analogues and has intrinsic ATPase activity, thus functioning as an energy-dependent efflux pump[113]. Transport requires hydrolysable ATP, and it has been shown in inside-out canalicular membrane vesicles. This transporter has been found to be a possible carrier for ATP from the inside to the outside of the cell (i.e. into the bile). This protein, known as a drug pump for organic cations seems to function also as a channel for exit of ATP[114]. Furthermore, this protein has been thought to function as a volume-regulated chloride channel[115], and might act as a channel for other anions[114].

Secretion of ATP through the gp-170 could be the expression of an autocrine function of the hepatocytes, due to the presence of purinergic receptors on the biliary domain of the cell, together with other enzymes involved in nucleotide degradation and purine conservation (ecto-ATPase, 5′-nucleotidase, Na-dependent nucleoside transport system, AMPase, nucleotidases). It is likely, though not yet demonstrated, that all these ectoenzymes in the canaliculus are associated with unidirectional transport, which maintains the physiological pool of purines, pyrimidines and amino acids. However, it is not certain if this carrier (gp-170) has a specific function in the absence of toxic drugs and chemotherapeutics; in this case, the p-glycoprotein could pump endogenous peptides that resemble drugs and act as a drug pump in the presence of these molecules, specifically creating an ATP gradient (electrochemical) between the inside and outside of the cell as the driving force for pumping molecules in the 300–990 M_r range[114].

Ethinyloestradiol, phalloidin and α-naphthylisothiocyanate (ANIT) administration can induce alterations of tight junction structure and function, as already mentioned[116]. Phalloidin administration in experimental conditions increases paracellular permeability for insulin, sucrose and polyethylene glycol in a manner similar to that observed for bile duct ligation. This again demonstrates the tight interrelationship of different mechanisms in inducing intrahepatic cholestasis[75,117].

A more obvious pathogenetic mechanism responsible for cholestasis is represented by *intracanalicular precipitation of biliary compounds*, due to decreased Na,K-ATPase activity on the sinusoidal domain of the hepatocytes; it is well known that changes in the activity of this enzyme are often associated with parallel effects on bile flow, especially on *bile acid-independent flow (BAIF)*. This phenomenon can be encountered in hypothyroid rats[37,118] (decreased pump activity secondary to low levels of thyroxine hormone), or adrenalectomized rats[119] or after administration of protoporphyrin, even though in this latter condition the precise mechanism underlying the decreased bile flow is not yet known[120,121]. Cholestasis in neonates with hypopituitarism can be antagonized by the administration of cortisone or thyroid hormones[122].

Other cholestatic compounds can act through the modification of membrane permeability, by decreased Na,K-ATPase activity and the consequent dissipation of Na gradient through the membrane, and through bile canaliculus precipitation of cholephilic compounds[123]: two substances included in this group are lithocholic acid and chlorpromazine (Fig. 3). These substances can at the same time alter membrane sodium pump and subcellular structures and functions of hepatocytes. However, a selective inhibition of this pump, such as after ouabain-like compound administration, might not be sufficient on its own to affect the driving forces for bile flow. Lithocholic acid in rats induces formation of deposits in small bile ductules, soluble with EGTA, a Ca^{2+}-chelating agent[2,3].

This mechanism seems to operate in spontaneous clinical conditions, such as virus A-induced cholestatic cholangiolytic hepatitis and in non-A–non-B chronic active hepatitis, which are characterized by specific alterations of bile ducts[124]. These cholestatic phenomena, due to obliteration and infiltration of bile ductules, might represent an immunological response, since a factor capable of inducing cholestasis, once injected into rats, has been isolated from serum and lymphocytes of these patients[2,3,125]. According to observations some years ago[1,4] cholestatic hepatitis affected all ages and both sexes, representing 15.2% of all cases (40 out of 263); 40% were HBV-positive. In those patients, cholestatic phenomena were sometimes clear, in some others they were less evident. In cholestatic hepatitis the course is generally prolonged[126-128].

The last pathogenetic mechanism is represented by the *mechanical obstruction and disruption of cholangioles and interlobular bile ducts*, including three types of lesions or three subgroups (Table 1). Considering ductular infiltration and disruption, the most common diseases are represented by primary biliary cirrhosis and several types of cholangitis (Figs 6–8).

Biliary atresia and primary sclerosing cholangitis, when located inside the liver, cholestatic forms of viral hepatitis and vanishing bile duct syndrome are less common. More specifically, in *vanishing bile duct syndrome*[129] there is an occlusion of small intrahepatic bile ducts; this syndrome, also called *duct paucity* or *ductopenia*, can occur after liver transplantation, or more commonly during primary liver cirrhosis. Among the second subgroup there are some benign diseases, such as sarcoidosis, or malignant diseases, such as Hodgkin's disease or multinodular carcinoma, characterized by *portal tract invasion*, when (only in some cases) cholestasis is present in the early stages, while in other cases cholestasis may be evident in more advanced stages, often with extrahepatic obstacles, due to compression of the biliary tree[130]. In the third subgroup, cholestasis occurs in rare cases, due to *congenital hypoplasia of lymph vessels* (Aagenaes's syndrome); in this malformative condition cholestasis is recurrent. Beginning during infancy, it is associated with lymphoedema of the lower limbs and progresses slowly towards cirrhosis. From a histological point of view there is a giant cell hepatitis with fibrosis in portal tracts and typical aspects of intrahepatic cholestasis[131,132].

GENERAL PATHOGENETIC MECHANISMS

Molecules, mainly drugs, capable of inducing intrahepatic cholestasis, as represented in Table 2, may act through two principal mechanisms, either

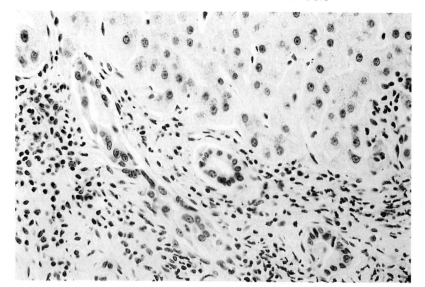

Fig. 6 Primary biliary cirrhosis (XII mechanism). In the portal space it is possible to observe a few biliary ductules, with some degeneration and mild inflammation. Unilamellar hepatocellular structures show, in some degree, pseudoductular features (×375)

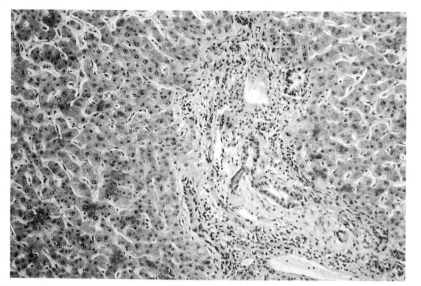

Fig. 7 Bacterial chronic cholangitis (XII mechanism). Biliary proliferation with periductal oedema, large flogistic proliferation and fibrosis can be seen in the portal space (×93)

toxicity or *hypersensitivity*. *Toxicity* may be due to two types of mechanism, either direct or indirect (see Table 3). Carbon tetrachloride and acetaminophen are the best examples for *direct hepatotoxins*, whereas *indirect hepatotoxins* may be represented by several drugs which interfere with

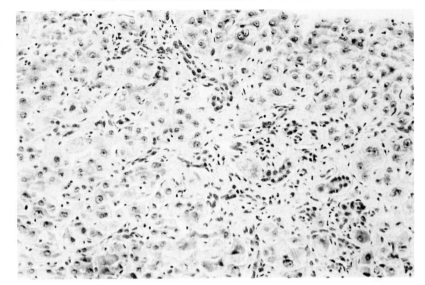

Fig. 8 Cholestatic cholangiolytic hepatitis (XII mechanism). In the periportal zone it is possible to observe proliferations of bile ductules along young connective tissue and initial mild fibrosis, together with small intraparenchymal spots of necrosis. (× 234)

Table 2 Principal drugs responsible for cholestatic hepatitis

Penicillin	Meprobamate
Erythromycin laurylsulphate	Ethchlorvynol
Trimethoprim-sulphamethoxazole	Rifampin
Diphenylhydantoin	Nitrofurantoin
Carbamazepine	Para-aminosalicylic acid
Phenindione	Indomethacin
6-Mercaptopurine	Naproxen
Sulphonylureas	Disulfiram
Ibuprofen	Ketoprofen
Sulindac	Papaverine
Imipramine	Disopyramide
Haloperidol	Diazepam

Table 3 Patterns of drug-induced cholestasis

		Hypersensitivity	
	Toxic mechanism	Idiosyncrasy	Sensitization
Latency	Some days	1 week–1 year	1–5 weeks
Rechallenge	Normal	Variable	Shorter response
Hypersensitivity reactions	No	No	Yes
Eosinophilia	No	No	Yes
Autoimmunity signs	No	No	Yes
Hepatocellular necrosis	Zonal	Diffuse	Diffuse
Inflammation	Mild (PMN)	Variable	Moderate (eosinophils, lymphomonocytes)
Granulomas	No	No	Sometimes

metabolic functions of liver cells, without directly damaging their structures[133-135]. In direct toxicity, damage may be foreseen; it is reproducible in animals and is independent of genetic predisposition. The severity of damage, furthermore, is in proportion to the dose of the drug, and aggression is directly against its cellular structures (involving proteins and/or DNA) through denaturative and lipoperoxidative processes at the level of the membrane of the cell and its intracellular organelles[134]. The molecule may be dangerous by itself or through one or more of its metabolites.

The *indirect hepatotoxins* may function through selective interaction with some molecules essential for the integrity of hepatocytes, with interferences of metabolic, enzymatic and secretory functions of the cell. A good example is represented by some C-17α-alkyl-substituted steroids which can alter the bile secretory mechanisms, including a cholestatic syndrome[136].

More specifically, the so-called *C-17β-conjugated* compounds, or D-ring glucuronide conjugates (oestradiol, oestriol, ethinyloestradiol, testosterone) represent a unique cholestatic class of agents which act through a competition with bile acid (taurocholate in particular) receptor sites located on the canalicular domain of the hepatocyte[136]. Defects in ATP-dependent bile acid transport may underlie various inheritable and acquired forms of cholestasis. Studies on the effects of cholestatic drugs, hormones and chemicals on this system (cyclosporine, FK-506 and long-chain hydrophobic peptides, such as angiotensin inhibitors) have been performed recently; ethinyloestradiol selectively inhibited ATP-dependent bile acid transport but not the other processes[19,136]. However, pathogenetic mechanisms responsible for the onset of cholestatic syndrome after oestrogen administration *in vivo*, and in humans in particular, are not yet fully defined[2-5].

The second principal mechanism inducing intrahepatic cholestasis is based on *hypersensitivity*, which can be distinguished in two forms, either *metabolic idiosyncrasy* or *acquired immunological sensitization*. In the case of the former it is possible to observe either an increased or extremely weak response towards the same molecules in different subjects[137-140]. Primaquine, for example, can lead to a severe haemolytic anaemia in patients affected by erythrocytic glucose-6-phosphate-dehydrogenase deficiency.

The anticoagulant drug, warfarin, represents another good example: some subjects demonstrate weak sensitivity because of an alteration in the receptor for the drug[140,141].

Acquired metabolic sensitization may occur in patients who are already immunologically sensitized to the molecule and suffer a kind of pharmacological allergy. In an unforeseen manner some molecules may lead to liver damage, including associated or prevalent cholestatic syndromes. This acquired hypersensitivity generally occurs during a free interval of 1-5 weeks, and it is believed that the molecule, either by itself or one of its metabolites acting as a hapten, constitutes a new antigenic molecule conjugating itself with some constituents of the hepatocellular membrane; an immunological reaction may subsequently occur[135]. This has been recently observed after the administration of procainamide for 6 weeks in humans, with the onset of an intrahepatic cholestatic jaundice[142]. The cholestatic syndrome, in this case, can happen when the canalicular membrane or the secretory apparatus

Table 4   Patients with drug-induced cholestasis out of 85 patients with drug-induced liver damage (6150 controlled cases)

Pharmacological class	Sex	Age	Drug
Analgesic–antipyretics	F	61	Phenacetin
Antibiotics	F	50	Rifampin
	M	43	Rifampin
	M	55	Rifampin
Hypoglycaemic agents	M	42	Sulphonylureas
	M	49	Sulphonylureas
	M	60	Sulphonylureas plus phenformin
	F	55	Sulphonylureas plus phenformin
Psychotropic drugs	F	70	Chlorpromazine
Steroid hormones	F	49	Oral contraceptives
Sulphonamides	F	37	Sulphamethoxypyridazine
Antithyroid drugs	F	78	Methimazole
Cathartics	F	50	Oxyphenisatin acetate

is damaged[141]. The interval between administration of the drug and the appearance of a cholestatic syndrome depends on whether the molecule acts by itself or through its metabolites[143,144]. Typical examples are represented by rifampin and halothane, which lead to jaundice 2–3 weeks following administration. Rifampin seem to induce a dose-dependent and foreseen decrease in bile acid and BSP uptake from the hepatocytes[145,146]. Furthermore, it seems to activate the microsomal drug-metabolizing system (MDMS), with consequent modulating action of biotransformation and potential toxicity of other drugs, such as isoniazid[131,141,147].

The mechanism of immunological sensitization is commonly accepted[141,143,144], even if the precise nature of the immunological response is not fully understood[139]. However, it is necessary to consider that the same molecules, especially drugs, are sometimes able to aid in inducing a direct cytotoxic effect, and later indirect immunological damage, as happens with halothane, which always seems to act through its metabolites[148,149]. It is not always possible to distinguish between these two pathogenetic mechanisms, since the same molecules are sometimes able to induce cholestatic syndromes in different ways[150].

Finally, it is important to consider the particular susceptibility shown by patients, already affected by liver disease, towards some drugs – for example azathioprine, which can produce a cholestatic syndrome more commonly than in other subjects[151,152].

PERSONAL EXPERIENCE

In our recent review of 6150 patients affected by liver damage, who had all undergone liver biopsy, we reported a series of 85 patients affected by drug-induced liver damage[12]. Among them, only 13 patients presented typical aspects of a cholestatic syndrome as reported in Table 4. Of these 13 patients, a female patient showed a cholestatic syndrome after administration of phenacetin, even if this drug generally induces toxic and not cholestatic damage.

Rifampin was administered to three other patients, inducing a cholestatic syndrome for several months after withdrawal of the drug. In other patients, the cholestatic syndrome was due to oral hypoglycaemic agents, contraceptive pills, laxatives or antithyroid drugs. Methizamide, in our experience, induced a cholestatic syndrome lasting some weeks after withdrawal of the treatment[12], even if some other authors reported a more prolonged free interval between the withdrawal of the drug and the onset of the cholestatic syndrome[153]. The cholestatic syndrome disappeared in a few weeks with good prognosis, except for one patient who was treated with chlorpromazine: the cholestatic syndrome worsened with time, even after withdrawal of the drug, progressing towards biliary cirrhosis.

CONCLUSIONS

Cholestasis defines a phenomenon in which the principal feature is represented by increased serum levels of bile acids, often associated with raised serum alkaline phosphatase, γ-GT and conjugated bilirubin, in the presence of itching and eventually jaundice. Cholestasis can occur in a series of conditions, during liver metabolic congenital disorders, acquired diseases or drug administration. This syndrome can represent the essential or principal sign in several cases, while in others it is only a simple complication during the course of severe liver diseases. Whatever the role played by cholestasis in the course of the disease, it can induce a series of functional and/or morphological alterations both in the liver and in other organs and tissues.

The principal steps at which pathogenetic mechanisms may be involved are at least 12, according to the most recent findings, most of them on the basis of experimental research.

Even if several conditions are not yet definitively known, these steps really constitute a continuous line along the metabolic pathway of bile acids and other biliary constituents. Several conditions are rare, while others are acquired and frequent, such as cholestatic syndromes which characterize the course of alcoholic hepatitis, primary biliary cirrhosis, cholangitis and drug-induced liver damage. In the last case, two principal mechanisms are involved: toxicity, direct and indirect, and hypersensitivity, the latter on the basis of idiosyncrasy or acquired immunological sensitization. However, also in the case of drug-induced cholestasis, more than one mechanism may be responsible in provoking an alteration in bile acid uptake and bile driving forces, for example during the administration of ethinyloestradiol; moreover, some other drugs, such as chlorpromazine, acting by itself or through its metabolites, may induce a cholestatic syndrome, on the basis of both toxic and immunological (sensitization) mechanisms.

In the case of drug-induced cholestasis, as for other types of cholestasis, the mechanism is often not influential in determining the course and prognosis of the disease. These can be predictable, in the case of toxic injuries, on the basis of the amount of drug administered. In the case of drug-induced cholestasis due to an imunologically abnormal response, the occurrence and course of the syndrome are often unpredictable, especially in the case of little-known drugs, and for pharmacological associations not often used in clinical practice.

ACKNOWLEDGEMENTS

This work was supported by a grant from MURST (Ministero dell'Universita' e della Ricerca Scientifica e Tecnologica) (Rome, Italy); financial support was also provided by the Italian Liver Foundation (Florence, Italy).

References

1. Sellinger M, Boyer JL. Physiology of bile secretion and cholestasis. In: Popper H, Schaffner F, editors. Progress in liver diseases, Vol. 9. New York: Grune & Stratton; 1990:237–59.
2. Gleeson D, Boyer JL. Intrahepatic cholestasis. In: McIntyre N, Benhamou J-P, Bircher J, Rizzetto M, Rodes J, editors. Oxford textbook of clinical hepatology, Vol. 2. Oxford: Oxford University Press; 1991:1087–107.
3. Oelberg D, Lester R. Cellular mechanisms of cholestasis. Annu Rev Med. 1986;37: 297–317.
4. Reichen J, Simon FR. Cholestasis. In: Arias IM, Jakoby DM, Popper H, Schachter D, Schafritz DA, editors. The liver. Biology and pathobiology. New York: Raven Press; 1988:1105–24.
5. Coleman R. Biochemistry of bile secretion. Biochem J. 1987;244:249–61.
6. Murphy GM. Serum bile acids: old and new. In: Setchell KDR, Kritchevsky D, Nair P, editors. The bile acids: chemistry, physiology and metabolism, Vol. IV. New York: Plenum Press; 1988:379–404.
7. van Berge Henegouwen GP, Brandt KH, Eyssen H et al. Sulphated and unsulphated bile acids in serum, bile and urine of patients with cholestasis. Gut. 1976;17:861–89.
8. Boyer JL. New concepts of mechanisms of hepatocyte bile formation. Physiol Rev. 1980;60:303–26.
9. Meier-Abt PJ. Cellular mechanisms of intrahepatic cholestasis. Drugs. 1990;40(Suppl. 3):84–97.
10. Nathanson MH, Boyer JL. Mechanisms and regulation of bile secretion. Hepatology. 1991;14:551–66.
11. Meier PJ. The bile salt secretory polarity of hepatocytes. J Hepatol. 1989;9:124–9.
12. Gentilini P, Baronti E, La Villa G et al. Il fegato. Fisiopatologia, clinica e terapia, Vol. I. Torino: UTET; 1991:387–426.
13. Chiarantini E, Arcangeli A, Mazzanti R et al. Ethinyl estradiol induced cholestasis. In: Gentilini P, Popper H, Sherlock S et al., editors. Problems in intrahepatic cholestasis. 2nd International Symposium, Florence 1978. Karger: Basel; 1979:102–10.
14. Boelsterli UA, Rakhit G, Balazs T. Modulation by S-adenosyl-L-methionine of hepatic Na/K-ATPase, membrane fluidity, and bile flow in rats with ethinyl estradiol-induced cholestasis. Hepatology. 1983;3:12–17.
15. Berr F, Simon FR, Reichen J. Ethinyl estradiol impairs bile salt uptake and Na/K pump function of rat hepatocytes. Am J Physiol. 1984;247:G437–G443.
16. Arias IM, Adachi Y, Tran T. Ethinyl estradiol cholestasis: a disease of the sinusoidal domain of the hepatocyte plasma membrane. Hepatology. 1983;3:872A.
17. Stacey NH. Effects of ethinyl estradiol on substrate uptake and efflux by isolated rat hepatocytes. Biochem Pharmacol. 1986;35:2495–500.
18. Bossard R, Stieger B, O'Neill B et al. Ethinylestradiol (EE) induces multiple canalicular membrane transport alterations in rat liver. J Hepatol. 1992;16(Suppl. 1):S7.
19. Romanelli RG, Gatmaitan Z, Arias IM. The effect of ethinyl estradiol on non-bile acid

organic anion transport in canalicular membrane vesicles from normal and mutant (TR−) rats. Hepatology. 1992;16:259A.

20. Goldsmith MA, Jones AL, Underdown BJ et al. Alterations in protein transport events in rat liver after estrogen treatment. Am J Physiol. 1987;253:G195–200.

21. Popper HJ, Szanto PB. Intrahepatic cholestasis (cholangiolitis). Gastroenterology. 1956;31:683–700.

22. Clarke AE, Maritz VM, Denborough MA. Phenothiazines and jaundice. Aust NZ J Med. 1972;4:376–82.

23. Carey MC, Hirom PC, Small DM. A study of physicochemical interactions between biliary lipids and chorpromazine hydrochloride. Bile-salt precipitation as a mechanism of phenothiazine-induced bile secretory failure. Biochem J. 1976;153:519–31.

24. Farrell GC. Drug-induced liver disease. In: Gitnick G, editor. Current hepatology, Vol. 11. St. Louis, Mosby-Year Book; 1990:86–128.

25. Sherlock S. Primary biliary cirrhosis. Clinical evaluation and treatment policies. Scand J Gastroenterol. 1982;77:63–74.

26. Utili R, Tripodi MF, Abernathy CO et al. Effects of bile salt infusion on chlorpromazine-induced cholestasis in the isolated perfused rat liver. Proc Soc Exp Biol Med. 1992;199: 49–53.

27. Keeffe EB, Blankenship N, Scharschmidt BF. Alteration of rat liver plasma membrane fluidity and ATPase activity by chlorpromazine hydrochloride and its metabolites. Gastroenterology. 1989;74:222–31.

28. Whitington PF. Cholestasis associated with parenteral nutrition in infants. Hepatology. 1985;5:693–6.

29. Zahavi I, Shaffer EA, Gall DG. Total parenteral nutrition-associated cholestasis: acute studies in infant and adult rabbits. J Pediatr Gastroenterol Nutr. 1985;4:622–7.

30. Duffy MC, Boyer JL. Pathophysiology of intrahepatic cholestasis and biliary obstruction. In: Ostrow, editor. Bile pigments and jaundice. New York: Marcel Dekker; 1986: 333–72.

31. Blitzer BL, Ratoosh SL, Donovan CB. Amino acid inhibition of bile acid uptake by isolated rat hepatocytes; relationship to dissipation of transmembrane Na^+ gradient. Am J Physiol. 1983;245:G399–403.

32. Quigley EM, Marsh M, Shaffer JL et al. Hepatobiliary complications of total parenteral nutrition. Geriatr Nurs Home Care. 1993;104:286–301.

33. Klaassen CD, Watkins JB. Mechanisms of bile formation, hepatic uptake and biliary excretion. Pharmacol Rev. 1984;36:1–67.

34. Javitt NG, Emerman S. Effect of sodium taurolithocholate on bile flow and bile acid excretion. J Clin Invest. 1968;47:1002–14.

35. Kakis G, Phillips MJ, Yousef IM. The respective roles of membrane cholesterol and of sodium potassium adenosine triphosphatase in the pathogenesis of lithocholate-induced cholestasis. Lab Invest. 1989;43:73–81.

36. Schwenk M, Schwarz LR, Greim H. Taurolithocholate inhibits taurocholate uptake by isolated hepatocyte at low concentrations. Naunyn-Schmiedeberg Arch Pharmacol. 1977;298:175–9.

37. Kakis G, Yousef IM. Pathogenesis of lithocholate- and taurolithocholate-induced intrahepatic cholestasis in rats. Gastroenterology. 1978;75:595–607.

38. Scholmerich J, Becher MS, Schmidt K et al. Influence of hydroxylation and conjugation of bile salts on their membrane damaging properties. Studies on isolated hepatocytes and lipid membrane vesicles. Hepatology. 1984;4:661–6.

39. Oelberg DG, Sackman JW, Dubinsky WA et al. Mechanisms of bile acid induced hemolysis. Gastroenterology. 1984;86:1198A.

40. Combettes L, Berthon B, Doucet E et al. Cholestatic bile acids permeabilize the endoplasmic reticulum of rat hepatocytes and neuroblastoma cells to calcium. Hepatology. 1988;8:1259A.

41. Layden TJ, Boyer JL. Taurolithocholate induced cholestasis; taurocholate but not taurodehydrocholate reverses cholestasis and bile canalicular membrane injury. Gastroenterology. 1977;73:120–8.

42. Strasberg SM, Kay RM, Ilson RG et al. Taurolithocholic acid and chlorpromazine cholestasis in rhesus monkey. Can J Physiol Pharmacol. 1979;57:1138–47.

43. Oelberg DG, Dubinsky WP, Adcock EW et al. Calcium binding by lithocholic acid

derivatives. Am J Physiol. 1984;247:G112–15.
44. Van der Meer R, Vonk RJ, Kuipers F. Cholestasis and the interactions of sulfated glyco- and taurolithocholate with calcium. Am J Physiol. 1988;254:G644–9.
45. Kawahara H, French SW. Role of cytoskeleton in canalicular contraction in cultured differentiated hepatocytes. Am J Pathol. 1990;136:521–32.
46. Desmet VT. Current problems in diagnosis of biliary disease and cholestasis. Semin Liver Dis. 1986;6:233–45.
47. Schaffner F, Popper H. Classification and mechanism of cholestasis. In: Wright R, Millward-Sadler GH, Alberti KGMM et al., editors. Liver and biliary disease. Pathophysiology, diagnosis, management, 2nd edn. London: Baillière Tindall–WB Saunders; 1985: 359–86.
48. Gordon LM, Sauerheber RD, Esgate JA et al. The increase in bilayer fluidity of rat liver plasma membranes achieved by the local anesthetic benzyl alcohol affects the activity of intrinsic membrane enzymes. J Biol Chem. 1980;255:4519–27.
49. Davis RA, Kern F Jr, Showalter R et al. Alterations of hepatic Na^+/K^+-ATPase and bile flow by estrogen: effects on liver surface membrane lipid structure and function. Proc Natl Acad Sci USA. 1978;75:4130–4.
50. Mills PR, Meier PJ, Smith DJ et al. The effect of changes in the fluid state of rat liver plasma membrane on the transport of taurocholate. Hepatology. 1987;7:61–6.
51. Smith DJ, Gordon ER. Membrane fluidity and cholestasis. J Hepatol. 1987;5:362–5.
52. Smith DJ, Gordon ER. Role of liver plasma membrane fluidity in the pathogenesis of estrogen-induced cholestasis. J Lab Clin Med. 1988;112:679–85.
53. Ishak K, Irey N. Hepatic injury associated with phenothiazines, clinicopathologic and follow up study of 36 patients. Arch Pathol. 1972;93:283–304.
54. Van Dyke RW, Scharschmidt BF. Effects of chlorpromazine on Na^+/K^+-ATPase pumping and solute transport in rat hepatocytes. Am J Physiol. 1987;253:G613–21.
55. Kukongviriyapan V, Stacey NH. Chemical-induced interference with hepatocellular transport. Role in cholestasis. Chem.-Biol. Interact. 1991;77:245–61.
56. Ziegler K, Frimmer M, Mullner S et al. 3'-isothiocyanobenzamido-^{3}H-cholate, a new affinity label for hepatocellular membrane proteins responsible for the uptake of both bile acids and phalloidin. Biochim Biophys Acta. 1984;773:11–22.
57. Frimmer M, Ziegler K. The transport of bile acids in liver cells. Biochim Biophys Acta. 1988;947:75–99.
58. Phillips DJ, Poucell S, Oda M. Biology of disease. mechanism of cholestasis. Lab Invest. 1986;54:593–608.
59. Bellentani S, Hardison WGM, Marchegiano P et al. Bile acid inhibition of taurocholate uptake by rat hepatocytes: role of OH groups. Am J Physiol. 1987;252:G339–44.
60. Blitzer BL, Bueler RL. Kinetic and energetic aspects of the inhibition of taurocholate uptake by Na^+-dependent amino acids: studies in rat liver plasma membrane vesicles. Am J Physiol. 1985;249:G120–40.
61. Moseley RH. Mechanisms of bile formation and cholestasis: clinical significance of recent experimental work. Am J Gastroenterol. 1986;81:731–5.
62. Fricker G, Landmann L, Meier PJ. Bile duct ligation reverses the bile salt secretory polarity of rat hepatocytes. Hepatology. 1987;7:1106A.
63. Kloppel TM, Hoops TC, Gaskin D et al. Uncoupling of the secretory pathways for IgA and secretory component by cholestasis. Am J Physiol. 1987;253:G232–40.
64. Miyai K, Richardson AL, Mayr W et al. Subcellular pathology of rat liver in cholestasis and choleresis induced by bile salts. I. Effects of lithocholic, 3-β-hydroxy-5-cholenic, cholic and dehydrocholic acids. Lab Invest. 1977;36:249–58.
65. Van der Sluijs P, Meijer DKE. Binding of drugs with a quaternary ammonium group to $α_1$ acid glycoprotein and asialo $α_1$ acid glycoprotein. J Pharmacol Exp Ther. 1985;234: 703–7.
66. Cohen KL, Rubin PE, Echevazzia RE. alpha-1-antitrypsin deficiency, emphysema and cirrhosis in an adult. Ann Intern Med. 1973;78:227–32.
67. Jeppsson JO, Larsson C, Eriksson S. Characterization of alpha-1-antitrypsin in the inclusion bodies from the liver in alpha-1-antitrypsin deficiency. N Engl J Med. 1975,293:576–9.
68. Schaffner F. Cholestassi in chronic hepatitis. In: Gentilini P, Popper H, Teodori U, editors. Chronic hepatitis. Basel: Karger; 1976:77–8.

69. Goldfischer S, Moore CL, Johnson AB *et al.* Peroxisomal and mitochondrial defects in the cerebro hepato renal syndrome. Science. 1973;182:62–4.
70. Bowen P, Lee CSN, Zellweger H *et al.* A familial syndrome of multiple congenital defects. Bull Johns Hopkins Hosp. 1964;114:402–14.
71. Kelley RI. The cerebrohepatorenal syndrome of Zellweger, morphologic and metabolic aspects. Am J Med Genet. 1983;16:503–17.
72. Alagille D. Syndromic paucity of interlobular bile ducts (Alagille syndrome or arteriohepatic dysplasia): review of 80 cases. J Pediatr. 1987;110:195–200.
73. Riley CA, Cotlier E, Jensen PS *et al.* Arteriohepatic dysplasia: a benign syndrome of intrahepatic cholestasis with multiple organ involvement. Ann Intern Med. 1979;91: 520–7.
74. Perrault B. Paucity of interlobular bile ducts. Dig Dis Sci. 1981;26:481–7.
75. Dubin M, Maurice M, Feldmann G *et al.* Phalloidin-induced cholestasis in the rat: relation to changes in microfilaments. Gastroenterology. 1978;75:450–5.
76. Thibault N, Claude JR, Ballet F. Actin filament alteration as a potential marker for cholestasis: a study in isolated rat hepatocyte couplets. Toxicology. 1992;73:269–79.
77. Weber AM, Tuchweber B, Yousef I *et al.* Severe familial cholestasis in North American Indian children — a microfilament dysfunction. Gastroenterology. 1981;81:653–62.
78. Phillips MJ, Oda M, Make E *et al.* Microfilament dysfunction as a possible cause of intrahepatic cholestasis. Gastroenterology. 1975;69:48–58.
79. Watanabe N, Tsukada N, Smith CR *et al.* Motility of bile canaliculi in the living animals: implications for bile flow. J Cell Biol. 1991;13:1069–80.
80. Watanabe S, Phillips MJ. Ca^{2+} causes active contraction of bile canaliculi: direct evidence from microinjection studies. Proc Natl Acad Sci USA. 1984;81:6164–8.
81. Durand-Schneider A-M, Bouanga J-C, Feldmann G *et al.* Microtubule disruption interferes with the structural and functional integrity of the apical pole in primary cultures of rat hepatocytes. Eur J Cell Biol. 1991;56:260–8.
82. Gores GJ, Herman B, Lemasters JJ. Plasma membrane bleb formation and rupture: a common feature of hepatocellular injury. Hepatology. 1990;11:690–8.
83. Kacich RL, Renston RH, Jones AL. Effects of cytochalasin D and colchicine on the uptake, translocation and biliary secretion of horse radish peroxidase and ^{14}C sodium taurocholate in the rat. Gastroenterology. 1983;85:385–94.
84. Kawahara H, Marceau N, French SW. Effect of agents which rearrange the cytoskeleton *in vitro* on the structure and function of hepatocytic canaliculi. Lab Invest. 1989;60: 692–704.
85. Dubin M, Maurice M, Feldmann G *et al.* Influence of colchicine and phalloidin on bile secretion and hepatic ultrastructure in the rat. Gastroenterology. 1980;79:646–54.
86. Katagiri K, Nakai T, Hoshino M *et al.* Tauro-β-muricholate preserves choleresis and prevents taurocholate-induced cholestasis in colcicine-treated rat liver. Gastroenterology. 1992;102:1660–7.
87. DeVos R, De Wolf-Peters C, Desmet V *et al.* Progressive intrahepatic cholestasis (Byler's disease): case report. Gut. 1975;16:943.
88. Linarelli LG, Williams CN, Phillips MJ. Byler's disease: fatal intrahepatic cholestasis. J Pediatr. 1972;81:484–92.
89. Scholmerich J, Baumgartner U, Miyai K *et al.* Tauroursodeoxycholate prevents taurolithocholate-induced cholestasis and toxicity in rat liver. J Hepatol. 1990;10:280–3.
90. Vial JD, Simon FR, MacKinnon AM. Effect of bile duct ligation on the ultrastructural morphology of hepatocytes. Gastroenterology. 1976;70:85–92.
92. Pflugl G, Kallen J, Schirmer T *et al.* X-ray structure of a decameric cyclophilin-cyclosporin crystal complex. Nature. 1993;361:91–3.
93. Stone BG, Udani M, Sanghvi A *et al.* Cyclosporin A-induced cholestasis. The mechanism in the rat model. Gastroenterology. 1987;93:344–51.
94. Galan AI, Roman ID, Munoz ME *et al.* Inhibition of biliary lipid and protein secretion by cyclosporine in the rat. Biochem Pharmacol. 1992;44:1105–13.
95. Rotolo FS, Branum GD, Bowers GA *et al.* Effect of cyclosporine on bile secretion in rats. Am J Surg. 1986;151:35–40.
96. Cadranel JF, Erlinger S, Desruenne M *et al.* Chronic administration of cyclosporin A induces a decrease in hepatic excretory function in man. Dig Dis Sci. 1992;37:1473–6.

97. Kallinowski B, Theilmann L, Zimmermann R et al. Effective treatment of cyclosporine-induced cholestasis in heart-transplanted patients treated with ursodeoxycholic acid. Transplantation. 1991;51:81128–9.
98. Ziegler K, Frimmer M. Cyclosporin A protects liver cells against phalloidin. Potent inhibition of the inward transport of cholate and phallotoxins. Biochim Biophys Acta. 1984;805:174–80.
99. Ziegler K, Frimmer M. Cyclosporin A and a diaziridine derivative inhibit the hepatocellular uptake of cholate, phalloidin and rifampicin. Biochim Biophys Acta. 1986;855:136–42.
100. Arias IM. Cyclosporin, the biology of the bile canaliculus, and cholestasis. Gastroenterology. 1993;104:1558–60.
101. Kadmon M, Klunemann C, Bohme M et al. Inhibition by cyclosporine A of adenosine triphosphate-dependent transport from the hepatocyte into bile. Gastroenterology. 1993;104:1507–14.
102. Muller M, Ishikawa T, Berger U et al. ATP-dependent transport of taurocholate across the hepatocyte canalicular membrane mediated by a 110-kDa glycoprotein binding ATP and bile salts. J Biol Chem. 1991;266:18920–6.
103. Nishida T, Gatmaitan Z, Che M et al. Rat liver canalicular membrane vesicles contain an ATP-dependent bile acid transport system. Proc Natl Acad Sci USA. 1991;88:6590–4.
104. Stieger B, O'Neill B, Meier PJ. ATP-dependent bile-salt transport in canalicular rat liver plasma-membrane vesicles. Biochem J. 1992;284:67–74.
105. Kobayashi K, Sogame Y, Hara H et al. Mechanism of glutathione S-conjugate transport in canalicular and basolateral rat liver plasma membrane. J Biol Chem. 1990;265:7737–41.
106. Schaub T, Ishikawa T, Keppler D. ATP-dependent leukotriene export from mastocytoma cells. FEBS Lett. 1991;279:83–6.
107. Kobayashi K, Sogame Y, Hayashi K et al. ATP stimulates the uptake of S-dinitrophenylglutathione by rat liver plasma membrane vesicles. FEBS Lett. 1988;240:55–8.
108. Akerboom TPM, Narayanaswami V, Kunst M et al. ATP-dependent S-(2,4-dinitrophenyl)-glutathione transport in canalicular plasma membrane vesicles from rat liver. J Biol Chem. 1991;266:13147–52.
109. Nishida T, Gatmaitan Z, Roy-Chowdhury J et al. Two distinct mechanisms for bilirubin glucuronide transport by rat bile canalicular membrane vesicles: demonstration of defective ATP-dependent transport in rats (TR⁻) with inherited conjugated hyperbilirubinemia. J Clin Invest. 1992;90:227–32.
110. Kitamura T, Jansen P, Hardenbrook C et al. Defective ATP-dependent bile canalicular transport of organic anions in mutant (TR⁻) rats with conjugated hyperbilirubinemia. Proc Natl Acad Sci USA. 1990;87:3557–61.
111. Nishida T, Hardenbrook C, Gatmaitan Z et al. ATP-dependent organic anion transport system in normal and TR⁻ rat liver canalicular membranes. Am J Physiol. 1992;262:G629–35.
112. Arias IM, Che M, Gatmaitan Z et al. The biology of bile canaliculus. Hepatology. 1993;17:318–29.
113. Mazzanti R, Gatmaitan Z, Croop JM et al. Quantitative image analysis of rhodamine 123 transport by adriamycin – sensitive and resistant NIH 3T3 and human hepatocellular carcinoma (Alexander) cells. J Cell Pharmacol. 1990;1:50–6.
114. Valverde MA, Diaz M, Sepulveda FV et al. Volume-regulated chloride channels associated with the human multidrug resistance P-glycoprotein. Nature. 1992;355:830–3.
115. Abraham EH, Prat AG, Gerweck L et al. The multidrug resistance (mdr1) gene product functions as an ATP channel. Proc Natl Acad Sci USA. 1993;90:312–16.
116. Krell H, Hoeke H, Pfaff E. Development of intrahepatic cholestasis by α-naphthylisothiocyanate in rats. Gastroenterology. 1982;82:507–14.
117. Elias E, Hruban Z, Wade JB et al. Phalloidin induced-cholestasis — a microfilament mediated change in junctional complex permeability. Proc Natl Acad Sci USA. 1980;77:2229–33.
118. Layden TJ, Boyer JL. The effect of thyroid hormone on bile salt-independent bile flow and Na/K-ATPase activity in liver plasma membranes enriched in bile canaliculi. J Clin Invest. 1976;57:1009–18.
119. Miner PB, Sutherland E, Simon FR. Regulation of hepatic sodium plus potassium

activated adenosine triphosphatase activity by glucocorticoids in the rat. Gastroenterology 1980;79:212–21.

120. Avner DL, Larsen R, Berenson MM. Inhibition of liver surface membrane Na+/K+-adenosine triphosphatase Mg2+-adenosine triphosphatase and 5′-nucleotidase activities by protoporphyrin. Gastroenterology. 1983;850:700–6.

121. Avner DL, Randall GL, Brenson MM. Protoporphyrin-induced cholestasis in the isolated in situ perfused rat liver. J Clin Invest. 1981;67:385–94.

122. Herman SP, Baggenstoss AH, Cloutier MD. Liver dysfunction and histologic abnormalities in neonatal hypopituitarism. J Pediatr. 1975;87:892–5.

123. Van Dyke RW, Scharschmidt BF. Effects of chlorpromazine on Na+/K+-ATPase pumping and solute transport in rat hepatocytes. Am J Physiol. 1987;253:G613–21.

124. Gentilini P, Surrenti C, Chiarantini E. Virus and drug induced cholestasis. Acta Gastroenterol Belg. 1979;42:369–89.

125. Popper H, Schaffner F. Cholestasis. In: Berk JE, editor. Gastroenterology, 4th edn. Philadelphia: WB Saunders; 1985:2697–731.

126. Gordon SC, Reddy KR, Schiff L et al. Prolonged intrahepatic cholestasis secondary to acute hepatitis A. Ann Intern Med. 1984;101:635–7.

127. Maddrey C, Boitnott JK. Drug-induced chronic hepatitis and cirrhosis. In: Popper H, Schaffner S, editors. Progress in liver diseases, Vol. VI. New York: Grune & Stratton, 1979:595–603.

128. Marbert UA, Shefer S, Leevy CM. Studies of the influence of immunological and serological factors from patients with cholestasis due to alcoholic or viral hepatitis on biliary function in the rat. Eur J Clin Invest. 1984;14:346–53.

129. Hubscher SG, Lumley MA, Elias E. Vanishing bile duct syndrome: a possible mechanism for intrahepatic cholestasis in Hodgkin's lymphoma. Infirm Can. 1993;17:70–7.

130. Birrer MJ, Young RC. Differential diagnosis of jaundice in lymphoma patients. Semin Liver Dis. 1987;7:269–77.

131. Aagenaes O. Hereditary recurrent cholestasis with lymphoedema: two new families. Acta Paediatr Scand. 1974;63:465–71.

132. Aagenaes O, Sigstad H, Bjorn-Hansen R. Lymphoedema in hereditary recurrent cholestasis from birth. Arch Dis Child. 1970;45:690–5.

133. George J, Farrell GC. Drug-induced liver disease. In: Gitnick G, editor. Current hepatology, Vol. 13. St Louis: Mosby; 1993:105–57.

134. Zimmerman HJ, Lewis JH. Drug-induced cholestasis. Med Toxicol. 1987;2:112–60.

135. Mitchell JR, Jollow DJ. Metabolic activation of drugs to toxic substances. Gastroenterology. 1975;68:392–410.

136. Vore M. Estrogen cholestasis. Membranes, metabolites, or receptors. Gastroenterology. 1987;93:643–9.

137. Mitchell JR, Jollow DJ, Potter WZ et al. Acetaminophen-induced hepatic necrosis. I. Role of drug metabolism. J Pharmacol Exp Ther. 1973;187:185–94.

138. Zimmerman HJ, Maddrey WC. Toxic and drug-induced hepatitis. In: Schiff L, Schiff ER, editors. Diseases of the liver, 6th edn. Philadelphia: Lippincott; 1987:591–667.

139. Zimmerman HJ. Hepatotoxicity; the adverse effect of drugs and other chemicals on the liver. New York: Appleton-Century-Crofts; 1978.

140. Klassen CD. Principles of toxicology. In: Gilman AG, Goodman LS, Rall TW et al., editors. Goodman and Gilman's The Pharmacological basis of therapeutics, 7th edn. New York: Macmillan; 1985:1592–604.

141. Read EA. The liver and drugs. In: Wright R, Millward-Sadler GH, Alberti KGMM et al., editors. Liver and biliary disease. London: Baillière Tindall; 1985:1003–31.

142. Chuang LC, Tunier AP, Akhtar N et al. Possible case of procainamide-induced intrahepatic cholestatic jaundice. Ann Pharmacother. 1993;27:434–7.

143. Klatskin G. Toxic and drug-induced hepatitis. In: Schiff L, editor. Diseases of the liver, 4th edn. Philadelphia: Lippincott; 1975:604–710.

144. Ockner RK. Drug-induced liver disease. In: Zakim D, Boyer JL, editors. Hepatology. Philadelphia: WB Saunders; 1982;691–722.

145. Kenwright S, Levi AJ. Sites of competition in the selective hepatic uptake of rifamycin-SV, flavaspidic acid, bilirubin and bromosulphthalein. Gut. 1974;15:220–7.

146. Galeazzi R, Lorenzini I, Orlandi F. Rifampicin-induced elevation of serum bile acids in

man. Dig Dis Sci. 1980;25:108–14.

147. Pessayre D, Mazel P. Induction and inhibition of hepatic drug metabolizing enzymes by rifampin. Biochem Pharmacol. 1976;25:943–8.

148. Cousins MJ, Sharp JH, Gourlay GK et al. Hepatotoxicity and halothane metabolism in an animal model with application for human toxicity. Anesth Intens Care. 1979;7:9–24.

149. Neuberger JM, Tredger JM, Davis M. Oxidative metabolism of halothane in the production of hepatocyte membrane neoantigens. In: Davis M, editor. Drug reactions and the liver. London: Pitman Medical; 1981:245–54.

150. Crantock L, Prentice R, Powell L. Cholestatic jaundice associated with captopril therapy. J Gastroenterol Hepatol. 1991;6:528–30.

151. Gentilini P. Corticosteroids and immunosuppressive drugs in chronic evolutive hepatitis treatment. Pharmacol Res Commun. 1971;3:287–308.

152. Gentilini P. Fegato e farmaci: aspetti di farmacologia clinica e di patologia iatrogena. Riv med Svizz Ital. 1979;3:103–18 (1st part); 4:161–75 (2nd part).

153. Findor J, Bruch Igartua E, Sorda J et al. Jaundice caused by methimazole. Acta Gastroenterol Latinoam. 1991;21:115–119.

24
S-Adenosylmethionine and the liver

J. M. MATO, L. ALVAREZ, J. MINGORANCE, C. DURÁN, P. ORTIZ and M. A. PAJARES

INTRODUCTION

During the past few years convincing evidence has been produced on the pathological consequences of methionine metabolism alterations. In this chapter we will present a summary of major advances in this area.

The first step in methionine breakdown is the formation of S-adenosylmethionine (SAMe), a process catalysed by SAMe-synthetase, also called methionine adenosyl transferase[1]. In this unusual reaction the adenosyl moiety of ATP is transferred to methionine, forming a sulphonium ion through the binding of the 5'-carbon atom of the ribose with the sulphur atom of methionine (Fig. 1). The tripolyphosphate formed as the result of the transfer of the adenosyl moiety of ATP is further hydrolysed to inorganic phosphate and pyrophosphate, making the synthesis of SAMe irreversible under physiological conditions[2]. In mammals this is the preferred pathway for methionine metabolism, since the transamination pathway, although it exists, is not a quantitatively important route even after methionine loading[3-5].

In an adult individual 6–8 g of SAMe are produced daily, the majority in the liver where it is also consumed[6,7]. Although SAMe can be decarboxylated for polyamine synthesis, most of it is used in transmethylation reactions, the process by which methyl groups are added to compounds[1]. The presence of a sulphonium ion in the molecule of SAMe makes it a 'high-energy' reagent, which can easily transfer its small methyl group to a large variety of acceptor substrates, including nucleic acids, proteins, phospholipids, catecholamines and a long list of small molecules. The transmethylation reactions that probably occur in normal individuals have been listed, and the relative demand of each on the available SAMe has been estimated[6,7].

All transmethylation reactions produce S-adenosylhomocysteine (SAH), a potent competitive inhibitor of transmethylation reactions (Fig. 2). In the normal rat liver the value of the ratio SAMe/SAH is around 5–7[8,9], and it has been determined that when this ratio is about 4 a variety of methyltransferases are inhibited by 10–60%[10]. Of all the enzymes that use SAMe, glycine methyltransferase is the most abundant and accounts for about 1% of liver

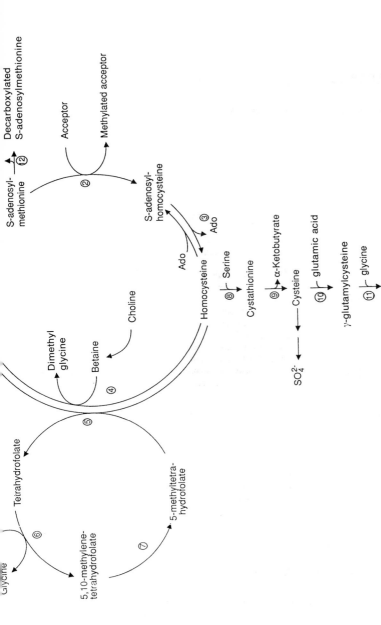

Fig. 1 Relevant reactions of liver methionine metabolism and related metabolic pathways. (1) *S*-adenosyl-L-methionine synthetase, also called methionine-adenosyltransferase; (2) transmethylation reactions; (3) *S*-adenosyl-L-homocysteine hydrolase; (4) betaine–homocysteine methyltransferase; (5) 5-methyltetrahydrofolate-homocysteine methyltransferase, also called methionine synthase; (6) serine oxidase; (7) 5,10-methylene-tetrahydrofolate reductase; (8) cystathionine β-synthase; (9) γ-cystathionase; (10) γ-glutamylcysteine synthetase; (11) glutathione synthetase; (12) *S*-adenosyl-L-methionine decarboxylase

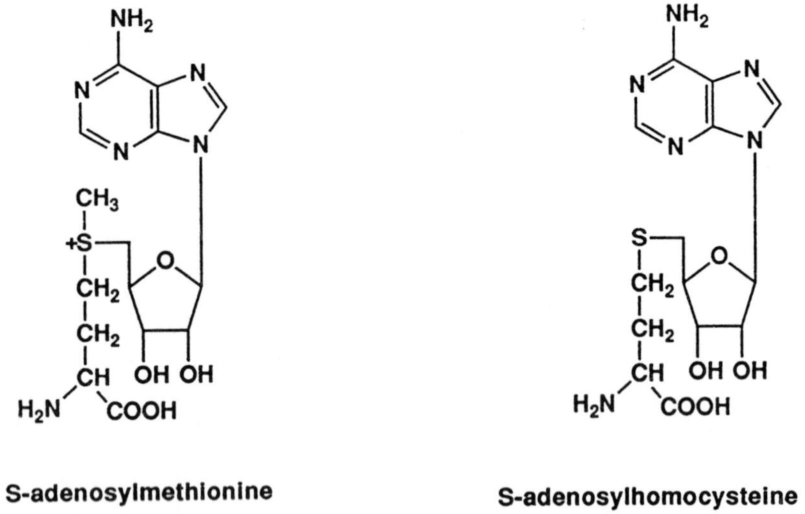

S-adenosylmethionine

S-adenosylhomocysteine

Fig. 2 Structure of S-adenosyl-L-methionine and S-adenosyl-L-homocysteine

cytosolic protein. This enzyme catalyses the synthesis of sarcosine from SAMe and glycine, which in turn is rapidly converted again to glycine. The function of this enzyme is to remove excess methyl groups, and thus it seems as a means of regulating the SAMe/SAH ratio[11]. SAH levels are maintained low by being further converted into adenosine and homocysteine, through the action of a hydrolase that cleaves the thioether bond of SAH. *In vivo*, adenosine is rapidly transformed into inosine, and homocysteine is also quickly removed, to be converted into either cystathionine and its derivatives (cysteine, glutathione, taurine, inorganic sulphate, etc.), by the transsulphuration pathway, or used again for the resynthesis of methionine. An accumulation of SAH produces a drastic reduction in the SAMe/SAH ratio with marked alterations of cellular behaviour such as lymphocyte function, chemotaxis or ion transport[10,12,13]. These effects have been interpreted as being due to the accumulation of SAH, which leads to a strong inhibition of phospholipid methylation, the process by which phosphatidylethanolamine is converted into phosphatidylcholine. However, this interpretation might be an oversimplification of the results, and inhibition of other methyltransferases might also be involved (see citations in ref. 13).

STRUCTURE OF LIVER SAMe-SYNTHETASE

Human and rat liver SAMe-synthetase have been cloned and sequenced[14–17]. The deduced amino acid sequences correspond to proteins with M_r values of 43 647 and 43 697 for the human and rat liver enzymes respectively[15,17]. A cDNA clone for rat liver SAMe-synthetase has been shown, by Northern analysis, to detect a single mRNA species of about 3.4 kb in both rat and human liver, but it did not hybridize with RNA from rat kidney, spleen, heart, testis or brain[15]. Similarly, a cDNA clone for human liver SAMe-synthetase has been shown to detect, by Northern analysis, a single mRNA species in both human and rat liver, but did not hybridize with RNA from human kidney, spleen, ganglion or gall-bladder[17]. This agrees with the high homology found (89% in the coding region) between rat and human liver SAMe-synthetase cDNA sequences, and with the observation that rat liver and kidney SAMe-synthetase DNA sequences are different[15,17,18]. The cDNA clone for rat kidney SAMe-synthetase has been shown to detect two mRNA species, of about 3.4 and 3.8 kb, in kidney, brain and testis, but did not hybridize with liver[18]. The occurrence of only one mRNA species coding for this protein in human and rat liver has been confirmed by primer extension analysis. This finding excludes the possibility of an alternative transcription site in the liver, as it has been proposed to take place in rat kidney to explain the presence, by Northern analysis, of two mRNA species[18]. Moreover, by Southern analysis, the existence of only one gene coding for human liver SAMe-synthetase has been demonstrated[17]. In summary, these results appear to indicate the existence of two different genes for SAMe-synthetase in mammals, one expressed specifically in the liver and a second gene expressed in non-hepatic tissues. Two SAMe-synthetase genes have also been identified in plants and yeast[19-21]. Moreover, an extensive similarity exists among bacteria, yeast, plant and mammalian SAMe-synthetases[14-21], indicating that the primary structure of this enzyme has been well preserved during evolution.

For a long time it has been known that the rat liver cytosol contains different forms of SAMe-synthetase, which were called α (M_r 200 kDa), β (M_r 110 kDa) and γ (M_r 190 kDa)[22-27]. More recently it has been shown that only the α and β forms are present in the normal adult rat liver[27,28]. Both forms, when analysed by SDS-PAGE, show a single polypeptide band with M_r of about 48 kDa. Tryptic peptide mapping of both forms presents the same profile on HPLC, and antibodies against the β form (low-M_r form) are able to recognize both SAMe-synthetases[27]. Moreover, the incubation of the α form (high-M_r form) in the presence of high concentrations of LiBr, converts this form into the low-M_r form[28]. These results indicate that the high-M_r form is a tetramer and the low-M_r form is a dimer of the same subunit. Similarly, in humans, two forms of SAMe-synthetase, with M_r of about 200 and 110 kDa, have also been found, by gel filtration chromatography, in liver extracts from normal and cirrhotic adult individuals[29]. Moreover, an active monomeric form of the enzyme has been found, by gel filtration, in the liver extract from one cirrhotic patient[30].

SAMe-SYNTHETASE REGULATION

The oxido/reduction state of sulphydryl groups of the enzyme, whose sequence contains 10 Cys residues[15], influences its kinetic properties and aggregation state. The presence of two accessible sulphydryl groups in the native enzyme is important in maintaining the activity of both forms of the enzyme[30,31]. This modification causes a loss of the enzyme activity in both the high- and low-M_r forms. Additionally, oxidation of sulphydryl groups leads to the dissociation of the high-M_r to the low-M_r form, whereas no modification of the low-M_r SAMe-synthetase was observed. One of the modified sulphydryl groups, localized at Cys-150, seems to be responsible for an 80% reduction in the activity in both SAMe-synthetase forms after N-ethylmaleimide treatment. Cys-150 is located close to the consensus sequence for the ATP-binding site, and its modification by N-ethylmaleimide can be partially protected by including the enzyme substrates (methionine) or analogues of the substrates (AMP-PNP) in the incubation mixture. This residue is conserved in the liver and kidney enzyme from both human and rat origin. These results are related to those observed with the *Escherichia coli* enzyme, where N-ethylmaleimide modification of Cys-90 of the sequence also leads to the dissociation of the enzyme to form an inactive dimer[32]. These results indicate the importance of sulphydryl groups in maintaining SAMe-synthetase activity and structure.

Modulation of rat liver SAMe-synthetase activity by the GSH/GSSG ratio was shown after the observation that both forms of the enzyme are inhibited by GSSG, and GSH has no effect on the enzyme activity although it protects from the inhibitory effect of GSSG. Moreover, inhibition of enzyme activity was correlated with dissociation of both SAMe-synthetases to a monomer. Since no incorporation of [^{35}S]GSSG has been observed with either of the enzyme forms, the available data obtained in the presence of GSSG seem to suggest that oxidation leads to the formation of an intrasubunit disulphide. In summary, both the activity and aggregation state of the enzyme are regulated by the GSH/GSSG ratio[34].

LIVER DAMAGE AND METHIONINE METABOLISM ALTERATION

In vivo experiments carried out by the injection to rats of buthionine sulphoximine (BSO), a molecule that inhibits γ-glutamylcysteine synthetase and therefore glutathione synthesis[35], have shown that a 30% reduction in the GSH concentration goes parallel with a 40% reduction of SAMe and a 60% reduction of liver SAMe-synthetase activity[36]. Alteration in these parameters is accompanied by a reduction in the number of mitochondria, mitochondrial swelling and degeneration, with rupture of membrane architecture and increased density. Moreover, loss and vacuolization of smooth endoplasmic reticulum and a reduction and degeneration of the rough endoplasmic reticulum is also observed after BSO treatment. These effects of BSO on liver structure are similar to those observed in mouse muscle, lung and epithelial cells after exposure to the drug[37-39]. The effect of BSO on liver structure, GSH levels and SAMe-synthetase activity is almost completely prevented by administration of a monoethylester of glutathione, a permeable derivative of GSH[40]. Indeed, these experiments have shown the existence of a correlation between the hepatic levels of GSH and liver SAMe-synthetase activity[36].

Similarly, CCl_4 administration to rats results in induction of hepatic fibrosis, a 60% reduction of hepatic SAMe-synthetase activity and a 45% depletion of liver GSH[41]. Reduction of SAMe-synthetase and of GSH is prevented by SAMe treatment. Moreover, the attenuation by SAMe of these parameters is associated with a reduction in the formation of fibrous tissue and a decrease in the number of rats that developed cirrhosis[41].

In this context it has been shown that SAMe prevents intracellular GSH depletion by GSH-depleting drugs, such as heroin, methadone, paracetamol and ethanol, in rat and human hepatocytes[42]. Moreover, a protective effect of SAMe has been described[42-45] as a reduction of the release of intracellular enzymes induced *in vivo* and *in vitro* by paracetamol, thioacetamide, heroin, methadone, ethanol and CCl_4. Interestingly, CCl_4- and BSO-induced SAMe-synthetase deficiency does not produce any significant modification of hepatic levels of SAMe-synthetase mRNA[41], indicating that this defect in SAMe-synthetase is due to inactivation of the enzyme (e.g. by formation of an inactive monomer) or to increased degradation, and not to a defective synthesis.

Impaired hepatic synthesis and utilization of SAMe has also been observed in other forms of liver injury. Thus, hepatic SAMe depletion and a reduction in the tetrameric form of SAMe-synthetase has been detected in galactosamine-induced liver injury in rats[29,46]. In addition, in this model the administration of SAMe protects from the hepatotoxic effect of galactosamine[46]. Similarly, in alcohol-induced liver injury in baboons there is a depletion of hepatic SAMe and a reduction in GSH levels. The depletion of hepatic SAMe and GSH in alcohol-induced liver injury in baboons is improved by the administration of exogenous SAMe. Furthermore, in the baboon model SAMe attenuates ethanol-induced liver injury, as shown by a smaller increase in plasma aspartate transaminase and glutamic dehydrogenase activities, fewer ethanol-induced megamitochondria and a smaller increase in mito-chondrial mass[47].

Enhanced lipid peroxidation resulting from the production of oxygen free radicals is a well-known consequence of chronic ethanol consumption[48]. Metabolism of these highly reactive species depends on the liver availability of the free-radical scavenger GSH, which is depleted in alcoholic states[49]. In an attempt to replenish GSH or to prevent free-radical cellular damage, ethanol administration to rats also induces an increase of methionine catabolism, which in turn leads to a reduction of the methylation ratio (SAMe/SAH ratio) and therefore of transmethylation reactions[50].

Other studies have also demonstrated a fall in methionine synthase activity induced by ethanol administration[50-52]. The mechanism for this effect is not clear but, similar to SAMe-synthetase, this enzyme is known to be sensitive to inhibition by free radicals and therefore by conditions that reduce GSH levels. Ethanol also induces an increase in the activity of betaine–homocysteine methyltransferase[51], the alternative pathway for homocysteine remethylation (see Fig. 1). Although this is an attempt to compensate for the inhibition of methionine synthase by ethanol, such an effect seems to be inefficient, as the methyl groups so transferred to form methionine are still rapidly lost[50] as CO_2. In summary, it seems likely that the increased catabolism of methionine at the expense of methylation reactions is motivated by a need to synthesize hepatic GSH to counteract the damaging oxidant effects of ethanol. Such adaptation results, however, in a deficiency of the methylation ratio (SAMe/SAH ratio) and therefore in the ability to replenish liver GSH levels[50].

In liver biopsy specimens from chronic liver disease patients (both of alcoholic and non-alcoholic origin) there is roughly a 35% depletion of GSH, higher levels of GSSG[54] and, in cirrhotics, approximately a 50% reduction of SAMe-synthetase activity[55]. SAMe-synthetase deficiency in human cirrhosis seems to be due to a specific decrease in the activity of the tetrameric form of the enzyme without affecting the dimeric form[29], indicating a higher susceptibility of the tetramer to inactivation in these patients (e.g. by formation of an inactive monomer). In fact, similar SAMe-synthetase mRNA levels have been detected in normal liver and in biopsies from patients with alcoholic cirrhosis[17], suggesting that the reduction of SAMe-synthetase activity found in these patients is not due to a deficiency synthesis of the enzyme. SAMe treatment attenuates the depletion of hepatic GSH, lowers the levels of GSSG in alcoholic and non-alcoholic liver disease[54], and improves the clearance of plasma methionine after its systemic administration to alcoholic cirrhotics[53], which suggests that SAMe administration may prevent SAMe-synthetase inactivation in patients with liver injury.

In an acute model of paracetamol-induced hepatotoxicity, exogenous SAMe has also been found to improve survival and diminish liver injury[56]. Moreover, in this model SAMe was as effective as N-acetylcysteine in reducing paracetamol-induced liver and plasma GSH depletion. Pretreatment with BSO, which inhibits GSH synthesis and potentiates paracetamol hepatotoxicity without known effects on the metabolism of the drug, abrogates the beneficial effect of N-acetylcysteine and SAMe on survival and on their capacity to restore GSH levels[56,57]. Methionine is less effective than N-acetylcysteine or SAMe in preventing liver injury, which agrees with the observation that in this model the conversion of methionine to SAMe is also impaired (Corrales, F. and Mato, J.M., unpublished).

The above results support a model where liver GSH, which derives from SAMe by the trans-sulphuration pathway (Fig. 1), is depleted and GSSG levels increase as a result of liver injury. This reduction of the GSH/GSSG ratio leads to SAMe-synthetase dissociation and inactivation, which in turn produces a further decrease in GSH and a still greater inactivation of SAMe-synthetase. The addition of exogenous SAMe, which has been shown to be taken up by hepatocytes[47,58], may break this vicious cycle by bypassing the deficit in SAMe synthesis. This would lead to an increase in GSH levels and to the prevention of SAMe synthetase inactivation, despite the existence of liver injury. These results also suggest that a reduction of SAMe-synthetase and depletion of GSH levels are important concomitants of different forms of liver injury *in vivo*.

The above results also suggest that liver SAMe-synthetase deficiency should not in itself be a cause of liver injury, but might be a risk factor for the development of liver disease, due to the lower capacity of the organ to respond to a higher demand of GSH under certain conditions, such as prolonged and heavy use of alcohol, exposure to toxic drugs or chemicals, autoimmune processes, infections with certain viruses or inborn metabolic errors. Indeed, there is evidence indicating that GSH depletion below a threshold level is necessary for toxicity due to oxidative stress[59,60]. These results point to the clinical relevance of alterations of liver methionine metabolism that lead to moderately depleted GSH levels, and to the clinical value of correcting these deficiencies. Sustaining this view is the observation that in cirrhotic patients methionine clearance deficiency correlates with the severity of liver disease[61]. The possible beneficial effect of long-term SAMe treatment on the appearance and management of clinical complications in chronic liver diseases, such as bleeding from oesophageal varices or brain damage secondary to liver dysfunction, has, however, not yet been examined. At the very least SAMe deserves further study in the treatment of cirrhosis because of these reports, and because of other studies indicating that it may reduce the formation of fibrous tissue in the diseased liver.

Acknowledgements

Work at the authors' laboratory was supported by Fondo de Investigaciones Sanitarias, Dirección General de Investigación Científica ·y Técnica, and Europharma.

References

1. Cantoni GL. Biochemical methylations: selected aspects. Ann Rev Biochem. 1975;44: 435–41.
2. Mudd SH. The adenosyltransferases. In: Boyer PD, editor. The enzymes, 3rd edn. New York: Academic Press; 1973: vol. 8, part A; 121–43.
3. Gahl WA, Bernardini I, Finkelstein JD et al. Transsulfuration in an adult with hepatic methionine adenosyltransferase deficiency. J Clin Invest. 1988;81:390–7.
4. Wu G, Thompson JR. Is methionine transaminated in skeletal muscle? Biochem J. 1989;257:281–4.
5. Cooper AJL. Methionine transamination in vivo. Biochem J. 1989;262:689–91.
6. Mudd SH, Poole JR. Labile methyl balances for normal humans on various dietary regimens. Metabolism. 1975;24:721–35.
7. Mudd SH, Ebert MH, Scriver CR. Labile methyl group balances in the human: the role of sarcosine. Metabolism. 1980;29:707–20.
8. Hoffman DR, Cornatzer WE, Duerre JA. Relationship between tissue levels of S-adenosylmethionine, S-adenosylhomocysteine, and transmethylation reactions. Can J Biochem. 1979;57:56–65.
9. Hoffman DR, Marion DV, Cornatzer WE et al. S-adenosylmethionine and S-adenosylhomocysteine metabolism in isolated rat liver: effects of L-methionine, L-homocysteine and adenosine. J Biol Chem. 1980;255:10822–7.
10. Cantoni GL, Richards HH, Chiang PK. Inhibitors of S-adenosylhomocysteine hydrolase and their role in the regulation of biological methylations. In: Usdin E, Borchardt RT, Creveling CR, editors. Transmethylation. New York: Elsevier–North Holland, 1979: 155–64.
11. Cook RJ, Wagner C. Glycine N-methyltransferase is a folate binding protein. Proc Natl Acad Sci USA. 1984;81:3631–4.
12. Garcia Castro I, Mato JM, Vasanthakumar G et al. Paradoxical effects of adenosine and adenosine analogs on neutrophil chemotaxis. J Biol Chem. 1983;258:4345–9.
13. Mato JM, Alemany S. What is the function of phospholipid methylation? Biochem J. 1983;212:1–10.
14. Horikawa S, Ishikawa M, Ozasa H et al. Isolation of a cDNA encoding the rat liver S-adenosylmethionine synthetase. Eur J Biochem. 1989;184:497–501.

15. Alvarez L, Asuncion M, Corrales F *et al.* Analysis of the 5' non-coding region of rat liver *S*-adenosylmethionine synthetase mRNA and comparison of the M_r deduced from the cDNA sequence and the purified enzyme. FEBS Lett. 1991;290:142–6.
16. Horikawa S, Tsukada K. Molecular cloning and nucleotide sequence of cDNA encoding the human liver *S*-adenosylmethionine synthetase. Biochem Int. 1991;25:81–90.
17. Alvarez L, Corrales F, Martin-Duce A *et al.* Isolation of a full-length cDNA coding for human liver *S*-adenosylmethionine synthetase. Tissue-specific gene expression and analysis of mRNA levels in hepatopathies. Biochem J. 1993;293:481–6.
18. Horikawa S, Sasuga J, Shimizu K *et al.* Molecular cloning and nucleotide sequence of cDNA encoding the rat kidney *S*-adenosylmethionine synthetase. J Biol Chem. 1990;265:13683–6.
19. Markham GD, De Parasis J, Gatmaitan J. The sequence of met K, the structural gene for *S*-adenosylmethionine synthetases in *Saccharomyces cerevisiae*. J Biol Chem. 1984;259:14505–7.
20. Thomas D, Surdin-Kerjan Y. SAMe 1, the structural gene for one of the *S*-adenosylmethionine synthetases in *Saccharomyces cerevisiae*. J Biol Chem. 1987;262:16704–9.
21. Thomas D, Rothstein R, Rosenberg N *et al.* SAMe 2 encodes the second methionine *S*-adenosyl transferase in *Saccharomyces cerevisiae*. Mol Cell Biol. 1988;8:5132–9.
22. Liau MC, Lin GW, Hulbert BC. Partial purification and characterization of tumor and liver *S*-adenosylmethionine synthetases. Cancer Res. 1977;37:427–35.
23. Liau MC, Chang CF, Berlanger L *et al.* Correlation of isozyme patterns of *S*-adenosylmethionine synthetase with fetal stages and pathological states of the liver. Cancer Res. 1977;39:162–9.
24. Kunz GL, Hoffman JL, Chia C-S *et al.* Separation of rat liver methionine adenosyltransferase isozymes by hydrophobic chromatography. Arch Biochem Biophys. 1980;202:565–71.
25. Sullivan DM, Hoffman JL. Fractionation and kinetic properties of rat liver and kidney methionine adenosyltransferase isozymes. Biochemistry. 1983;22:1636–41.
26. Okada G, Teraoka H, Tsukada K. Multiple species of mammalian *S*-adenosylmethionine synthetase. Partial purification and characterization. Biochemistry. 1981;20:934–40.
27. Cabrero C, Puerta J, Alemany S. Purification and comparison of two forms of *S*-adenosyl-L-methionine synthetase from rat liver. Eur J Biochem. 1987;170:299–304.
28. Cabrero C, Alemany S. Conversion of rat liver *S*-adenosyl-L-methionine synthetase from high-M_r form to low-M_r form by LiBr. Biochim Biophys Acta. 1988;952:277–81.
29. Cabrero C, Martin-Duce A, Ortiz P *et al.* Specific loss of the high-molecular weight form of *S*-adenosyl-L-methionine synthetase in human liver cirrhosis. Hepatology. 1988;8:1530–4.
30. Corrales F, Cabrero C, Pajares MA *et al.* Role of sulphydryl groups in *S*-adenosylmethionine synthesis. Hepatology. 1990;11:216–22.
31. Pajares MA, Corrales F, Ochoa P *et al.* The role of cysteine-150 in the structure and activity of rat liver *S*-adenosyl-L-methionine synthetase. Biochem J. 1991;274:225–9.
32. Markham GD, Satishchandran C. Identification of the reactive groups of *S*-adenosylmethionine synthetase. J Biol Chem. 1988;263:866–72.
33. Pajares MA, Duran C, Corrales F *et al.* Modulation of rat liver *S*-adenosylmethionine synthetase activity by glutathione. J Biol Chem. 1992;267:17589–605.
34. Pajares MA, Corrales F, Durán C *et al.* How is rat liver *S*-adenosylmethionine synthetase regulated? FEBS Lett. 1992;309:1–4.
35. Griffith OW, Meister A. Potent and specific inhibition of glutathione synthesis by buthionine sulfoximine (*S*-n-butyl-homocysteine sulfoximine). J Biol Chem. 1979;239:538–48.
36. Corrales F, Ochoa P, Rivas C *et al.* Inhibition of glutathione synthesis in the liver leads to *S*-adenosyl-L-methionine synthetase reduction. Hepatology. 1991;14:528–33.
37. Martensson J, Meister A. Mitochondrial damage in muscle occurs after marked depletion of glutathione and is prevented by giving glutathione monoester. Proc Natl Acad Sci USA. 1989;86:471–5.
38. Martensson J, Jain A, Frayer W *et al.* Glutathione metabolism in the lung: inhibition of its synthesis leads to lamellar body and mitochondrial defects. Proc Natl Acad Sci USA. 1989;86:5296–300.
39. Martensson J, Steinherz R, Jain A *et al.* Glutathione ester prevents buthionine sulfoximine-induced cataracts and lens epithelial cell damage. Proc Natl Acad Sci USA. 1989;86:8727–31.
40. Anderson ME, Powri F, Puri RN *et al.* Glutathione monoethyl ester: preparation, uptake

by tissues, and conversion to glutathione. Arch Biochem Biophys. 1985;239:538–48.
41. Corrales F, Giménez A, Alvarez L et al. S-adenosylmethionine treatment prevents carbon tetrachloride-induced S-adenosylmethionine synthetase inactivation and attenuates liver injury. Hepatology. 1992;16:1022–7.
42. Jover R, Ponsoda X, Gómez-Lechón MJ et al. S-adenosyl-L-methionine prevents intracellular glutathione depletion by GSH-depleting drugs in rat and human hepatocytes. In: Mato JM, Lieber CS, Kaplowitz N et al., editors. Methionine metabolism: molecular mechanism and clinical and clinical implications. Madrid: CSIC Press; 1992:153–60.
43. Stramentinoli G, Pezzoli C, Galli-Kienle M. Protective role of S-adenosyl-L-methionine against acetaminophen induced mortality in mice. Biochem Pharmacol. 1979;28:3567–71.
44. Tsuji M, Kodama K, Oguchi K. Protective effects of S-adenosyl-L-methionine against CCl$_4$-induced hepatotoxicity in cultured hepatocytes. Jpn J Pharmacol. 1990;52:209–14.
45. Osada J, Aylagas H, Sánchez-Vegazo I et al. Effect of S-adenosyl-L-methionine on thioacetamide-induced liver damage. Toxicol Lett. 1986;32:97–106.
46. Stramentinoli G, Gulano M, Ideo G. Protective role of S-adenosyl-L-methionine on liver injury induced by D-galactosamine in rats. Biochem Pharmacol. 1978;27:1431–3.
47. Lieber CS, Casini A, De Carli LM et al. S-adenosyl-L-methionine attenuates alcohol-induced liver injury in the baboon. Hepatology. 1990;11:165–71.
48. Sáez GT, Bannister WH, Bannister JV. Free radicals and thiol compounds: the role of glutathione against free radical toxicity. In: Viña J, editor. Glutathione: metabolism and physiological functions. Boca Raton, FL: CRC Press; 1990:237–54.
49. Shaw S, Jayatilleke E, Lieber CS. Hepatic lipid peroxidation. Potentiation by chronic alcohol feeding and attenuation by methionine. J Lab Clin Med. 1981;98:417–25.
50. Trimble KC, Molloy A, Scott JM et al. The effect of ethanol on one-carbon metabolism: increased methionine catabolism and lipotrope methyl group wastage. In: Mato JM, Lieber CS, Kaplowitz N et al., editors. Methionine metabolism: molecular mechanism and clinical implications. Madrid: CSIC Press; 1992:46–58.
51. Finkelstein JD, Cello JP, Lyle WE. Ethanol-induced changes in methionine metabolism in rat liver. Biochem Biophys Res Commun. 1974;61:525–31.
52. Barak AJ, Beckenhauer HC, Tuma DJ et al. Effects of prolonged ethanol feeding on methionine metabolism in rat liver. Biochem Cell Biol. 1987;63:230–3.
53. Corrales F, Puerta J, Moreno J et al. Methionine intolerance in alcoholic cirrhosis: effects of S-adenosyl-L-methionine treatment. In: Mato JM, Lieber CS, Kaplowitz N et al., editors. Methionine metabolism: molecular mechanism and clinical implications. Madrid: CSIC Press; 1992:227–32.
54. Vendemiale G, Altomare E, Trizio T et al. Effects of oral S-adenosyl-L-methionine on hepatic glutathione in patients with liver disease. Scand J Gastroenterol. 1989;24:407–15.
55. Martin-Duce A, Ortiz P, Cabrero C et al. S-adenosyl-L-methionine synthetase and phospholipid methyltransferase are inhibited in human cirrhosis. Hepatology. 1988;8:65–8.
56. Bray GP, Tredger JH, Williams R. S-adenosylmethionine protects against acetaminophen hepatotoxicity in two mouse models. Hepatology. 1992;15:297–301.
57. Wong BK, Corcoran GB. N-Acetylcysteine stereoisomers as in vivo probes of the role of glutathione in drug detoxification. In: Viña J, editor. Glutathione: metabolism and physiological functions. Boca Raton, FL: CRC Press; 1990:256–62.
58. Traver J, Varela I, Mato JM. Effect of exogenous S-adenosylmethionine on phosphatidylcholine synthesis by isolated rat hepatocytes. Biochem Pharmacol. 1984;33:1562–4.
59. Van de Straat R, de Vries J, Debets AJ et al. The mechanism of prevention of paracetamol-induced hepatotoxicity by 3,4-dialkyl substitution. The roles of glutathione depletion and oxidative stress. Biochem Pharmacol. 1987;36:2065–70.
60. Lauterburg BH, Velez ME. Glutathione deficiency in alcoholics: risk factor for paracetamol hepatotoxicity. Gut. 1988;29:1153–7.
61. Marchesini G, Bugianesi E, Bianchi G et al. Defective methionine metabolism in cirrhosis: relation to severity of liver disease. Hepatology. 1992;16:149–55.

25
Effects of *S*-adenosylmethionine (SAMe) on experimental liver fibrosis

J. CABALLERÍA, A. GIMÉNEZ, F. CORRALES, R. DEULOFEU,
L. ALVAREZ, A. PARÉS, M. A. PAJARES, M. GASSÓ, M. RUBIO,
J. M. MATO and J. RODÉS

INTRODUCTION

Methionine metabolism is impaired in patients with liver damage[1]. Methionine is converted into *S*-adenosylmethionine (SAMe) by enzyme SAMe-synthetase. Normal hepatic SAMe levels and SAMe utilization are necessary for the production of detoxifying agents and for maintaining normal membrane fluidity of hepatocytes[2]. A delay in the clearance of plasma methionine after its systemic administration to patients with liver diseases has been observed[3] and is probably related to the reduction of SAMe synthetase activity described in human liver cirrhosis[4,5] and in experimental models of liver injury[6,7]. In chronic liver disease SAMe administration could produce a beneficial effect by preventing SAMe synthetase inactivation and restoring normal methionine metabolism.

Liver fibrosis is common in most chronic liver diseases regardless of their aetiology. It is the leading cause of morbidity and mortality from hepatic disease. Despite the differential therapeutic approaches proposed in the past few years there is no established therapy for the fibrogenesis of hepatic cirrhosis[8]. The purpose of this study was to assess the effects of SAMe treatment on liver collagen deposition and on parameters of liver collagen synthesis in an experimental model of CCl_4-induced liver fibrosis.

MATERIALS AND METHODS

The study was performed in male Wistar rats weighing about 250 g fed a standard diet *ad libitum* (Purina Chow A03, Panlab lab, Barcelona, Spain). The animals were induced to cirrhosis by intraperitoneal injection of 0.5 ml of carbon tetrachloride diluted 1 : 1 in vegetable oil twice a week throughout the study. Half of the rats received a daily intramuscular injection of 3 mg/kg bodyweight of SAMe from the beginning of the study. SAMe was kindly provided by Europharma (Madrid, Spain). Sets of five to seven rats of each group were killed by cardiac puncture and exsanguination after 3, 6 and 9 weeks of treatment. Two additional groups of rats, a control group and another that received only SAMe were also studied at week 9. The liver was rapidly removed, weighed and cut into pieces. Liver samples were fixed in 4% formaldehyde solution and embedded in paraffin for histological examination and collagen measurement. Liver samples were also frozen in liquid nitrogen and kept at $-70°C$ until prolyl hydroxylase (PHase) activity determination was performed. Samples of the liver of rats studied after 9 weeks of treatment were immediately processed for determination of SAMe levels, SAMe-synthetase activity, SAMe-synthetase messenger RNA (mRNA) levels and glutathione (GSH) concentration. The experiments followed the criteria set by our institutions for the care and use of laboratory animals.

For histological analysis, 4 μm thick sections were stained with haematoxylin and eosin, Masson's trichrome and reticulin stain, and coded for blind reading. Liver condition was classified as normal liver, steatotis, fibrosis or cirrhosis.

Hepatic collagen concentration was determined by the method of Lopez de Leon and Rojkind[9] validated by Jiménez et al.[10], based on the selective capacity of two dyes, Sirius Red and Fast Green to bind to collagen and non-collagenous proteins respectively. Briefly, after staining, 15 μm liver slices were eluted in 0.1% NaOH : methanol (1 : 1 v : v) and the absorbance of the eluted colours was read in a spectrophotometer (Hitachi 150-20, Hitachi Ltd, Tokyo, Japan) at 630 nm (maximal absorbance for Fast Green) and 540 nm (maximal absorbance for Sirius Red). Results were expressed as μg collagen/mg total protein in the liver, according to colour equivalences estimated previously. Intra-assay and inter-assay coefficients of variation were 4% and 10%, respectively.

Hepatic PHase activity was measured in liver homogenates according to the method of Hutton et al.[11] with slight modifications described previously[12]. This method measured the tritiated water formed when tritiated proline (40 Ci/mmol, Amersham International, UK) present in the substrate is hydroxylated to hydroxyproline. In brief, the frozen liver specimens were homogenized in 0.5 ml of an ice-cold solution of sucrose 0.25 mol/l, EDTA 10 μmol/l, dithiothreitol 1 mmol/l, phenyl methyl sulphone fluoride 50 μg/ml, 0.1% (wt/vol) Triton X-100 and Tris-HCl buffer 50 mmol/l, adjusted to pH 7.2 at 4°C in an Elvehem-Potter Teflon–glass homogenizer (B. Braun-Biotech, Barcelona, Spain). The homogenates were centrifuged at 500g for 5 min, and aliquots of the supernatants were taken for the enzyme assays by measuring the formation of tritium-labelled water in 3,4-(n)-[^{3}H]proline-labelled polypeptide substrate prepared from 9-day-old chick embryos. The reaction mixture consisted of the following: 100 μl [^{3}H]proline-labelled substrate; 100 μl tissue homogenate; and 800 μl Tris-HCl buffer at pH 7.2, which contained ferrous ammonium sulphate 1 mmol/l, detanuralized BSA 2 g/l, catalase 0.4 g/l, α-ketoglutarate 2 mmol/l, dithiothreitol 0.1 mmol/l and ascorbic acid 50 mmol/l. The reaction was incubated aerobically for 30 min at 30°C and stopped by the addition of 0.1 ml of 50% trichloracetic acid. The tritiated water produced was separated by vacuum distillation and counted in a scintillation counter (1217 Rackbeta LKB Wallac, Sweden). Total protein concentration in homogenates was measured by the method of Bradford[13], and results were expressed as counts per minute per milligram of protein in homogenate. Intra-assay and inter-assay coefficients of variation were 7% and 10%, respectively.

For SAMe-synthetase determination, liver samples were homogenized in 4 vol of 10 mmol/l Tris-HCl at pH 7.5, containing sucrose 0.3 mol/l, 0.1% β-mercaptoethanol, benzamidine 1 mmol/l and PMSF 0.1 mmol/l. The homogenate was centrifuged for 20 min at 10 000g; the supernatant was again centrifuged for 1 h at 100 000g. SAMe synthetase activity was measured in the last supernatant, as described earlier[4].

SAMe levels were determined in liver samples which were immediately deproteinized by homogenization in 10% trichloracetic acid dissolved in 0.05 N HCl containing 20 000 dpm [^{3}H-methyl]SAMe. Extraction and HPLC analysis were performed as described previously[14]. Aliquots of total liver RNA isolated by the guanidium thiocyanate method[15] were used for measuring the SAMe-synthetase mRNA by Northern blot[7].

GSH concentration was determined by the method of Hissin[16]. Approximately 250 mg of liver were homogenized on ice in 3.75 ml of 0.1 mol/l sodium phosphate, 0.005 mol/l EDTA buffer at pH 8, and 1 ml of 25% H_3PO_4. The homogenate was centrifuged at 100 000g for 30 min to obtain the supernatant for GSH assay. The supernatant was processed as described previously, and samples of the final solution were transferred to a quartz cuvette and fluorescence at 420 nm was determined with excitation at 350 nm[7].

Results are expressed as mean $\pm$ SEM. Statistically significant differences between groups were estimated with one-way analysis of variance and the Newman–Keuls test was performed for multiple comparisons. A p value 0.05 or less was considered significant.

RESULTS

The liver biopsy specimens of the rats studied at 3 weeks showed normal liver, mild or moderate steatosis, or mild deposition of collagen fibres in the sinusoids. These changes were similar in CCl_4 and in CCl_4 + SAMe-treated rats. By contrast, at 6 weeks the liver of all the CCl_4-treated rats showed marked fibrosis whereas the liver of the CCl_4 + SAMe rats only showed minimal changes similar to those of the rats studied at 3 weeks. The differences were even more evident in the rats receiving treatment for 9 weeks. Three of six rats of the CCl_4 group and only one of seven rats of the CCl_4 + SAMe group had cirrhosis. The remaining rats of the CCl_4 group had marked fibrosis, and the remaining rats of the CCl_4 + SAMe group showed less prominent collagen septa.

The hepatic collagen content increased progressively according to the duration of the process of induction to cirrhosis, and was significantly higher

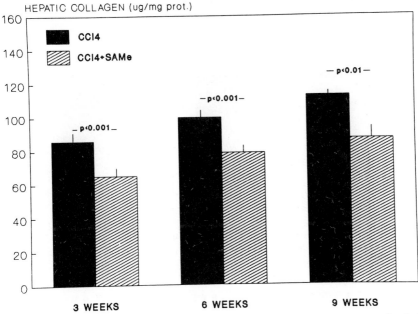

Fig. 1 Hepatic collagen concentration in CCl_4 and in CCl_4 + SAMe-treated rats after 3, 6 and 9 weeks of treatment

Table 1 Hepatic prolyl hydroxylase activity, collagen content, SAMe-synthetase activity, SAMe mRNA levels, and SAMe and glutathione concentrations in rats studied after 9 weeks of CCl_4 treatment

	Control	SAMe	CCl_4	CCl_4 + SAMe
Prolyl hydroxylase (cpm/mg protein)	194.5 ± 33.7	134.8 ± 37.3	489.9 ± 52.8^a	361.0 ± 26.5^b
Collagen (μg/mg protein)	49.9 ± 1.9	51.1 ± 3	112.8 ± 5.9^a	86.7 ± 2.8^b
SAMe synthetase (pmol/min per mg protein)	109.8 ± 17.6	123.4 ± 16.2	42.8 ± 11.9^a	107.2 ± 13.5
SAMe mRNA (arbitrary units)	2.3 ± 0.2	2.7 ± 0.4	2.2 ± 0.1	3.1 ± 0.3
SAMe (nmol/g tissue)	42.9 ± 0.9	44.2 ± 6.4	38.1 ± 5.2	54.8 ± 7.5
GSH (μmol/g tissue)	6.59 ± 0.4	6.05 ± 0.37	3.63 ± 0.34^a	5.45 ± 0.34

The values are expressed as mean $\pm$ SEM. The significance of differences between groups was determined by one-way ANOVA and the Newman-Keuls test.
[a] $p < 0.05$ CCl_4-treated rats vs the other three groups.
[b] $p < 0.05$ CCl_4 + SAMe-treated rats vs control group.

in the CCl_4 group than in the CCl_4 + SAMe group in the three periods of the study (3 weeks: 85.9 ± 2.2 vs $65 \pm 2\,\mu$g/mg protein, $p < 0.001$; 6 weeks: 99.7 ± 4.1 vs $78.7 \pm 1.8\,\mu$g/mg protein, $p < 0.001$; and 9 weeks: 112.8 ± 5.9 vs $86.7 \pm 2.8\,\mu$g/mg protein, $p < 0.01$) (Fig. 1, Table 1).

Similarly, the PHase activity was higher in the CCl_4 group than in the CCl_4 + SAMe group at 3 weeks (399.6 ± 30 vs 284.9 ± 48 cpm/mg protein,

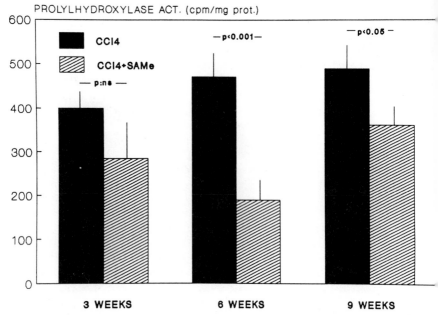

Fig. 2 Hepatic prolyl hydroxylase activity in CCl_4 and in CCl_4 + SAMe-treated rats after 3, 6 and 9 weeks of treatment

p: n.s.), at 6 weeks (471.4 $\pm$ 53.5 vs 189.2 $\pm$ 25 cpm/mg protein; $p < 0.01$), and at 9 weeks (489.9 $\pm$ 52.8 vs 361 $\pm$ 26.5 cpm/mg protein, $p < 0.05$) (Fig. 2, Table 1).

Table 1 shows the activity of SAMe-synthetase, GSH and SAMe concentrations and SAMe-synthetase mRNA levels obtained from controls and CCl_4-treated animals. The group of controls and the group of rats receiving only SAMe had similar mean SAMe-synthetase activity (110 $\pm$ 17.6 and 123 $\pm$ 16.2 pmol/min per mg protein) which was significantly lower in the CCl_4 group (42.8 $\pm$ 11.9 pmol/min per mg protein). The CCl_4-induced SAMe-synthetase reduction was corrected with SAMe treatment (107 $\pm$ 13.5 pmol/min per mg protein). Despite the marked reduction of SAMe-synthetase in the CCl_4-treated group the levels of SAMe and the steady-state levels of SAMe-synthetase mRNA were not different in the CCl_4-treated group compared with the control and the CCl_4 + SAMe-treated groups. The mean GSH concentration was 6.6 $\pm$ 0.4 μmol/g tissue in the control group and only 3.6 $\pm$ 0.34 μmol/g tissue in the CCl_4-treated group. The CCl_4-induced GSH reduction was also corrected by SAMe (5.45 $\pm$ 0.35 μmol/g tissue).

DISCUSSION

The results of the current study indicate that in a rat model of CCl_4-induced liver damage, SAMe administration reduces liver fibrosis and fibrogenesis as demonstrated by smaller increases in hepatic collagen content and in prolyl hydroxylase activity in rats receiving SAMe simultaneously to CCl_4 in comparison with those that only received CCl_4. As a consequence of the reduction of liver fibrosis, SAMe administration in CCl_4-injured rats results in less liver damage and after 9 weeks of CCl_4 treatment, the number of animals developing cirrhosis was lower in the group simultaneously receiving SAMe. Furthermore, SAMe treatment also produces a normalization of SAMe-synthetase activity and GSH concentration. Our results agree with the observation that CCl_4-induced hepatotoxicity in cultured rat hepatocytes is attenuated by the addition of SAMe to the medium[17] and with several reports indicating that different forms of liver injury are favourably influenced by SAMe treatment[18].

The possible antifibrotic properties of SAMe have recently been evaluated by Casini et al.[19] incubating human fibroblasts with different concentrations of SAMe. The addition of SAMe to the cultures of fibroblasts in concentrations which can be found in vivo induced a marked decrease in collagen synthesis with no adverse effects on cell proliferation and viability. The results of the present study suggest that, in an experimental model of liver fibrosis, SAMe also has a beneficial effect in vivo. Moreover, more recent experiments carried out in our laboratory (unpublished results) confirm these results and show that the administration of SAMe after 3 and 6 weeks from the beginning of CCl_4 injury also produces a normalization of hepatic SAMe synthetase activity and GSH levels and a significant reduction of liver fibrosis.

Methionine metabolism is impaired in a variety of cases of experimental liver injury, such as damage induced by galactosamine, alcohol and CCl_4. In these situations there is a defect of SAMe synthetase activity[6,7]. The normal levels of SAMe synthetase mRNA observed, suggest that the reduced SAMe-synthetase activity in CCl_4-treated rats might be due to an inactivation of the enzyme. Hepatic GSH, which is derived from SAMe via the transsulphuration pathway, is also depleted as a consequence of liver damage[7,20]. GSH appears to protect against SAMe-synthetase inactivation by preventing oxidation of sulphydryl groups. Thus, the depletion of GSH leads to inactivation of SAMe-synthetase activity, which in turn produces a further decrease in GSH and still greater inactivation of SAMe synthetase[21]. The administration of exogenous SAMe may lead to an increase of GSH levels[22] and to the prevention of SAMe-synthetase inactivation, and consequently, to an attenuation of liver damage.

Our results suggest that a reduction of SAMe synthesis, a depletion of GSH levels or both play an important role in the pathogenesis of liver fibrosis in vivo. The mechanisms of the protective effects of SAMe in the development of liver fibrosis are not known. SAMe deficiency produces an impairment of important transmethylation[2] and transsulphuration pathways[23,24] that, among other effects, alter the integrity and fluidity of membranes, and reduce the protection against toxic agents, leading to cellular necrosis and, as a final consequence, to fibrosis. Thus, normalization of methionine metabolism could prevent or attenuate the damage produced by different hepatotoxins.

Several reports have shown that SAMe administration has a beneficial effect in various chronic liver diseases including alcoholic and non-alcoholic cirrhosis[18,20] and cholestasis[25]. Changes in collagen metabolism are a common feature of chronic liver diseases and play an important role in the progression of the disease. Thus, the reduction of fibrosis could be one of the mechanisms to explain the effect of SAMe on these diseases. Although clinical studies are necessary, the attenuation of fibrogenesis in CCl_4-induced liver injury by SAMe administration provides a rationale for the use of SAMe in the treatment of fibrotic liver disease.

Acknowledgements

This study was supported in part by grants from Fondo de Investigaciones Sanitarias de la Seguridad Social (91/0357) and from Europharma (Madrid, Spain).

References

1. Corrales F, Alvarez L, Pajares MA et al. Impairment of methionine metabolism in liver diseases. Drug Invest. 1992;4(Suppl. 4):8–13.
2. Chawla RK, Bonkonwsky HL, Galambos JT. Biochemistry and pharmacology of S-adenosyl-L-methionine and rationale for its use in liver disease. Drugs. 1990;40(Suppl 3): 98–110.
3. Kinsell LW, Harper HA, Marton HC et al. Rate of dissapearance from plasma of intravenously administered methionine in patients with liver damage. Science. 1947;106: 589–90.
4. Martin-Duce A, Ortiz P, Cabrero C et al. S-adenosyl-L-methionine synthetase and phospholipid methyltransferase are inhibited in human cirrhosis. Hepatology. 1988;8:65–8.
5. Marchesini G, Bugianesi E, Bianchi G et al. Defective methionine metabolism in cirrhosis: relation to severity of liver disease. Hepatology. 1992;16:149–55.
6. Lieber CS, Casini A, DeCarli LM et al. S-Adenosyl-L-methionine attenuates alcohol-induced liver injury in the baboon. Hepatology. 1990;11:165–72.
7. Corrales F, Giménez A, Alvarez L et al. S-adenosylmethionine treatment prevents carbon tetrachloride-induced S-adenosylmethionine synthetase inactivation and attenuates liver injury. Hepatology. 1992;16:1022–7.
8. Brenner DA, Alcorn JM. Therapy for hepatic fibrosis. Semin Liver Dis. 1990;10:75–83.
9. Lopez de Leon A, Rojkind M. A simple micromethod for collagen and total protein determination in formalin-fixed, paraffin-embedded sections. J Histochem Cytochem. 1985;8:737–43.
10. Jiménez W, Parés A, Caballería J et al. Measurement of fibrosis in needle liver biopsies: evaluation of a colorimetric method. Hepatology. 1985;5:815–18.
11. Hutton JJ, Tappel AL, Underfriend S. A rapid assay for collagen proline hydroxylase. Anal Biochem. 1966;16:384–94.
12. Torres-Salinas M, Parés A, Caballería J et al. Serum procollagen type III peptide as a marker of hepatic fibrogenesis in alcoholic hepatitis. Gastroenterology. 1986;90:1241–6.
13. Bradford AE. A rapid and sensitive method for the quantitation of microgram quantities of protein utilizing the principle of protein-dye binding. Anal Biochem. 1976;72:248–54.
14. Cabrero C, Martin-Duce A, Ortiz P et al. Specific loss of the high-molecular-weight form of S-adenosyl-L-methionine synthetase in human liver cirrhosis. Hepatology. 1988;8: 1530–4.
15. Chomczynski P, Sacchi N. Single-step method of RNA isolation by acid guanidinium thiocyanate-phenol-chloroform extraction. Anal Biochem. 1987;162:156–9.
16. Hissin PJ, Hill R. A fluorimetric method for determination of oxidized and reduced glutathione in tissues. Anal Biochem. 1976;74:214–26.
17. Tsuji M, Kodama K, Oguchi K. Protective effects of S-adenosyl-L-methionine against CCl_4-

induced hepatotoxicity in cultured hepatocytes. Jpn J Pharmacol. 1990;52:209–14.
18. Friedel HA, Goa KL, Benfield P. S-adenosyl-L-methionine: a review of its pharmacological properties and therapeutic potential in liver dysfunction and affective disorders in relation to its physiological role in cell metabolism. Drugs. 1989;38:389–416.
19. Casini A, Banchetti E, Milani S et al. S-adenosylmethionine inhibits collagen synthesis by human fibroblasts in vitro. Methods Find Exp Clin Pharmacol. 1989;11:331–4.
20. Vendemiale G, Altomare E, Trizio T et al. Effects of oral S-adenosyl-L-methionine on hepatic glutathione in patients with liver disease. Scand J Gastroenterol. 1989;24:407–15.
21. Corrales F, Ochoa P, Rivas C et al. Inhibition of glutathione synthesis in the liver leads to S-adenosyl-L-methionine synthetase reduction. Hepatology. 1991;14:528–33.
22. Jover J, Ponsoda X, Fabra R et al. S-adenosyl-L-methionine prevents intracellular glutathione depletion by GSH-depleting drugs in rat and human hepatocytes. Drug Invest. 1992;4(Suppl. 4):46–53.
23. Mato JM, Corrales F, Martin-Duce A et al. Mechanisms and consequences of the impaired trans-sulphuration pathway in liver disease: Part I. Biochemical implications. Drugs. 1990;40(Suppl. 3):58–64.
24. Pisi E, Marchesini G. Mechanisms and consequences of the impaired trans-sulphuration pathway in liver disease: Part II. Clinical consequences and potential for pharmacological intervention in cirrhosis. Drugs. 1990;40(Suppl. 3):65–72.
25. Frezza M, Terpin M. The use of S-adenosyl-L-methionine in the treatment of cholestatic disorders. A meta-analysis of clinical trials. Drug Invest. 1992;4(Suppl. 4):101–8.

26
Rationale for the use of ademetionine (SAMe) in chronic cholestatic liver disease

R. NACCARATO and A. FLOREANI

HEPATIC METABOLISM OF ADEMETIONINE (SAMe)

Ademetionine (SAMe) is a naturally occurring molecule distributed throughout the body tissues, including the liver. It acts as a methyl group donor and as an enzyme activator in a number of biochemical reactions, including enzymatic transmethylation and trans-sulphuration reactions and also in the synthesis and metabolism of hormones, neurotransmitters, nucleic acids, phospholipids, proteins and drugs[1]. Methionine is metabolized in the liver, where it is converted into S-adenosyl-L-methionine by SAMe-synthetase. The two major pathways initiated by SAMe are transmethylation and trans-sulphuration.

Transmethylation

The liver is the most important site of transmethylation reactions, since up to 85% of all transmethylation reactions occur in this organ[2]. SAMe regulates several physiological functions associated with membranes (Table 1). The most important of these functions is the methylation of phospholipids, mainly phosphatidylethanolamine (PE) to phosphatidylcholine (PC) in hepatic microsomes. The PC formed by this reaction is rich in polyunsaturated fatty acids and acts as a preferred substrate for some membrane-associated enzymes. It is known that protein methylation modulates Na^+/Ca^{2+}

Table 1 SAMe and methylation of cellular membranes

1. Methylation of phospholipids (phosphatidylethanolamine to phosphatidylcholine)
2. Regulation of N-methylation of phospholipids by drugs and hormones
3. Methylation of membrane proteins
4. Regulation of membrane enzymes

Table 2 Classification of intrahepatic cholestasis

Biochemical abnormalities
Cholestasis of pregnancy
Benign idiopathic recurrent cholestasis

Bile duct damage
Primary biliary cirrhosis
Primary sclerosing cholangitis
Graft-versus-host disease

Hepatocyte damage
Viral (HAV, HBV, HDV, HCV, CMV, EBV)
Autoimmune
Toxic (drugs, hormones, toxic compounds)

exchange activity in cardiac sarcolemmal vesicles[3]. SAMe also regulates the activity of Na^+-K^+-ATPase which is present in the plasma membrane of all animal cells including hepatocytes[4]. Finally SAMe increases Na^+/H^+ exchange activity, increasing the fluidity of the colonic membrane[5,6].

Trans-sulphuration

By means of this pathway glutathione and sulphated compounds are synthesized via homocysteine and cysteine. Evidence exists for the impairment of the trans-sulphuration pathway in patients with liver cirrhosis[7,8]. The consequences of this impaired trans-sulphuration pathway include:

1. impaired hepatic metabolism of amino acids;
2. reduced synthesis of several compounds: glutathione, taurine, choline, carnitine, creatinine which may cause fatty liver, myopathy and retinal dysfunction;
3. nutritional deficiencies.

CHRONIC CHOLESTATIC LIVER DISEASES AND SAMe METABOLISM

Cholestasis is a clinical and biochemical syndrome usually characterized by itching and elevation of the serum alkaline phosphatase and bile salts; jaundice may be a late event. It results from a generalized impairment in the secretion of bile and specific defects in organic anion secretion[9]. From the clinical point of view several conditions may cause cholestasis (Table 2). The pathophysiology and biochemical mechanisms in these conditions are different, but as a practical approach it seems meaningful to differentiate between biochemical mechanisms, bile duct damage and hepatocyte damage.

Biochemical mechanisms

These are exemplified by intrahepatic cholestasis of pregnancy. This condition typically occurs during the last trimester of pregnancy in women congenitally hypersensitive to the oestrogen load produced by the placenta[10]. Oestrogens alter membrane lipid composition mainly by inducing an accumulation of cholesteryl ester which in turn induces an altered cholesterol/phospholipid ratio[11]. The major consequence is the suppression of $Na^+–K^+$-ATPase activity. Stramentinoli et al.[12–14] demonstrated that SAMe protects against oestrogen-induced cholestasis in rats and produces an increase in biliary methylated derivatives of oestrogen which are metabolically inert. These authors suggest that SAMe might act by means of a decreased bioavailability of oestrogen.

Another hypothesis may be made; that is that an important factor in oestrogen-induced cholestasis is decreased oestriol sulphation relative to D-ring glucuronidation in the liver[15]. If this were the case, SAMe would act by improving cholestasis through the trans-sulphuration mechanism.

Bile duct damage

This type of cholestasis is exemplified by two conditions: primary biliary cirrhosis (PBC) and primary sclerosing cholangitis (PSC). The mechanism of cholestasis is inflammatory, immunologically mediated damage occurring in the bile duct epithelium. Progressive loss of bile ducts then takes place, together with chronic inflammation of the portal tracts and ductular proliferation, until the 'vanishing bile duct syndrome' develops. Hepatocyte damage follows when the inflammation extends beyond the limiting plate to periportal areas and is subsequent to the cholestasis. Cholestasis induces a variety of effects on hepatocytes including increased junctional permeability, depression of canalicular contractility, inhibition of membrane-associated enzymes and bile acid hepatotoxicity[16].

The rationale for the use of SAMe in these conditions is to restore a consequence of reduced activity of the enzyme SAMe synthetase: transmethylation and trans-sulphuration. In particular, the former reaction is involved in the biosynthesis of membrane phospholipids which play an important role in many intracellular events by preserving plasma membrane fluidity. Nevertheless, in both PBC and PSC medical therapy directed against immunological damage remains a major long-term objective and SAMe should be considered only for minor purposes.

Hepatocyte damage

Intrahepatic cholestasis as a result of hepatocyte lesions is due to several conditions including viruses, alcohol, drugs and toxic compounds. Moreover, some experimental models may explain the rationale of SAMe in this type of cholestatic damage.

Alcohol

The main pathway of ethanol metabolism involves its conversion by alcohol dehydrogenase (ADH). A second pathway, that of peroxisomal catalase, can

Table 3 Uncontrolled clinical trials with SAMe in intrahepatic cholestasis of pregnancy

Author	Patients	Days	Dose/day	Route	Bile acids	ALT	Itching
Lafuenti, 1988[26]	10	15	1800 mg	p.o.	=	↓	↓
Bonfirraro, 1990[33]	9	15	800 mg	i.v.	↓	↓	↓
Catalino, 1992[25]	55	10–30	800 mg	i.v.	↓	↓	↓

also oxidize ethanol but its quantitative role in humans is unknown. The third pathway utilizes the microsomal ethanol oxidizing system (MEOS) and is particularly active at relatively high blood ethanol levels[17]. Alcohol-induced toxicity leads to alterations in microtubules, mitochondria and plasma membranes. They are related to several mechanisms, including acetaldehyde toxicity, production of free radicals, lipid peroxidation and glutathione depletion. Lieber et al.[18] demonstrated that long-term ethanol consumption in baboons resulted in a significant reduction of hepatic SAMe concentration. Moreover, SAMe-synthetase is markedly reduced in cirrhotic patients (either of alcoholic or non-alcoholic aetiology)[19]. Patients with alcoholic liver disease show decreased levels of glutathione both in plasma and in the liver[20-22].

In the baboon model SAMe administration attenuates ethanol-induced liver damage (a minor increment in transaminase levels, a reduced number of megamitochondria)[19]. In humans, oral SAMe administration restores hepatic glutathione depletion in patients with both alcoholic and non-alcoholic liver disease[23].

On the basis of these data it seems that SAMe may play an encouraging role in the treatment of chronic alcoholic liver disease.

Paracetamol

Paracetamol hepatotoxicity following overdose is the most common cause of fulminant hepatic failure in the United Kingdom. The use of SAMe as an antidote has recently been evaluated in two mouse models. In C5B16 mice, deaths were abolished by SAMe given within 1 h of 3.3 mmol/kg body weight acetaminophen, and reduced if given 2–5 h after acetaminophen administration. Mixed disulphate/tosylate salt of SAMe abolished mortality in C3H mice given 2 mmol/kg body weight of acetaminophen[24]. In both mouse models SAMe reduced depletion of plasma and liver glutathione, liver damage and release of AST after acetaminophen administration. Pretreatment with buthionine sulphoximine, which inhibits glutathione synthesis, abolished the beneficial effect of SAMe on survival and the plasma glutathione level.

CLINICAL TRIALS

Intrahepatic cholestasis of pregnancy

Three uncontrolled trials (Table 3) and three controlled trials (Table 4) are reported in the literature. The uncontrolled trials were carried out on small numbers of patients, except one[25] which included 55 patients. The duration

Table 4   Placebo-controlled clinical trials with SAMe in intrahepatic cholestasis of pregnancy

Author	Patients	Days	Dose/day	Route	Bile acids	ALT	Itching
Frezza, 1984[27]	18	20	800 mg	i.v.	↓	↓	↓
			200 mg	i.v.	=	=	=
Frezza, 1990[30]	30	18	800 mg	i.v.	↓	↓	↓
Ribalta, 1991[28]	18	20	800 mg	i.v.	=	=	=

Table 5   Placebo-controlled clinical trials with SAMe in intrahepatic cholestasis of liver disease

Author	Patients	Days	Dose/day	Route	Symptoms	Liver biochemistry
Giannuoli, 1986[34]	20	14	800 mg	i.v.	↓	—
Cacciatore, 1989[35]	18	14	800 mg	i.v.	↓	—
Frezza, 1990[30]	220	14	1600 mg	p.o.	↓	↓
Manzillo, 1992[31]	343	14	800 mg	i.v.	↓	↓
	68	60	1600 mg	p.o.	—	↓

of treatment ranged from 10 to 30 days and the dosage was at least 800 mg/day. Two studies showed a significant amelioration of itching and of bile acid and ALT serum levels. One study[26] failed to demonstrate an amelioration of the same parameters, except for ALT.

The three controlled studies were performed on 18, 6 and 18 patients respectively. The duration of treatment ranged from 7 to 20 days and the daily dosage from 200 to 900 mg. In one study[27] the dosage of 200 mg/day failed to produce a significant reduction in bile acid and ALT, although statistical significance was reached with a daily dosage of 800 mg/day.

Nevertheless, another trial[28] did not show a significant reduction in symptoms and liver enzymes.

Intrahepatic cholestasis of liver diseases

Intrahepatic cholestasis is an accompanying feature of acute and chronic liver disease involving bile secretion impairment at hepatocyte level and/or at intrahepatic bile duct level. In a retrospective multicentric survey, 35% of a cohort of 2520 patients who presented over 2 years with newly diagnosed chronic liver disease, had intrahepatic cholestasis involving abnormal levels of serum bilirubin and alkaline phosphatase[29].

Four controlled double-blind trials, SAMe vs placebo, have been carried out in intrahepatic cholestasis of liver diseases (Table 5). Two of these were performed in large series of patients[30,31]. In the first trial[30] only chronic liver disease patients (26% chronic active hepatitis, 68% cirrhosis, 6% primary biliary cirrhosis) were enrolled. Unfortunately, neither the aetiology of chronic active hepatitis nor of cirrhosis was specified. Subjective symptoms (pruritus, fatigue, and a feeling of being unwell) significantly improved in patients treated with SAMe vs those treated with a placebo. Moreover, serum markers of cholestasis (bilirubin and alkaline phosphatase, except GGT) decreased after SAMe administration, and their values were significantly lower than the corresponding values in the placebo group.

The second trial[31] consisted of patients with acute hepatitis (25.3%), with chronic hepatitis (27%), with cirrhosis (38%) and with PBC (9.3%). Unfortunately, in this trial also, the aetiology of the acute and chronic hepatitis was not specified. The design of the study randomly assigned either intravenous SAMe (800 mg/day) or a placebo during the first 2 weeks of therapy. Responders were defined according to the following parameters:

1. pruritus – patients who experienced complete resolution of the symptom at the end of treatment;
2. biochemical parameters – patients whose serum levels showed either a 50% reduction versus baseline or returned to reference values.

According to these criteria, 60% of patients with chronic liver diseases who received SAMe were classified as responders compared with 34% who received a placebo. During the subsequent phase of the study a further significant decrease in cholestasis indices was observed in the SAMe group compared with the placebo group.

CONCLUSIONS

The rationale for the use of SAMe in chronic cholestatic liver disease may be summarized as follows: (1) increased bioavailability of sulphates; (2) modification of hepatocyte membrane fluidity; (3) recovery of glutathione depletion; (4) inactivation of cholestatic oestrogen metabolites. Several preclinical studies support these items. Moreover, the majority of clinical studies (including uncontrolled and controlled clinical trials) have already demonstrated the efficacy of SAMe in controlling symptoms and in decreasing liver enzymes in intrahepatic cholestasis of liver disease.

To obtain a global assessment of the therapeutic efficacy of this compound, a meta-analysis of six controlled clinical trials of SAMe in the symptomatic treatment of intrahepatic cholestasis of liver disease and pregnancy was carried out[32]. The results confirm that SAMe is more effective than a placebo in resolving pruritus and reducing or normalizing the biochemical variables of cholestasis and hepatocellular necrosis in this condition. At present the therapeutic effects of SAMe should be regarded as symptomatic; nevertheless, long-term clinical trials on the effect of SAMe administration and on survival are needed in intrahepatic cholestasis.

References

1. Finkelstein JD. Methionine metabolism in mammals. J Nutr Biochem. 1990;1:228–37.
2. Mudd SH, Poule SR. Labile methyl balances for normal humans on various dietary regimens. Metabolism. 1975;24:721–35.
3. Panagia V, Okumura K, Makino N et al. Stimulation of Ca^{++}-pump in rat heart sarcolemma by phosphatidylethanolamine N-methylation. Biochim Biophys Acta. 1986;856:383–7.
4. Pascale R, Daino R, Garcea R et al. Inhibition by ethanol of rat liver plasma membrane (Na$^+$,K$^+$) ATPase: protective effect of S-adenosyl-L-methionine, L-methionine, and N-acetylcysteine. Toxicol Appl Pharmacol. 1989;97:216–29.

5. Brasitus TA, Dudeja PK, Worman HJ et al. The lipid fluidity of rat colonic brush-border membrane vesicles modulates Na^+-H^+ exchange and osmotic water permeability. Biochim Biophys Acta. 1986;855:16–24.

6. Dudeja PK, Foster ES, Brasitus TA. Regulation of Na^+-H exchange by transmethylation reactions in rat colonic brush border membranes. Biochim Biophys Acta. 1986;859:61–8.

7. Horowitz JH, Rypins EB, Henderson JM et al. Evidence for impairment of transsulfuration pathway in cirrhosis. Gastroenterology. 1981;81:668–75.

8. Chawla RK, Lewis FW, Kutner MH et al. Plasma cysteine, cystine and glutathione in cirrhosis. Gastroenterology. 1984;87:770–6.

9. Gleeson D, Boyer JL. Intrahepatic cholestasis. In: McIntyre N, Benhamou J-P, Bircher J et al., editors. Oxford textbook of clinical hepatology. Oxford: Oxford University Press; 1991:1088–107.

10. Reyes H. The enigma of intrahepatic cholestasis of pregnancy: lesson from Chile. Hepatology. 1982;2:87–96.

11. Schreiber AJ, Simon FR. Estrogen-induced cholestasis: clues to pathogenesis and treatment. Hepatology. 1983;3:607–13.

12. Stramentinoli G, Gualano M, Rouagnati P et al. Influence of S-adenosyl-L-methionine on irreversible binding by ethynil estradiol to rat liver microsomes and its implication in bile secretion. Biochem Pharmacol. 1979;28:981–4.

13. Stramentinoli G, Gualano M, Di Padova C. Effect of S-adenosyl-L-methionine on ethynyl estradiol-induced impairment of bile flow in female rats. Experientia. 1977;33:1361–2.

14. Stramentinoli G, Di Padova G, Gualano M et al. Ethynyl estradiol-induced impairment of bile secretion in the rat: protective effects of S-adenosyl-L-methionine and its implication in estrogen metabolism. Gastroenterology. 1981;80:154–8.

15. Vore M. Estrogen cholestasis: membranes, metabolites, or receptors? Gastroenterology. 1987;93:643–9.

16. Schaffner F. Cholestasis. In: Millward-Sadler GH, Wright R, Arthur MJP, editors, Wright's liver and biliary disease, 3rd edn. Philadelphia: W.B. Saunders; 1992:371–89.

17. Lieber CS. Interaction of alcohol with other drugs and nutrients. Implication for the therapy of alcoholic liver disease. Drugs. 1990;40:23–44.

18. Lieber CS, Casini A, De Carli LM et al. S-adenosyl-L-methionine attenuates alcohol-induced liver injury in the baboon. Hepatology. 1990;11:165–72.

19. Cabrero C, Duce AM, Ortiz P et al. Specific loss of the high-molecular weight form of S-adenosyl-L-methionine synthetase in human liver cirrhosis. Hepatology. 1988;8:1530–4.

20. Lauterburg BH, Velez ME. Glutathione deficiency in alcoholics: risk factor for paracetamol hepatotoxicity. Gut. 1988;29:1153–7.

21. Poulsen HE, Ranek L, Andreasen PB. The hepatic glutathione content in liver disease. Scand J Clin Lab Invest. 1981;41:573–6.

22. Jewell SA, Di Monte D, Gentile A et al. Decreased hepatic glutathione in chronic alcoholic patients. J Hepatol. 1986;3:1–6.

23. Vendemiale G, Altomare E, Trizio T et al. Effects of oral S-adenosyl-L-methionine on hepatic glutathione in patients with liver disease. Scand J Gastroenterol. 1989;24:407–15.

24. Bray GP, Tredger JM, Wiliams R. S-Adenosylmethyionine protects against acetaminophen hepatotoxicity in two mouse models. Hepatology. 1992;15:297–301.

25. Catalino F, Scarponi S, Cesar F et al. Efficacy and safety of intravenous S-adenosyl-L-methionine therapy in the management of intrahepatic cholestasis of pregnancy. Drug Invest. 1992;4(Suppl. 4):78–82.

26. Lafuenti G, Plotti G, Nicolanti G et al. Valutazione delle modificazioni di parametri clinici e biochimici in gravide con colestasi in terapia con S-adenosyl-L-methionine per os. Giorn It Ost Gin. 1988;5:356–61.

27. Frezza M, Pozzato G, Chiesa L et al. Reversal of intrahepatic cholestasis of pregnancy in women after high dose S-adenosyl-L-methionine administration. Hepatology. 1984;4:274–8.

28. Ribalta J, Reyes H, Gonzales M et al. S-adenosyl-L-methionine in the treatment of patients with intrahepatic cholestasis of pregnancy: a randomized, double-blind, placebo-controlled study with negative results. Hepatology. 1991;13:1084–9.

29. Bortolini M, Almasio P, Bray G et al. Multicentre survey of the prevalence of intrahepatic cholestasis in 2520 consecutive patients with newly diagnosed chronic liver disease. Drug Invest. 1992;4(Suppl. 4):83–9.

30. Frezza M, Surrenti C, Manzillo G *et al.* Oral *S*-adenosylmethionine in the symptomatic treatment of intrahepatic cholestasis. A double-blind, placebo-controlled study. Gastroenterology. 1990;99:211–15.
31. Manzillo G, Piccinino F, Surrenti G *et al.* Multicentre double-blind placebo-controlled study of intravenous and oral *S*-adenosyl-L-methionine (SAMe) in cholestatic patients with liver disease. Drug Invest. 1992;4(Suppl. 4):90–100.
32. Frezza M, Terpin M. The use of *S*-adenosyl-L-methionine in the treatment of cholestatic disorders. A meta-analysis of clinical trials. Drug Invest. 1992;4(Suppl. 4):101–8.
33. Bonfirraro G, Chieffi O, Quinti R *et al.* *S*-Adenosyl-L-methionine (SAMe)-induced amelioration of intrahepatic cholestasis of pregnancy. Results of an open study. Drug Invest. 1990;2:125–8.
34. Giannuoli G, Tinè F, Malizia G *et al.* *S*-Adenosylmethionine for treatment of pruritus in compensated chronic liver disease. A pilot study. Hepatology. 1986;6:1110.
35. Cacciatore L, Varriale A, Cozzolino G *et al.* *S*-Adenosylmethionine (SAMe) in the treatment of pruritus in chronic liver disease. Acta Ther. 1989;15:363–71.

27
Bile acids and the liver

G. PAUMGARTNER and U. BEUERS

PHYSIOLOGICAL ASPECTS

Bile acids represent the largest fraction of all substances that are transported by the liver from blood to bile[1]. As physiological detergents they play an important role in biliary secretion and intestinal absorption of lipids.

Bile acids are taken up into the hepatocyte mainly by a sodium-dependent transport system which is located in the basolateral membrane[1-3]. They are secreted into bile presumably by an ATP-dependent and a membrane potential-driven transport mechanism in the canalicular membrane[3,4]. At high bile acid loads vesicular transport of bile acids may also play a role[5,6].

Canalicular bile acid secretion is responsible for bile acid-dependent bile formation and is the rate-limiting step in hepatocellular transport of bile acids. Each bile acid molecule secreted into the bile canaliculus osmotically obligates a certain volume of water which enters the canaliculus mainly via a paracellular pathway through the tight junctions[1-3].

PATHOPHYSIOLOGICAL ASPECTS

Under physiological conditions, intracellular concentrations of bile acids are low and no bile acid toxicity is observed. However, when canalicular secretion is impaired or bile acid loads exceed the excretory capacity, intracellular accumulation of bile acids may occur which may damage the liver cell.

The toxic effects of bile acids are mainly related to their detergency and lipophilicity[7]. Depending on these properties bile acids can solubilize membrane lipids, alter cell permeability and cause liver injury.

Research on bile acid hepatotoxicity has a long history. In 1960 Holsti demonstrated that feeding of lithocholic acid to rabbits leads to liver cirrhosis[8]. In 1966 Javitt showed that taurolithocholic acid induces cholestasis in rats[9]. In 1972 Greim and co-workers found a correlation between the intrahepatic concentration of dihydroxy bile acids and hepatocellular injury in patients with biliary obstruction[10]. In 1975 Morrissey and colleagues demonstrated that chenodeoxycholic acid is hepatotoxic in the baboon[11]. In

1976 Herz and co-workers showed that even the hydrophilic bile acid taurocholic acid causes cholestasis when it is infused in the isolated perfused rat liver at rates exceeding its apparent excretory transport maximum[12]. More hydrophobic bile acids such as taurochenodeoxycholic acid exhibit this phenomenon at much lower infusion rates[13].

Lithocholic acid (LCA), deoxycholic acid (DCA), and chenodeoxycholic acid (CDCA) exhibit the greatest toxic potential of the physiological bile acids[7]. Since the DCA pool is depleted when the enterohepatic circulation is interrupted, CDCA is the major hydrophobic bile acid under cholestatic conditions[14].

Ursodeoxycholic acid (UDCA), a dihydroxy bile acid like CDCA or DCA, is less hydrophobic than CDCA or DCA. Its lipophilicity, however, is sufficient to ensure conservation in the enterohepatic circulation. It has been recognized for a decade that UDCA may exert hepatoprotective effects in the experimental animal[15,16]. When taurine-conjugated UDCA (TUDCA) is administered simultaneously with one of the more hydrophobic bile acids in the bile fistula rat it can overcome the cholestatic effect of these bile acids[13] (Fig. 1), an effect recently also shown for the trihydroxy bile acid tauro-β-muricholic acid[17]. In isolated human hepatocytes, injury induced by glycin-conjugated CDCA (GCDCA) can be diminished by addition of UDCA[18]. Hepatotoxic effects of hydrophobic bile acids were inhibited by UDCA conjugates in the rat *in vivo*, as well as in rat hepatocytes *in vitro*[19,20]. Recently, Poo and co-workers could demonstrate that in the experimental model of the bile duct-ligated rat UDCA treatment inhibited the development of fibrosis and portal hypertension[21].

THERAPEUTIC ASPECTS

UDCA has been used for therapy of liver diseases for a long time. In ancient China, dried bile of the black bear called 'Yutan', which mainly contains UDCA[22] has been an established remedy for treatment of hepatobiliary diseases for centuries[13]. In 1957, UDCA was introduced for the treatment of a variety of gastrointestinal complaints in Japan. In 1976 the first two controlled studies on the therapeutic effects of UDCA in chronic hepatitis were published in Japan[23,24]. In 1981 Leuschner and co-workers used UDCA for dissolution of gallstones in patients with chronic hepatitis, and observed that serum liver tests improved[25]. In 1986 and 1987 the first pilot studies of UDCA treatment in primary biliary cirrhosis (PBC) were reported[26,27] (Fig. 2). A large randomized controlled study by Poupon and colleagues has shown that UDCA in a daily dose of 13–15 mg/kg body weight improves clinical symptoms, serum liver tests, and liver histology in patients with PBC[28], and also prolongs the time to liver transplantation or death in these patients after a period of 4 years[29]. Preliminary data on other ongoing controlled trials[30–32] confirm the beneficial effect of UDCA in PBC. Similarly, it has been shown that UDCA improves serum liver tests[33–36] and liver histology[36] in patients with primary sclerosing cholangitis.

What are the underlying mechanisms for these beneficial effects of UDCA

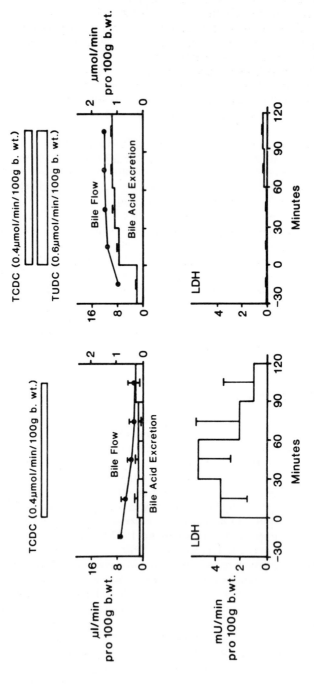

Fig. 1 Effects of bile acids on bile formation and hepatocellular integrity in the rat. Changes in bile flow rate (closed circles, upper panel), biliary bile salt secretion (open bars, upper panel), and LDH release (open bars, lower panel) in rats infused with TCDCA alone (left panels) or TCDCA and TUDCA simultaneously (right panels). Values are means ± SD. TUDCA co-administration prevents TCDCA-induced decrease of bile flow and increase of LDH release and stimulates bile salt excretion. (Reproduced from ref. 13 with permission)

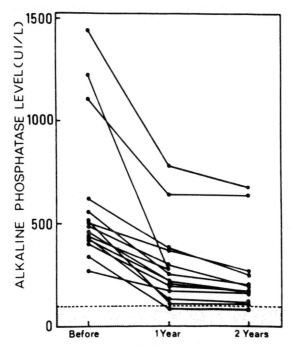

Fig. 2 Changes of serum alkaline phosphatase activities in 15 patients with PBC over 2 years of UDCA treatment (13–15 mg/kg daily). The dotted line indicates the upper limit of normal. (Reproduced from ref. 27 with permission)

in chronic cholestatic liver diseases? Several mechanisms have been suggested and will be discussed briefly:

1. Displacement of endogenous hydrophobic bile acids from the entero-hepatic circulation by competitive inhibition of ileal bile acid absorption by UDCA. This hypothesis, proposed by Poupon et al.[27,28], was based on observations in patients with PBC who showed a decrease in endogenous primary serum bile acids after periods of 6–24 months of UDCA treatment. In addition the ileal reabsorption of primary bile acids was inhibited in healthy controls[37] and patients with ileostomies[38,39]. On the other hand, decreases in serum levels or biliary levels of hydrophobic bile acids during short-term (1 month to 6 months) UDCA treatment of cholestatic liver disease were not observed in several studies at time-points when serum liver tests were markedly improved[35,40–42]. To investigate whether UDCA displaces endogenous hydrophobic bile acids from the bile acid pool at a time when the first effects on serum liver tests become apparent, we determined the pool size of CDCA and DCA, the major hydrophobic bile acids, in five patients with cholestatic liver disease (PBC, PSC) and four healthy controls before and 1 month after starting UDCA therapy (13–15 mg/kg daily)[14] (Fig. 3). Pool size, fractional turnover and synthesis rate of CDCA and DCA were

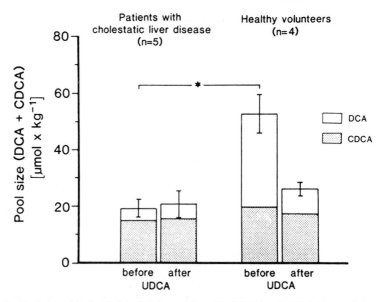

Fig. 3 Pool size of hydrophobic dihydroxy bile acids (CDCA + DCA) before and 1 month after the start of UDCA treatment (13–15 mg/kg daily) in five patients with chronic cholestatic liver disease and four healthy controls. Values are means ± SD. *$p < 0.02$. (Reproduced from ref. 14 with permission)

determined by an indicator dilution method using ^{13}C-labelled CDCA and [2]H-labelled DCA. Gas chromatography/mass spectrometry was employed for isotope ratio measurement in serum. In patients with cholestatic liver disease, marked improvement of cholestatic marker enzymes was observed after 1 month of treatment. UDCA had no effect on the pool size of CDCA in patients with cholestatic liver disease, a finding recently also reported by others[43,44], or in healthy volunteers (Fig. 3). Patients with cholestatic liver disease had a markedly reduced DCA pool before treatment. This small pool, amounting to only 14% of the DCA pool of healthy volunteers, was not further decreased by UDCA therapy. However, UDCA decreased the size of the DCA pool and increased the DCA fractional turnover in healthy volunteers[14]. Therefore, the observed improvement of liver tests during short-term treatment of patients with PBC or PSC cannot be explained by displacement of hydrophobic, potentially hepatotoxic bile acids from the enterohepatic circulation.

2. Dilution of endogenous hydrophobic bile acids by expansion of the bile acid pool with UDCA. Indirect evidence suggests that UDCA treatment leads to dilution of endogenous bile acids by expansion of the bile acid pool with UDCA. This assumption is based on determination of serum and biliary bile acid levels in patients with cholestatic liver disease during UDCA treatment as mentioned above[14,35,36,40–42], and was clearly shown in a controlled fashion by Poupon et al.[45]. Whether dilution of

endogenous hydrophobic bile acids with UDCA or the absolute level of UDCA *per se* in the circulation is of functional relevance for the beneficial effect of UDCA in cholestatic liver disease is not yet clear.

3. Stabilization of hepatocellular membranes by UDCA. In hepatocytes and erythrocytes *in vitro*, UDCA exerts a membrane-stabilizing effect against damaging effects of more hydrophobic bile acids[20,46]. Since effective bile acid concentrations were in a range which is merely reached in serum or in the hepatocyte *in vivo* the relevance of these findings remains unclear.

4. Immune modulation. It was first observed by Calmus *et al.* that aberrant expression of HLA class I molecules on hepatocellular membranes in patients with PBC was reduced by UDCA treatment[47]. This observation might be of importance since HLA class I molecules are target molecules for cytotoxic T lymphocytes which may damage hepatocytes in cholestatic liver disease. In four patients of our PSC trial we studied the hepatocellular expression of HLA class I molecules before and 12 months after start of therapy. In two patients treated with UDCA hepatocellular HLA class I expression almost completely disappeared after 1 year, whereas in two patients treated with placebo no changes were observed[36]. Since hepatocellular HLA class I expression is observed in cholestatic disease of different origins, and may even be induced by experimental bile duct ligation[48], it may be assumed that the observed effects of UDCA in patients with cholestatic liver disease may largely be a consequence of the improvement of cholestasis. *In vitro* studies have shown modulating effects of UDCA on functions of immunocompetent cells such as monocytes or lymphocytes[49]. The relevance of these interesting findings is yet unclear.

5. Stimulation of hepatocellular biliary secretion by UDCA. Hepatocellular secretion is regulated by a complex network of signals which are not yet fully elucidated. Cytosolic free Ca^{2+} $[Ca^{2+}]_i$ plays a key role in the regulation of secretion. Taurine-conjugated UDCA, the main form of UDCA in the rat, has recently been demonstrated to act as a potent hepatocellular Ca^{2+} agonist at physiological bile acid concentrations and to induce sustained $[Ca^{2+}]_i$ increases[50] in rat hepatocytes by mobilizing intra- and extracellular Ca^{2+} (Fig. 4). TUDCA (but not TCA or TCDCA) induced a sustained increase of vesicular exocytosis by Ca^{2+}-dependent mechanisms in the isolated perfused rat liver[51]. Vesicular exocytosis represents the final step of the transcytotic vesicular pathway which may be of functional importance for bile acid secretion in bile acid-loaded liver cells[5,6] and for targeting of transport proteins involved in bile formation (like the Cl^-/HCO_3^- exchanger) to the canalicular membrane[52]. This mechanism could lead to improved secretion of endogenous bile acids[53] and other cholephils[54] into bile under cholestatic conditions.

Hypercholeresis[55], partly explained by a cholehepatic shunt mechanism[56], is another phenomenon observed under UDCA treatment in the experimental animal. Indirect evidence suggests that this mechanism

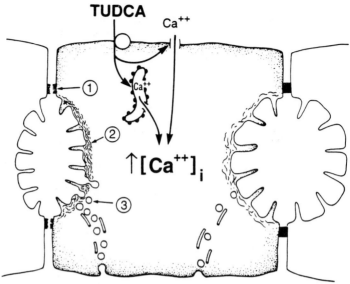

Fig. 4 Putative effects of TUDCA-induced cytosolic free Ca^{2+} $[Ca^{2+}]_i$ increase on hepatocyte bile formation. The figure shows a model of a liver cell in a hypothetical 'resting' state (right) and a hypothetical 'stimulated' state (left). TUDCA, presumably after carrier-mediated uptake into the hepatocyte, induces sustained increases of $[Ca^{2+}]_i$ by depleting intracellular microsomal IP_3-sensitive Ca^{2+} stores independently of IP_3 and inducing Ca^{2+} entry across the plasma membrane (see ref. 50). This $[Ca^{2+}]_i$ increase may affect bile formation by: (1) modulating the permeability of hepatocyte tight junctions, (2) mediating contraction of the canaliculus and extrusion of canalicular bile, and (3) activating vesicular exocytosis, the final step of the transcytotic vesicular pathway (see ref. 51). (Reproduced from ref. 60 with permission)

does not play a significant role in patients with cholestatic liver disease under UDCA treatment[41,57]. However, further studies in patients with cholestatic liver disease are awaited.

SUMMARY

Bile acids play a key role in normal hepatocellular function. Depending on their detergency, lipophilicity, and concentration in the hepatocyte, and other as yet unknown factors, they can exert choleretic or cholestatic, protective or toxic effects on the liver.

UDCA, a dihydroxy bile acid, has recently been introduced as a treatment for cholestatic liver disease[58,59]. In cholestasis which may be the consequence of a variety of noxious agents, bile acids are retained in the hepatocyte and in the systemic circulation. Hydrophobic bile acids may damage the hepatocyte and thus perpetuate and aggravate the cholestasis. A vicious cycle ensues which may lead to necrosis, fibrosis and secondary biliary cirrhosis of the liver. UDCA might interrupt this vicious cycle by acting as a hepatocellular Ca^{2+} agonist, thereby increasing hepatocellular secretion. In addition, dilution of the endogenous bile acid pool, stabilization of hepatocellular membranes, immune modulation, and other yet unknown effects may play a role in mediating the beneficial effects of UDCA. Future studies on the mechanism(s) of action of UDCA in cholestatic liver disease will help to further elucidate the complex functional relationships between bile acids and the liver.

References

1. Carey MC, Cahalane MJ. The enterohepatic circulation. In: Arias I, Jakoby BW, Popper H et al., editors. The liver – biology and pathobiology. New York: Raven Press; 1988: 573–616.
2. Nathanson MH, Boyer JL. Mechanisms and regulation of bile secretion. Hepatology. 1991;14:551–66.
3. Hofmann AF. The enterohepatic circulation of bile acids in health and disease. In: Sleisinger MH, Fordtran JS, editors. Gastrointestinal disease. Philadelphia: W. B. Saunders; 1993; 127–50.
4. Arias IM, Che M, Gatmaitan Z et al. The biology of the bile canaliculus. Hepatology. 1993;17:318–29.
5. Crawford JM, Berken CA, Gollan JL. Role of the hepatocyte microtubular system in the excretion of bile salts and biliary lipid: implications for intracellular vesicular transport. J Lipid Res. 1988;29:144–56.
6. Erlinger S. Role of intracellular organelles in the hepatic transport of bile acids. Biomed Pharmacother. 1990;44:409–16.
7. Schölmerich J, Becher MS, Schmidt K et al. Influence of hydroxylation and conjugation of bile salts on their membrane-damaging properties: studies on isolated hepatocytes and lipid membrane vesicles. Hepatology. 1984;4:661–6.
8. Holsti P. Cirrhosis of the liver induced in rabbits by gastric instillation of 3-monohydroxy-cholanic acid. Nature. 1960;186:250.
9. Javitt JB. Cholestasis in rats induced by taurolithocholate. Nature. 1966;210:1262–3.
10. Greim H, Trülzsch D, Czygan P et al. Mechanism of cholestasis. 6. Bile acids in human livers with or without biliary obstruction. Gastroenterology. 1972;63:846–50.
11. Morrissey KP, McSherry CK, Swarm RL et al. Toxicity of chenodeoxycholic acid in the nonhuman primate. Surgery. 1975;77:851–60.
12. Herz R, Paumgartner G, Preisig R. Inhibition of bile formation by high doses of taurocholate in the perfused rat liver. Scand J Gastroenterol. 1976;11:741–6.
13. Kitani K. Hepatoprotective effect of ursodeoxycholate in experimental animals. In: Paumgartner G, Stiehl A, Barbara L et al., editors. Strategies for the treatment of hepatobiliary diseases. Dordrecht: Kluwer; 1990:43–56.
14. Beuers U, Spengler U, Zwiebel FM et al. Effect of ursodeoxycholic acid on the kinetics of the major hydrophobic bile acids in health and in chronic cholestatic liver disease. Hepatology. 1992;15:603–8.
15. Krol T, Kitamura T, Miyai K et al. Tauroursodeoxycholate reduces ductular proliferation and portal inflammation in bile duct-ligated hamsters. Hepatology. 1983;3:881 (abstract)
16. Kitani K, Kanai S. Tauroursodeoxycholate prevents taurocholate induced cholestasis. Life Sci. 1982;30:515–23.
17. Kanai S, Ohta M, Kitani K et al. Tauro β-muricholate is as effective as tauroursodeoxy-cholate in preventing taurochenodeoxycholate-induced liver damage in the rat. Life Sci. 1990;47:2421–8.
18. Galle PR, Theilmann L, Raedsch R et al. Ursodeoxycholate reduces hepatotoxicity of bile salts in primary human hepatocytes. Hepatology. 1990;12:486–91.
19. Heuman DM, Mills AS, McCall J et al. Conjugates of ursodeoxycholate protect against cholestasis and hepatocellular necrosis caused by more hydrophobic bile salts. In vivo studies in the rat. Gastroenterology. 1991;100:203–11.
20. Heuman DM, Pandak WM, Hylemon PB et al. Conjugates of ursodeoxycholate protect against cytotoxicity of more hydrophobic bile salts: in vitro studies in rat hepatocytes and human erythrocytes. Hepatology. 1991;14:920–6.

21. Poo JL, Feldmann G, Erlinger S et al. Ursodeoxycholic acid limits liver histologic alterations and portal hypertension induced by bile duct ligation in the rat. Gastroenterology. 1992;102:1752–9.
22. Shoda M. Über die Ursodesoxycholsäure aus Bärengallen und ihre physiologische Wirkung. J Biochem. 1927;7:505–10.
23. Mijayi K, Akiyama T, Ito M et al. The effect of ursodeoxycholic acid on liver functions in patients with chronic liver disease. A double blind study in one institution and the study on the effect on hepatic blood flow. Rinsho to Kenkyu. 1976;53:1395–403.
24. Yamanaka M, Oto M, Obata H et al. The examination of the therapeutic efficacy of ursodeoxycholic acid on chronic hepatitis. A double blind study. Shindan to Chiryo. 1976;64:2150–7.
25. Leuschner U, Leuschner M, Sieratzki J et al. Gallstone dissolution with ursodeoxycholic acid in patients with chronic active hepatitis and two years follow-up. A pilot study. Dig Dis Sci. 1985;30:642–9.
26. Fisher MM, Paradine ME. Influence of ursodeoxycholic acid on biochemical parameters in cholestatic disease. Gastroenterology. 1986;90:1625 (abstract).
27. Poupon R, Chretien Y, Poupon RE et al. Is ursodeoxycholic acid an effective treatment for primary biliary cirrhosis? Lancet. 1987;1:834–6.
28. Poupon RE, Balkau B, Eschwege E et al. and the UDCA–PBC Study Group. A multicenter, controlled trial of ursodiol for the treatment of primary biliary cirrhosis. N Engl J Med. 1991;324:1548–54.
29. Poupon RE, Chretien Y, Balkau B et al. and the UDCA–PBC Study Group. Ursodeoxycholic acid therapy for primary biliary cirrhosis: a four year controlled study. Hepatology. 1992;16:91A (abstract).
30. Lindor KD, Baldus WP, Jorgensen RA et al. Ursodeoxycholic acid is beneficial therapy for patients with primary biliary cirrhosis. Hepatology. 1992;16:91A.
31. Heathcote EJL, Cauch K, Walker V et al. The Canadian multi-centre double blind randomized controlled trial of ursodeoxycholic acid in primary biliary cirrhosis. Hepatology. 1992;16:91A.
32. Combes B, Carithers RL, McDonald MF et al. Ursodeoxycholic acid therapy in patients with primary biliary cirrhosis. Hepatology. 1991;14:91A (abstract).
33. Stiehl A, Raedsch R, Rudolph G et al. Treatment of primary sclerosing cholangitis with ursodeoxycholic acid: first results of a controlled study. Hepatology. 1989;10:602 (abstract).
34. Chazouilleres O, Poupon R, Capron JP et al. Ursodeoxycholic acid for primary sclerosing cholangitis. J Hepatol. 1990;11:120–3.
35. O'Brien CB, Senior J, Renu-Arora JK et al. Ursodeoxycholic acid for the treatment of primary sclerosing cholangitis: a 36-month open pilot trial. Hepatology. 1991;14:838–47.
36. Beuers U, Spengler U, Kruis W et al. Ursodeoxycholic acid for treatment of primary sclerosing cholangitis: a placebo-controlled trial. Hepatology. 1992;16:707–14.
37. Marteau P, Chazouilleres O, Myara A et al. Effect of chronic administration of ursodeoxycholic acid on the ileal absorption of endogenous bile acids in man. Hepatology. 1990;12:1206–8.
38. Stiehl A, Raedsch R, Rudolph G. Acute effects of ursodeoxycholic and chenodeoxycholic acid on the small intestinal absorption of bile acids. Gastroenterology. 1990;98:424–8.
39. Eusufzai S, Ericsson S, Cederlund T et al. Effect of ursodeoxycholic acid treatment on ileal absorption of bile acids in man as determined by the SeHCAT test. Gut. 1991;32:1044–8.
40. Nakagawa M, Colombo C, Setchell KDR. Comprehensive study of the biliary bile acid composition of patients with cystic fibrosis and associated liver disease before and after UDCA administration. Hepatology. 1990;12:322–34.
41. Crosignani A, Podda M, Battezzati PM et al. Changes in bile acid composition in patients with primary biliary cirrhosis induced by ursodeoxycholic acid administration. Hepatology. 1991;14:1000–7.
42. Beuers U, Fischer S, Spengler U et al. Formation of iso-ursodeoxycholic acid during administration of ursodeoxycholic acid in man. J Hepatol. 1991;13:97–103.
43. Rudolph G, Endele R, Senn M et al. Effect of ursodeoxycholic acid on the kinetics of cholic acid and chenodeoxycholic acid in patients with primary sclerosing cholangitis. Hepatology. 1993;17:1028–32.
44. Mazzella G, Parini P, Bazzoli F et al. Ursodeoxycholic acid administration on bile acid

metabolism in patients with early stages of primary biliary cirrhosis. Dig Dis Sci. 1993;38: 896–902.

45. Poupon RE, Chretien Y, Poupon R *et al.* Serum bile acids in primary biliary cirrhosis: effect of ursodeoxycholic acid therapy. Hepatology. 1993;17:599–604.
46. Güldütuna S, Zimmer G, Imhof M *et al.* Molecular aspects of membrane stabilization by ursodeoxycholate. Gastroenterology. 1993;104:1736–44.
47. Calmus Z, Gane P, Rouger P *et al.* Hepatic expression of class I and class II major histocompatibility complex molecules in primary biliary cirrhosis: effect of ursodeoxycholic acid. Hepatology. 1990;11:12–15.
48. Innes GK, Nagafuchi Y, Fuler BJ *et al.* Increased expression of major histocompatibility antigens in the liver as a result of cholestasis. Transplantation. 1988;45:749–52.
49. Yoshikawa M, Tsujii T, Matsumara K *et al.* Immunomodulatory effects of ursodeoxycholic acid on immune responses. Hepatology. 1992;16:358–64.
50. Beuers U, Nathanson MH, Boyer JL. Effects of tauroursodeoxycholic acid on cytosolic Ca^{++} signals in isolated rat hepatocytes. Gastroenterology. 1993;104:604–12.
51. Beuers U, Nathanson MH, Isales CM *et al.* Tauroursodeoxycholic acid stimulates hepatocellular exocytosis and mobilizes extracellular Ca^{++}: associated mechanisms that are defective in cholestasis. J Clin Invest. 1993;92(In press).
52. Benedetti A, Strazzabosco M, Boyer JL. Cellular regulation of Cl^-/HCO_3^- exchange activity by HCO_3^-, cAMP and colchicine in isolated rat hepatocytes. Hepatology. 1990;12:887 (abstract).
53. Kitani K, Kanai S. Interactions between different bile salts in the biliary excretion of the rat. Chem Pathol Pharmacol. 1983;39:139–52.
54. Colombo C, Castellani MR, Balistreri WF *et al.* Scintigraphic documentation of an improvement in hepatobiliary excretory function after treatment with ursodeoxycholic acid in patients with cystic fibrosis and associated liver disease. Hepatology. 1992;15:677–84.
55. Dumont M, Erlinger S, Uchman S. Hypercholeresis induced by ursodeoxycholic acid and 7-ketolithocholic acid in the rat: possible role of bicarbonate transport. Gastroenterology. 1980;79:82–9.
56. Yoon YB, Hagey LR, Hofmann AF *et al.* Effect of side-chain shortening on the physiological properties of bile acids: hepatic transport and effect on biliary secretion of 23-norursodeoxycholate in rodents. Gastroenterology. 1986;90:837–52.
57. Knyrym K, Vakil N, Pfab R *et al.* The effects of intraduodenal bile acid administration on biliary secretion of ionized calcium and carbonate in man. Hepatology. 1989;10:134–42.
58. Hofmann AF. Bile acid hepatotoxicity and the rationale of UDCA therapy in chronic cholestatic liver disease: some hypotheses. In: Paumgartner G, Stiehl A, Barbara L *et al.*, editors. Strategies for the treatment of hepatobiliary diseases. Dordrecht: Kluwer; 1990: 13–34.
59. Poupon RE, Poupon R. Ursodeoxycholic acid for the treatment of cholestatic diseases. Prog Liver Dis. 1992;10:219–38.
60. Beuers U, Nathanson MH, Boyer JL. Effect of taurine-conjugated ursodeoxycholic acid on Ca^{++} homeostasis in isolated rat hepatocytes. In: Paumgartner G, Stiehl A, Gerok W, editors. Bile acids and the hepatobiliary system. Dordrecht: Kluwer; 1992:211–16.

28
Meta-analysis of the clinical results with UDCA in chronic liver diseases

S. BELLENTANI, F. MANENTI and A. FERRARI

INTRODUCTION

During the past 10 years ursodeoxycholic acid (UDCA or ursodiol) has been introduced in clinical practice, mainly in Europe, for the therapy of cholestatic liver diseases. Primary biliary cirrhosis (PBC) was the first chronic cholestatic liver disease where this type of therapy was firstly applied on a long-term basis[1,2]. Subsequently, after a fortuitous observation made by Leuschner that UDCA was able to reduce the level of ALT and AST in patients with chronic hepatitis (CH) and cholesterol gallstones[3] it was utilized also in patients with chronic hepatitis[4-14]. Usually, the modifications of serum biochemical indices of liver cytolysis (ALT and AST) and cholestasis (GGT and ALP) are considered, while, to date, few studies have explored the long-term efficacy of ursodiol on outcomes clinically more relevant than the reduction of serum liver enzymes, such as liver histology[14-19], reduction of life-threatening complications[20] or survival. As a consequence a critical revision of the published studies, through meta-analysis of the results derived from double-blind randomized (DBR) clinical trials (full papers and abstracts), as attempted in this chapter, is almost exclusively concerned with the efficacy of UDCA in lowering ALT, AST, AP, bilirubin and GGT, and a 'classical' meta-analysis of more relevant outcomes affecting the natural history of these two chronic liver diseases is impossible.

METHODS

Data source identification and study selection

Medline and *Index Medicus* were searched in order to select articles and abstracts published and conforming with necessary quality scoring. Abstracts were used to identify, whenever possible, subsequent published studies. Unpublished studies were not included in the final data pool. Only DBR clinical trials were further considered, while single-blind or open clinical

Table 1 Studies excluded on second review from meta-analysis

Reference	Disease	No. of patients	Published as	Exclusion rationale
1	PBC	15	Full paper	Open series
36	PBC	4	Full paper	Open series
35	PBC	9	Full paper	Open series
42	PBC	16	Abstract	Insufficient data rep.[a]
37	PBC	50	Abstract	Insufficient data rep.[a]
38	PBC	15	Full paper	Open series
39	PBC	3	Full paper	Open series
40	PBC	26	Abstract	Single blinded
41[b]	PBC	178	Abstract	Insufficient data rep.[a]
41[b]	PBC	222	Abstract	Insufficient data rep.[a]
44	PBC	88	Full paper	Insufficient data rep.[c]
3	CH	6	Full paper	Open series
49	CH	21	Full paper	Open series
45	CH	45	Full paper	Open series
46	CH	27	Full paper	Open series
47	CH	12	Full paper	Single blinded
12	CH	20	Abstract	Open series
51	CH	22	Full paper	Single blinded
6	CH	18	Full paper	Open series
14	CH	36	Abstract	Insufficient data rep.
50	CH	91	Letter	Insufficient data rep.

[a] Group mean without standard deviation or without absolute value
[b] Not cited on *Medline* and reported only by Simko et al.[41]
[c] Composite biochemical score was used

trials were excluded from this analysis. The effect size and p test for heterogeneity were performed according to standard procedures[21–25].

RESULTS

The most numerous studies on the therapeutic use of ursodiol in chronic liver diseases concerned PBC and CH (15 articles each). Among them only 13 (eight on PBC and five on CH) were DBR clinical trials, the other studies being either single-blind or open clinical trials. The latter studies were excluded from the analysis (see Table 1). In the 14 DBR clinical trials published and further considered, the admission and exclusion criteria, and the dosage of UDCA used (10–12 mg/kg) to treat the 794 and 287 patients with PBC and CH respectively, were quite homogeneous. The duration of treatment was variable, ranging from 1 to 48 months. To our knowledge, while writing this paper, six of the 15 DBR clinical trials (five on PBC and one on CH) are still published in the form of abstracts (see Tables 1 and 2) and the data relative to the effect of UDCA on serum ALT, AST, GGT, bilirubin or AP in five out of six of these abstracts are insufficient to calculate the effect size based on means and standard deviations. Therefore, we eventually used only eight full papers (four on PBC and four on CH) and one abstract (on PBC) to perform the meta-analysis. Three papers on PBC contained information on liver histology which was also analysed. Tables 1 and 2 list the studies excluded and included from meta-analysis, the criteria

Table 2 Studies and patient features included in meta-analysis

Reference	Site, country	Disease	No. of patients	Dosage UDCA (per day)
15	Single centre, Germany	PBC	18	10 mg/kg
36	Multicentre, Japan	PBC	41	600 mg
16	Multicentre, France–Canada	PBC	116	13–15 mg/kg
19	Multicentre, USA	PBC	149	10–12 mg/kg
18	Single centre, USA	PBC	14	10–12 mg/kg
13	Multicentre, Italy	CH	56	600 mg
8	Single centre, Italy	CH	26	450 mg
9	Single centre, Italy	CH	50	600 mg
11	Single centre, Italy	CH	29	450 mg

used for exclusion, the number of patients, the dosage of UDCA used and the duration of therapy.

Table 2 shows the study design and patient features of the nine DBR clinical trials (five on PBC and four on CH) utilized for the meta-analysis: the population included 338 patients with PBC and 161 with CH. All studies met the following criteria: they represented published (eight full papers and one abstract), randomized, double-blind clinical trials of UDCA therapy; they reported a group mean with standard deviation or standard error of the mean at baseline (placebo or no treatment) and treatment phases; they reported the number of drop-outs and used the same biochemical parameters as end-points to judge the efficacy of treatment.

Only two of the papers reported a questionable result in terms of improvement either of bilirubin in PBC[18] or of AST and ALT in CH[11]. The others showed a favourable outcome for all the biochemical parameters, with average variations in respect to the basal value during the 1–48 months of therapy ranging from -11% to $+20\%$ in the placebo and from -15% to -87% in UDCA-treated patients.

Using the meta-analysis techniques of Hedges and Olkin[23], the effect size and 95% confidence intervals (CI) for quantitative data of four biochemical indices analysed could be computed for each of the nine studies. The χ^2 test for heterogeneity of effect size was also calculated, and was significant for all the four biochemical indices considered. This confirmed that the data could be considered representative of homogeneous populations, and that the variance in effect sizes observed was no greater than could be expected from sampling error alone.

In three of the papers[15,16,19], the effect of ursodiol therapy on total bilirubin was also reported, but the data were not included in the calculation of effect size, because they failed the heterogeneity test (p for heterogeneity $= 0.04$). The data from individual studies relative to ALP, AST, ALT and GGT could be merged, and an overall effect size both for PBC and CH could be calculated. Figures 1 and 2 illustrate the effect sizes of these biochemical parameters and the overall effect size with 95% CI estimating upper and lower limits in PBC and CH respectively. When CI excludes zero, improvement (greater than 0) or deterioration (lower than 0) from placebo can be calculated. When CI includes 0, no difference between placebo and

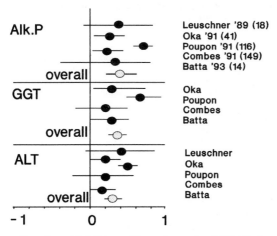

Fig. 1 Treatment effect size with 95% confidence intervals of UDCA therapy on alkaline phosphatase (Alk.P), alanine-transferase (ALT) and gamma-glutamyl-transpeptidase (GGT) in the five double-blind randomized clinical trials analysed on PBC (numbers of patients are reported in parentheses; UDCA on the right, placebo on the left)

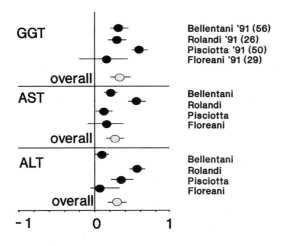

Fig. 2 Treatment effect size with 95% confidence intervals of UDCA therapy on ALT, AST and GGT in the four double-blind randomized clinical trials on CH analysed (numbers of patients are reported in parentheses; UDCA on the right, placebo on the left)

treatment can be determined. Only one study on CH[11] did not show a significant difference between UDCA and placebo. Using Cohen's definition of small (0,2), medium (0,5) and large (0,8) effect size[23], small effect size improvement with UDCA was seen for all the biochemical indices tested, both in PBC and CH. A somewhat higher effect size improvement with

Table 3 Reports on UDCA therapy in less common types of chronic cholestatic liver diseases

Reference	Disease
25	Primary sclerosing cholangitis
26	Primary sclerosing cholangitis
27	Cystic fibrosis
28	Intrahepatic cholestasis of pregnancy
29	Biliary atresia
30	Chronic intrahepatic cholestasis of infancy
31	Parenteral nutrition-associated cholestasis

UDCA, both in PBC and CH, was seen for biochemical markers of cholestasis (ALP and GGT) than for biochemical markers of liver necrosis (ALT and AST). Among the nine studies selected for meta-analysis, only four studies (three on PBC and one on CH) also reported data relative to the effect of ursodiol on liver histology[13,15,16,18]. The one on CH[13] revealed no effect of UDCA on liver histology after 1 year of treatment. For the other three on PBC[15,16,18] (for a total of 124 patients), on the basis of patients who improved and patients who deteriorated, the overall odds ratio calculated was 2.0 ± 0.7, suggesting that ursodiol treatment doubled the probability of improvement of liver histology in respect to placebo.

In all the other studies not considered for meta-analysis (see Table 1), the reduction of AST, ALT and GGT in UDCA-treated patients both in PBC and CH was similar; the percentage of reduction in respect to placebo ranged between 25% and 50%.

More limited experience is also available in other less common types of cholestatic liver diseases, such as primary sclerosing cholangitis[25,26], cystic fibrosis associated with cholestasis[27], acute cholestasis of pregnancy[28], biliary atresia[29], Alagille syndrome and idiopathic intrahepatic cholestasis[30], home parenteral nutrition-associated cholestasis[31]. All these studies, mainly including open clinical series, showed an improvement of biochemical indices of cholestasis and cytolysis in ursodiol-treated patients (Table 3).

DISCUSSION

The indications for the use of ursodiol in chronic liver diseases are growing year by year. UDCA has recently been used not only in cholestatic liver diseases[32-35], such as PBC[2,15,16,18-20,36-44], but also in chronic non-cholestatic liver diseases, such as chronic hepatitis[4-14,17,45-50], alcoholic liver diseases[50] and cirrhosis[7,17]. To extract the maximum amount of information from previous studies we chose meta-analysis. We selected only DBR clinical trials in order to strengthen our conclusions. Other authors[41,48] have recently performed meta-analysis on UDCA therapy in PBC and CH, by also including open clinical series, non-comparative, non-randomized or single-blind trials, and since this is not a common procedure for meta-analysis[22,23], their results should be interpreted with some caution. Nevertheless, their conclusions on the effect of UDCA on biochemical parameters and liver histology are similar to ours. Our results show that ursodiol treatment for a minimum of 3 months and a maximum of 24 months was effective in lowering the biochemical indices of liver function, both in PBC and CH, and that its efficacy was more pronounced on markers of cholestasis. However, according to Cohen's definition[24], the improvement of overall effect size in respect to placebo must be classified as small. We previously demonstrated[4] that one of the conditions to maintain the efficacy of ursodiol in lowering ALT, AST and GGT is to prolong therapy and that, after only 1 month from withdrawal of the drug, there is a rebound of these serum biochemical parameters to the baseline level. This is true both for CH and PBC. Therefore, in order to understand if the efficacy of long-term treatment with UDCA is not limited to a 'cosmetic' effect on serum transaminases, GGT and ALP, we tried to detect in the studies published some other stronger outcomes, such as quality of life, work performance, social participation, general well-being and mood, reduction of annoying symptoms such as pruritus, reduction of life-threatening complications, liver histology and survival. Unfortunately, life-threatening complications and liver histology were considered in only two and four out of the nine studies analysed. The reduction of life-threatening complications in patients treated with UDCA in respect to placebo was questionable in both studies[16,43]. More detailed results, based either on histology score or on descriptive information from improved and deteriorated liver histology, were reported in the other four articles. The one on CH[13] did not show any improvement. Meta-analysis of the other three on PBC[15,16,18] revealed an improvement of UDCA in respect to placebo after 9–24 months of therapy, with an odds ratio of 2.0 ± 0.7. All the other studies either did not consider other possible outcomes or did not present sufficient data to be evaluated by meta-analysis. We only can mention that eight out of the 14 patients on PBC reported a favourable effect of UDCA on pruritus and that Leuschner, in a recent abstract[20], suggested that UDCA could improve the prognosis of PBC during 10 years' therapy in 15 patients. Furthermore, two other observations suggest that: 1-UDCA is beneficial especially for early-stage (I and II) PBC patients while in later stages (III and IV) a higher percentage (40%) of patients showed a further increase of bilirubin and a worsening of pruritus[52]; 2-UDCA seems to have a higher efficacy in lowering AST, ALT and GGT in patients with CH and cirrhosis in respect to patients with only CH[17].

We conclude that, although data available are insufficient and often not sufficiently standardized, long-term administration of ursodiol (450–900 mg/day) improves routinely used laboratory liver function tests, especially ALP and GGT, markers of cholestasis, both in PBC and CH. Liver histology improved only in PBC, where a higher cholestatic component is present. We hope that in the future researchers in this field may reach a more homogeneous definition of end-points and outcomes, in order to answer the main questions of whether long-term treatment with UDCA may ultimately increase survival in patients with PBC or CH.

References

1. Poupon R, Chretien Y, Poupon RE et al. Is ursodeoxycholic acid an effective treatment for primary biliary cirrhosis? Lancet. 1987;1:834–6.

2. Poupon RE, Eschwege E, Poupon R and the UDCA–PBC Study Group. Ursodeoxycholic acid for treatment of primary biliary cirrhosis. Interim analysis of a double-blind multicenter randomized trial. J Hepatol. 1990;11:16–21.
3. Leuschner U, Leuschner M, Sieratzki J et al. Gallstone dissolution with ursodeoxycholic acid in patients with chronic active hepatitis and two years' follow-up. Dig Dis Sci. 1985;30:642–9
4. Bellentani S, Tabarroni G, Barchi T et al. Effect of ursodeoxycholic acid treatment on alanine aminotransferase and gamma-glutamyltranspeptidase serum levels in patients with hypertransaminasemia. J Hepatol. 1989;8:7–12.
5. Podda M, Ghezzi C, Battezzati PM et al. Effect of ursodeoxycholic acid in chronic liver disease. Dig Dis Sci. 1989;34:59S–65S.
6. Crosignani A, Battezzati PM, Setchell KDR et al. Effects of ursodeoxycholic acid on serum liver enzymes and bile acid metabolism in chronic active hepatitis: a dose response study. Hepatology. 1991;13:339–344.
7. Lirussi F, Beccarello A, Okolicsanyi L. Combination therapy of ursodeoxycholic acid and silymarin in non-cholestatic chronic liver disease. Eur J Clin Invest. 1991;21:13.
8. Rolandi E, Franceschini R, Cataldi A et al. Effects of ursodeoxycholic acid (UDCA) in serum liver damage indices in patients with chronic active hepatitis. A double-blind controlled study. Eur J Clin Pharmacol. 1991;40:473–6
9. Pisciotta G, Scialabba A, Montalto G et al. L'acido ursodeossicolico nel trattamento delle malattie croniche di fegato. Risultati a breve termine. Min Gastroenterol Dietol. 1991;37(1):29–33.
10. Podda M, Ghezzi C, Battezzati PM et al. Ursodeoxycholic acid and taurine as therapy for cholestatic liver disease. Hepatology. 1991;13(6):1257–9.
11. Floreani A, Chiaramonte M, Fabris P et al. Poor effect of ursodeoxycholic acid in anti-hepatitis C virus-positive chronic liver disease. Curr Ther Res. 1991;50(5):579–85.
12. Buzzelli G, Moscarella S, Focardi G et al. Ursodeoxycholic acid (UDCA) in chronic active hepatitis. Results of a controlled trial. J Hepatol. 1991;13(Suppl. 2):364.
13. Bellentani S, Manenti F, Tiribelli C, Podda M. Ursodeoxycholic acid (UDCA) in chronic hepatitis: a double-blind multicenter trial. Gastroenterology. 1991;100(5):A719.
14. Attili AF, Rusticali G, Carli L et al. Effect of ursodeoxycholic acid (UDCA) on serum enzymes and liver histology in patients with chronic active hepatitis (CAH). Am J Gastroenterol. 1991;86(9):362.
15. Leuschner U, Fischer H, Kurtz W et al. Ursodeoxycholic acid in primary biliary cirrhosis: results of a controlled double-blind trial. Gastroenterology. 1989;97:1268–74.
16. Poupon RE, Balkau B, Eschwege E et al. A multicenter, controlled trial of ursodiol for the treatment of primary biliary cirrhosis. N Engl J Med. 1991;324:1548–54.
17. Bellentani S, Podda M, Tiribelli C et al. Ursodiol in long-term treatment of hepatitis: a double-blind multicenter clinical trial. J Hepatol. (In press).
18. Batta AK, Salen G, Mirchandani R et al. Effect of long-term treatment with ursodiol on clinical and biochemical features and biliary bile acid metabolism in patients with primary biliary cirrhosis. Am J Gastroenterol. 1993;88:691–700.
19. Combes B, Charithers RL Jr, McDonald MF et al. Ursodeoxycholic acid therapy in patients with primary biliary cirrhosis. Hepatology. 1991;14(4):284.
20. Leuschner M, Guldutuna S, Leuschner U. Does ursodeoxycholic acid (UDCA) improve the prognosis of primary biliary cirrhosis (PBC)? J Hepatol. 1991;13(2):S138.
21. Beto JA, Bansal VK. Quality of life in treatment of hypertension. A meta-analysis of clinical trials. Am J Hypertens. 1992;5:125–33.
22. Boissel JP, Blanchard J, Panak E et al. Considerations for the meta-analysis of randomized clinical trials. Summary of a panel discussion. Contr Clin Trials. 1989;10:254–81.
23. Hedges LV, Olkin I. Statistical methods for meta-analysis. New York: Academic Press; 1985.
24. Cohen J. Statistical power analysis for the behavioral sciences. New York: Academic Press; 1969.
25. Chazouilleres O, Poupon R, Capron JP et al. Ursodeoxycholic acid for primary sclerosing cholangitis. J Hepatol. 1990;11:120–3.
26. Beuers U, Spengler U, Kruis W et al. Ursodeoxycholic acid for treatment of primary sclerosing cholangitis: a placebo-controlled trial. Hepatology. 1992;16:707–14.
27. Cotting J, Lentze MJ, Reichen J. Effects of ursodeoxycholic acid in patients with cystic

fibrosis and longstanding cholestasis. Gut. 1990;31:918–21.
28. Palma J, Reyes H, Ribalta J et al. Effects of ursodeoxycholic acid in patients with intrahepatic cholestasis of pregnancy. Hepatology. 1992;15:1043–7.
29. Ullrich D, Rating D, Schroter W et al. Treatment with ursodeoxycholic acid renders children with biliary atresia suitable for liver transplantation. Lancet. 1987;2:1324.
30. Balistrieri WF, A-Kader HH, Heubi JE et al. Ursodeoxycholic acid (UDCA) decreases serum cholesterol levels, ameliorates symptoms, and improves biochemical parameters in pediatric patients with chronic intrahepatic cholestasis. XI. International Bile Acid Meeting, 11–13 October, Freiburg, 1990:65.
31. Lindor KD, Burnes J. Ursodeoxycholic acid for the treatment of home parenteral nutrition-associated cholestasis. Gastroenterology. 1991;101:250–3.
32. James OFW. Ursodeoxycholic acid treatment for chronic cholestatic liver disease. J Hepatol. 1990;11:5–8.
33. Poupon R, Calmus Y. Ursodeoxycholic acid (UDCA) in the treatment of chronic cholestatic diseases. Biochimie. 1991;73:1335–8.
34. De Caestecker JS, Jazrawi RP, Petroni ML, Northfield TC. Ursodeoxycholic acid in chronic liver disease. Gut. 1991;32:1061–5.
35. Lotterer E, Bauer FE, Bircher J. Safety of ursodeoxycholic acid in chronic cholestasis. Hepatology. 1988;8:1416.
36. Batta AK, Salen G, Arora R et al. Effect of ursodeoxycholic acid on bile acid metabolism in primary biliary cirrhosis. Hepatology. 1989;10:414–19.
37. Hadziyannis SJ, Hadziyannis ES, Makris A. A randomized trial of ursodeoxycholic acid (UDCA) in primary biliary cirrhosis. Hepatology. 1989;10:580.
38. Matsuzaki Y, Tanaka N, Osuga T et al. Improvement of biliary enzyme levels and itching as a result of long-term administration of ursodeoxycholic acid in primary biliary cirrhosis. Am J Gastroenterol. 1990;85:105–13.
39. Perdigoto R, Wiesner RH. Progression of primary biliary cirrhosis with ursodeoxycholic acid therapy. Gastroenterology. 1992;102:1389–91.
40. Kehagioglou K. Effect of UDCA on the natural course of PBC. J Hepatol. 1991;13(2):S134.
41. Simko V, Michael S, Prego V. Effect of ursodeoxycholic acid (UDCA) in primary biliary cirrhosis (PBC): a meta-analysis (MA). Gastroenterology. 1993;104:A996.
42. O'Brien CB, Senior JR, Sternlieb JM et al. Ursodiol treatment of primary biliary cirrhosis. Gastroenterology. 1990;80:A617.
43. Oka H, Toda G, Ikeda Y et al. A multi-center double-blind controlled trial of ursodeoxycholic acid for primary biliary cirrhosis. Gastroenterol Jpn. 1991;25:774–80.
44. Battezzati PM, Podda M, Bianchi FB et al. Ursodeoxycholic acid for symptomatic primary biliary cirrhosis. Preliminary analysis of a double-blind multicenter trial. J Hepatol. 1993;17:332–8.
45. Osuga T, Tanaka N, Matsuzaki Y et al. Effect of ursodeoxycholic acid in chronic hepatitis and primary biliary cirrhosis. Dig Dis Sci. 1989;34(Suppl):49–51.
46. Ideo G, Bellati G, Bottelli R, Pedraglio E. Treatment of non-A–non-B chronic hepatitis with ursodeoxycholic acid: results from a prospective double blind controlled trial. In: Meeting Handbook, XI International Bile Acid Meeting (Poster Abstract No. 72), Freiburg, Germany: Falk symposium No. 58, 1990.
47. Podda M, Ghezzi C, Battezzati PM et al. Ursodeoxycholic acid, taurine, or a combination of the two for chronic hepatitis. Gastroenterology. 1990;98:1044–50.
48. Simko V, Michael S. Effect of ursodeoxycholic acid (UDCA) in chronic hepatitis (CH): a meta analysis (MA). Gastroenterology. 1993;104:A995.
49. Ohya T. Long-term administration of ursodeoxycholic acid in patients with chronic hepatitis. A comparison of the effect of two doses on liver function. Jpn Pharmacol Ther. 1985;13:271.
50. Puoti C, Pannullo A, Annovazzi G. Ursodeoxycholic acid and chronic hepatitis C infection. Lancet. 1993;341:1413–1414.
51. Plevris JN, Hayes PC, Bouchier AD. Ursodeoxycholic acid in the treatment of alcoholic liver disease. Eur J Gastroenterol Hepatol. 1991;3(9):653–6.
52. Kneppelhout JC, Mulder CJ, Van-Berge-Henegouwen GP et al. Ursodeoxycholic acid treatment in primary biliary cirrhosis with emphasis on late stage disease. Neth J Med. 1992;41:11–16.

29

S-Adenosyl-L-methionine (SAMe)-dependent nicotinamide methylation: a marker of hepatic damage

R. CUOMO, R. PUMPO, G. CAPUANO, G. SARNELLI and
G. BUDILLON

INTRODUCTION

Methylation reactions play an important role in human metabolism. Up to 85% of these reactions occur in the liver[1]. Methyl-deficient diets have been shown to induce liver cancer, and many carcinogenic substances can cause hypomethylation of DNA[2-7]. Methylation reactions are involved in the transformation of xenobiotics and of endogenous substances[8-11].

The primary biological methyl group donor is S-adenosyl-L-methionine (SAMe)[12,13]. The synthesis and liver concentration of SAMe, and many SAMe-dependent reactions may be deranged in experimental liver damage[14-17]. The activity of SAMe-synthetase is also reduced in human cirrhosis[18,19].

Nicotinamide (NAM), a vitamin used in the synthesis of hepatic nucleotides, is normally excreted in urine after methylation (Fig. 1) when administered in excess of body requirements[20,21]. The SAMe is also the co-substrate of NAM-methyltransferase.

The aim of this study was to use NAM to explore the efficiency of methylation reactions in human and experimental liver damage.

MATERIALS AND METHODS

Human study

Eleven healthy volunteers aged 25–60 years (six males) served as controls. Twenty patients aged 35–65 (14 males) with non-alcoholic cirrhosis attending our clinic entered the study. All patients had a biopsy-proven cirrhosis. According to Child's classification 12 subjects were class A and eight were class B. Child class C patients were excluded from the study to avoid

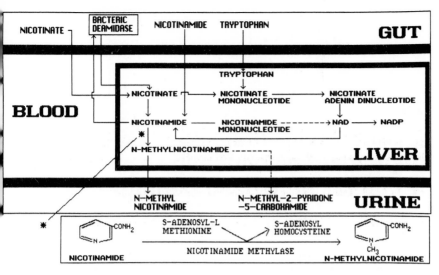

Fig. 1 Nicotinamide metabolic pathways

interference by ascites or impaired kidney function. All subjects and patients gave their informed consent to the study. All subjects and patients refrained from taking drugs or vitamin supplements in the 7 days prior to the study, and were on normal diets.

All subjects and patients were given an oral load of NAM (1.5 mg/kg body weight) after a 12-h fast. Controls and patients continued the fast for 5 h after oral load. Blood samples were taken at 0, 30, 60, 120 and 300 min. All serum samples were stored at $-20°C$ until analysis. Serum values of timed N-methylnicotinamide (NMN) concentration after an oral load of NAM were determined in each subject. The area between 0 and 300 min under the serum concentration vs time curve (AUC) was calculated using the trapezoidal rule.

Animal study

Twenty-four male Sprague-Dawley rats were used. The portal vein of each rat was cannulated and the liver was isolated and connected to a recirculating perfusion apparatus. The perfusion medium was a Krebs-Ringer bicarbonate buffer supplemented with 3% bovine serum albumin, 0.1% glucose and heparin 4 mg/ml. Metabolic stress was obtained by a pre-perfusion period of 10 min with saline alone rather than Krebs-Ringer medium immediately after the liver isolation.

Nicotinamide ($1.09\,\mu$mol/g of liver) with or without SAMe (1.0 mmol/l) was introduced in the perfusion medium 10 min after liver isolation. Medium samples (1 ml) were removed from the perfusion apparatus at 1, 3, 5, 10, 15 and 20 min to evaluate NMN concentration.

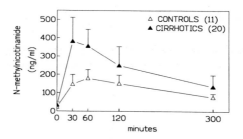

Fig. 2 Time-courses of NMN after NAM oral load (1.5 mg/kg body weight) (mean ± SD) in human healthy controls and patients with liver cirrhosis

Table 1 Serum N-methylnicotinamide after oral load of nicotinamide in controls and cirrhotic patients (Child A and B)

	Controls (11) (mean ± SD)	Cirrhotics (20) (mean ± SD)
ΔPeak (ng/ml)	168 ± 43	402 ± 95*
AUC (μg/ml × min)	36 ± 9	68 ± 18*

ΔPeak: difference between maximum and basal serum value of NMN; AUC: area under curve of NMN from 0 to 300 min; *$p < 0.01$ vs controls.

N-Methylnicotinamide assay

N-Methylnicotinamide was measured with a fluorimetric technique using an alkaline condensation reaction of NMN with methyl-ethylketone to form the fluorescent product[22,23]. In our experience the precision and accuracy of this method are greater than 90%.

The data for each group are expressed as mean ± SD. Statistical analysis was performed with the Mann–Whitney test.

RESULTS

Results in humans

The time-courses of NMN after NAM loads in controls and cirrhotic patients are reported in Fig. 2. Data on NMN serum kinetics are shown in Table 1. NMN production is significantly higher in cirrhotic patients than in controls ($p < 0.01$).

Results in rat

The results obtained in the animal study are shown in Figs. 3 and 4. Basal production of NMN by normal rat liver increases 3.5 and 4.5 times with NAM and NAM ± SAMe, respectively. The production of NMN in basal conditions and with NAM ± SAMe is significantly higher in the stressed

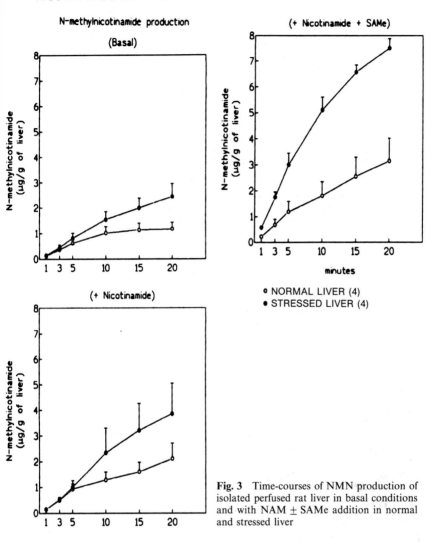

Fig. 3 Time-courses of NMN production of isolated perfused rat liver in basal conditions and with NAM ± SAMe addition in normal and stressed liver

than in the control liver ($p < 0.01$). The addition of SAMe to the perfusion medium significantly enhanced NMN production in stressed rat liver only ($p < 0.01$).

DISCUSSION

Despite evidence of a defective methylation of other endogenous and exogenous substances, our study shows that methylation of NAM is increased in human cirrhosis after oral load of the vitamin[18,24].

In humans the methylation of NAM could represent a dissipative pathway by which to eliminate this substance when administered in excess of body

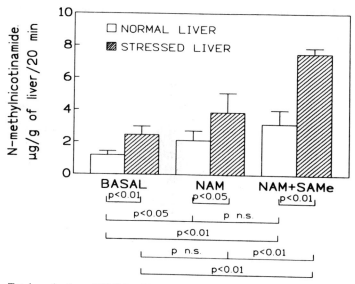

Fig. 4 Total production of NMN at 20 min perfusion of isolated rat liver in basal conditions and with NAM ± SAMe addition in normal and stressed liver

requirements. NAM methylation could be higher in cirrhotics than in healthy subjects because of the energy crisis of liver cells[25] that prevents the anabolic utilization of NAM for the synthesis of pyridine nucleotides. Finally, NAM methylation could use the available SAMe to the detriment of other metabolic pathways.

To verify these hypotheses we selected the experimental model of *in vitro* rat liver perfusion, with or without energy deficiency induced by metabolic stress (see Methods).

Significant increases of NMN production were observed in stressed rat liver with respect to the control. The addition of SAMe to the perfusion medium did not modify NAM methylation in the control liver, but further enhanced NAM methylation in the stressed liver. Therefore, the stress appears to induce a relative defect of SAMe availability.

In conclusion, the increase of NMN production observed in cirrhotics may be interpreted as a consequence of the energy crisis of the hepatic cell whereby it is unable to utilize efficiently NAM for pyridine nucleotide synthesis. Liver SAMe is preferably expended in the dissipative metabolism of NAM, and is thus unavailable for other metabolic requirements. Therefore, SAMe can be rationally proposed as adjuvant therapy in cirrhotic patients.

Acknowledgement

This study was supported by a grant from Ministero dell'Università e della Ricerca Scientifica (60%–1991).

References

1. Mudd SH, Poole JR. Labile methyl balances for normal humans on various dietary regimens. Metabolism. 1975;24:721–35.
2. Razin A, Riggs AD. DNA methylation and gene function. Science. 1980;218:604–10.
3. Felsenfeld G, McGee JD. Methylation and gene control. Nature. 1982;296:602–3.
4. Doerfler W. DNA methylation and gene activity. Annu Rev Biochem. 1983;52:93–124.
5. Boehm TL, Drahovsky D. Alterations of enzymatic methylation of DNA cytosines by chemical carcinogens: a mechanism involved in the initiation of carcinogenesis. J Natl Cancer Inst. 1983;71:429–33.
6. Aiba N, Nambu S, Inoue K et al. Hypomethylation of the c-myc oncogene in liver cirrhosis and chronic hepatitis. Gastroenterol Jpn. 1989;24(3):270–6.
7. Dietary methyl groups and cancer – Review article. Nutr Rev. 1986;44(8):278–80.
8. Cantoni GL. Biological methylation: selected aspects. Annu Rev Biochem. 1975;44:435–51.
9. Weisger RA, Jakoby WS. S-methylation: Thiol S-methyl-transferase. In: Jakoby WS, ed. Enzymatic basis of detoxication, Vol. II. San Diego, CA: Academic Press; 1980:131–40.
10. McFadden PN, Clarke S. Conversion of isoaspartyl peptides to normal peptides: implications for the cellular repair of damaged proteins. Proc Natl Acad Sci USA. 1987;48:2595–9.
11. Hirata F, Axelrod J. Phospholipid methylation and biological signal transmission. Science. 1980;209:1082–90.
12. Stramentinoli G. Pharmacological aspects of S-adenosyl-L-methionine: pharmacokinetics and pharmacodynamics. Am J Med. 1987;83:35–42.
13. Cantoni GL. Biological methylation: selected aspects. Annu Rev Biochem. 1975;44:435–51.
14. Lieber CS, Casini A, De Carli LM et al. S-Adenosyl-L-methionine attenuates alcohol-induced liver injury in the baboon. Hepatology. 1990;11:165–72.
15. Feo F, Pascale R, Garcea R et al. Effect of the variations in S-adenosyl-L-methionine liver content on fat accumulation and ethanol metabolism in ethanol-intoxicated rats. Toxicol Appl Pharmacol. 1986;83:331–41.
16. Cabrero C, Martin-Duce A, Ortiz P et al. Specific loss of the high-molecular-weight form of S-adenosyl-L-methionine synthetase in human liver cirrhosis. Hepatology. 1988;8:1530–4.
17. Stramentinoli G, Gulano M, Ideo G. Protective role of S-adenosyl-L-methionine on liver injury induced by D-galactosamine in rats. Biochem Pharmacol. 1978;27:1431–3.
18. Duce AM, Ortiz P, Cabrero C et al. S-Adenosyl-L-methionine synthetase and phospholipid methyltransferase are inhibited in human liver cirrhosis. Hepatology. 1988;8(1):65–8.
19. Gaull GE, Rassin DK, Solomon GE et al. Biochemical observations on so-called hereditary tyrosinemia. Pediatr Res. 1970;4:337–44.
20. Hankes LV. Nicotinic acid and nicotinamide. In: Tannenbaum SR, Walstra P, editors. Handbook of vitamins. New Jersey: L.J. Machlin; 1984:329–77.
21. Jenkes BH, McKee WR, Swendseid ME et al. Methylation main derivatives in plasma and urine after an oral dose of nicotinamide given to subject fed a low methionine diet. Am J Clin Nutr. 1987;46:496–502.
22. Clark BR. Fluorimetric quantitation of picomole amounts of N-methylnicotinamide and nicotinamide in serum. Methods Enzymol. 1980;66:5–8.
23. Clark BR, Halfem RM, Smith RA. A fluorimetric method for quantitation in the picomole range of methylnicotinamide and nicotinamide in serum. Anal Biochem. 1975;68:54–61.
24. Geubel AP, Mairlot MC, Buchet JP et al. Abnormal methylation capacity in human liver cirrhosis. Int J Clin Pharmacol Res. 1988;VIII(2):117–22.
25. Budillon G, Citarella C, Loguercio C et al. Hyperuricemia induced by fructose load in liver cirrhosis. Ital J Gastroenterol. 1992;24:373–7.

30
Effects of ademetionine (SAMe) and UDCA on bile acid metabolism and bile acid pool size in primary biliary cirrhosis

E. RODA, A. CIPOLLA, N. VILLANOVA, G. MAZZELLA, C. CERRÈ, C. POLIMENI and A. RODA

INTRODUCTION

Primary biliary cirrhosis (PBC) is a chronic progressive non-suppurative cholangiolytic cholestatic disorder that primarily affects middle-aged women. This disorder involves progressive destruction of the medium-sized interlobular bile ducts. No medical therapy has yet been shown to prolong survival; nevertheless this remains a major long-term objective.

The administration of ursodeoxycholic acid (UDCA), a bile acid used as a cholesterol gallstone dissolving agent, improves liver function test in patients with cholestatic liver diseases, such as PBC[1-3].

The mechanism by which UDCA improves liver function tests is still debated. UDCA reduces the concentration in bile of potentially hepatotoxic endogenous bile acids since these are replaced by the more hydrophilic and less detergent UDCA[4]. We have recently hypothesized that UDCA administration replaces endogenous bile acids in the enterohepatic circulation by increasing bile acid fractional turnover rate[3].

Growing clinical evidence has been gathered that indicates the utility of S-adenosyl-L-methionine administration (SAMe) as a potential therapeutic agent in patients with cholestasis[5,6].

The anticholestatic effect of SAMe has been related to the ability of the compound to restore hepatocyte membrane fluidity (through both methylation of membrane phospholipids and restoration of Na^+,K^+-ATPase activity) and to increase the availability of sulphated compounds through the trans-sulphuration pathway[7].

The aim of this study was to evaluate the effects of UDCA and of SAMe at high doses (given separately and then in combination) on biliary lipid metabolism in patients with PBC.

METHODS

Patients

The study was carried out in five patients (one male, four female, age 35–71 years), for whom the diagnosis of PBC (stage II–III) was histologically confirmed. All patients had increased levels of transaminases, alkaline phosphatases γ-glutamyltranspeptidases and had a positive antimitochondrial test. All patients gave written informed consent to the study which was performed in conformance with the 1975 Declaration of Helsinki.

Experimental design

Each patient received in a single-blind cross-over design SAMe (1600 mg/day p.o.), UDCA (10 mg/kg per day) and then UDCA + SAMe at the same dosages for 4 weeks. The sequence SAMe, UDCA and UDCA + SAMe was assigned using a random table.

The following parameters were evaluated before and after each treatment: serum liver function tests, cholesterol saturation index and biliary lipid percentage molar in bile; biliary bile acid pattern, biliary lipid outputs and bile acid pool size.

Biliary lipids

Gallbladder bile was obtained from each patient by intravenous administration of 4 μg of cerulein (Farmitalia, SpA, Milan, Italy) before biliary lipid secretion studies in order to induce a valid gallbladder contraction. From the samples obtained, 1 ml of dark duodenal juice was diluted with isopropyl alcohol, 1 ml was stored at $-20°C$, and the remainder was reinfused.

Biliary lipid secretion rate

Biliary lipid secretion rate was evaluated by the intestinal perfusional technique according to the method of Grundy and Metzger[8].

A triple-lumen tube was positioned with two proximal outlets adjacent to the ampulla of Vater and the third 10 cm distally. A liquid formula containing 43% of calories as fat, 15% as protein and 42% as carbohydrates was infused by a persistaltic pump at a rate of 2.6 ml/min. The caloric infusion rate was 3.4 cal/min. PEG 4000 was used as a dilution marker. This type of formula and these infusion rates were chosen in order to obtain a steady and valid gallbladder contraction throughout the study. After the first 4 h, which were allowed for stabilization of hepatic bile secretion, hourly samples were taken for 6 consecutive hours. Cholesterol[9], bile acids[10], and phospholipids[11] were measured by enzymatic colorimetric methods. PEG 4000 was measured according to the Hyden method[12] after precipitation of proteins and addition of a 33% solution of trichloroacetic acid. The rate of cholesterol secretion

Table 1 Serum liver function tests before and during treatment

	ALT	AST	Alk Ph	γ-GT	Bilirubin	Cholesterol-LDL
Before	109 ± 48	110 ± 53	531 ± 251	393 ± 244	2.1 ± 2.0	203 ± 40
SAMe	106 ± 59	102 ± 39	566 ± 288	252 ± 130**	1.7 ± 1.1	187 ± 42
UDCA	82 ± 45*	77 ± 44*	378 ± 210*	105 ± 51*	2.1 ± 1.9	178 ± 33**
UDCA + SAMe	79 ± 41*	71 ± 45*	368 ± 180*	82 ± 42*	1.9 ± 1.8	180 ± 42

*vs Before and vs SAMe $p < 0.05$, **vs Before $p < 0.01$.

was calculated taking into account the small amount of cholesterol measured into the infusate by the method of Abell et al.[13]. The cholesterol concentration in the infusate was always lower than that measured in hourly duodenal aspirates. The hourly outputs of biliary lipids were calculated according to the classic equation of Grundy and Metzger[8].

Total bile acid pool size was measured simultaneously with biliary outputs, as described by others[14]. The biliary bile acid pattern was determined by reverse-phase high-performance liquid chromatography (HPLC) according to the method of Van Berge Henegouwen[15], with minor modifications.

STATISTICAL ANALYSIS

The results are expressed as means ± SE. Statistical differences between groups were calculated using Student's t-test.

RESULTS

After 4 weeks of UDCA treatment an improvement of liver function tests was observed in all five patients studied, who also reported the improvement of pruritus and fatigue (Table 1). SAMe determined a significant reduction of γ-GT but not of transaminases and alkaline phosphatases (Table 1). The association of UDCA + SAMe improved all liver function tests, with a slight further reduction of γ-GT with respect to UDCA alone (Table 1).

Cholesterol saturation index (CSI) and percentage molar of cholesterol in bile were decreased after UDCA administration and after UDCA + SAMe, but not after SAMe alone (CSI: 1.28 ± 0.07 before, 1.10 ± 0.03 after UDCA, 1.17 ± 0.04 after SAMe, 1.11 ± 0.03 after SAMe + UDCA, before vs UDCA and vs UDCA + SAMe $p < 0.05$; cholesterol percentage molar: 7.2 ± 0.25 before, 4.7 ± 0.07 UDCA, 7.2 ± 0.26 SAMe, 4.6 ± 0.15 SAMe + UDCA, before vs UDCA, before vs SAMe + UDCA, $p < 0.05$) (Table 2).

The amount of primary bile acids (Table 3), cholic (CA) and chenodeoxycholic acid (CDCA) significantly decreased after UDCA and after UDCA + SAMe administration (CA percentage molar; 54.4 ± 5.7 before, 26.7 ± 5.4 UDCA, 26.1 ± 1.6 UDCA + SAMe, $p < 0.05$; CDCA percentage molar: 32.6 ± 2.1 before, 26.3 ± 1.2 UDCA, 25.1 ± 0.7 UDCA + SAMe, $p < 0.05$); the amount of UDCA increased in both treatments (UDCA percentage molar: 2.6 ± 1.5 before, 37.2 ± 1.7 UDCA, 40 ± 2 UDCA + SAMe, $p < 0.05$). UDCA + SAMe therapy slightly decreased deoxycholic acid (DCA) percent-

Table 2 Biliary lipid composition and cholesterol saturation index

Patients	Cholesterol (percentage molar)				Bile acids (percentage molar)				Phospholipids (percentage molar)				Saturation index (Carey)			
	B	U	S	S+U	B	U	S	S+U	B	U	S	S+U	B	U	S	S+U
1	6.5	4.4	6.3	4.4	76.1	78.5	75.1	78.5	17.4	17.1	18.5	17.1	1.12	1.01	1.04	1.05
2	7.4	4.8	7.2	4.7	78.7	78.0	73.5	78.2	13.9	17.2	19.3	17.1	1.48	1.09	1.15	1.12
3	8.0	4.7	7.8	5.0	74.3	80.3	73.8	78.5	17.7	15.0	18.4	16.2	1.34	1.21	1.27	1.23
4	7.2	4.8	7.2	4.7	77.1	78.0	72.0	77.4	15.7	17.2	19.7	17.9	1.36	1.09	1.13	1.08
5	6.9	4.6	7.7	4.1	73.1	77.5	74.3	80.2	20.0	17.9	17.9	15.7	1.09	1.08	1.28	1.07
Mean	7.2	4.7	7.2	4.6	75.8	78.5	73.7	78.6	16.9	16.9	18.8	16.9	1.28	1.10	1.17	1.11
± SE	0.25	0.07	0.26	0.15	0.99	0.49	0.51	0.46	1.02	0.49	0.32	0.36	0.07	0.03	0.04	0.03

B: Before; S: SAMe (1600 mg/day); U: UDCA (10 mg/kg per day); S + U: SAMe (1600 mg/day) + UDCA (10 mg/kg per day)
Cholesterol and bile acids: B vs U & S + U, U vs S, S vs S + U, S + U $p < 0.05$; Saturation index: B vs U and vs S + U $p < 0.05$

Table 3 Bile acid pool composition (percentage molar; mean $\pm$ SE)

	CA	CDCA	DCA	LCA	UDCA
Before	54.4 $\pm$ 5.7	32.6 $\pm$ 2.1	8.4 $\pm$ 2.7	2.0 $\pm$ 0.5	2.6 $\pm$ 1.5
UDCA	26.7 $\pm$ 5.4*	26.3 $\pm$ 1.2*	7.3 $\pm$ 5.5	2.5 $\pm$ 0.6	37.2 $\pm$ 1.7*
SAMe	51.0 $\pm$ 4.2	36.7 $\pm$ 3.2	7.3 $\pm$ 3.0	2.4 $\pm$ 0.9	2.6 $\pm$ 1.8
UDCA + SAMe	26.1 $\pm$ 1.6*	25.1 $\pm$ 0.7*	6.0 $\pm$ 0.4	2.8 $\pm$ 1.1	40.0 $\pm$ 2.0*

LCA: lithocholic acid; DCA: deoxycholic acid; CDCA: chenodeoxycholic acid; UDCA: urso-deoxycholic acid; CA: cholic acid
*$p < 0.05$ vs Before and vs SAMe

age molar when compared to basal values and to UDCA and SAMe given separately, this was, however, not statistically significant (DCA percentage molar: 8.4 $\pm$ 2.7 basal, 7.3 $\pm$ 5.5 UDCA, 7.3 $\pm$ 3 SAMe, 6.0 $\pm$ 0.4 UDCA + SAMe, p = n.s.).

Bile acid secretion (Table 4) increased during UDCA and UDCA + SAMe but was virtually unaffected by SAMe alone (bile acid secretion: 1066 $\pm$ 105 before, 1524 $\pm$ 86 UDCA, 1579 $\pm$ 111 UDCA + SAMe, $p < 0.05$, 970 $\pm$ 118 SAMe, p = n.s.).

CA pool size (Table 5) decreased after UDCA, remained unchanged both after SAMe and after UDCA + SAMe (CA pool size: 2.2 $\pm$ 0.11 before, 1.6 $\pm$ 0.09 UDCA, $p < 0.05$; 2.1 $\pm$ 0.08 SAMe, 2.3 $\pm$ 0.13 SAMe + UDCA, UDCA vs SAMe and vs UDCA + SAMe, $p < 0.05$).

CA turnover rate (Table 5) increased after UDCA and after UDCA + SAMe versus basal. It was unchanged after SAMe alone (CA turnover; 0.28 $\pm$ 0.04 basal, 0.83 $\pm$ 0.08 UDCA, 0.66 $\pm$ 0.04 UDCA + SAMe, $p < 0.05$; 0.32 $\pm$ 0.05 SAMe, p = n.s.).

CA synthesis (Table 5) increased after UDCA treatment; and a non-significant increase of CA synthesis was observed after UDCA + SAMe when compared to UDCA alone (CA synthesis: 0.62 $\pm$ 0.12 before, 1.31 $\pm$ 0.1 UDCA, 0.67 $\pm$ 0.11 SAMe, 1.57 $\pm$ 0.17; before vs UDCA and UDCA + SAMe, $p < 0.05$; UDCA vs SAMe, $p < 0.05$; SAMe vs UDCA + SAMe, $p < 0.05$).

DISCUSSION

This study shows that SAMe given orally to patients with PBC at the dosage of 1600 mg/day improves γ-GT. UDCA administration confirmed our previous results on LFT and bile acid metabolism in PBC patients[2,3]. Particularly, we observed a significant improvement in LFT and a reduced concentration in bile of primary bile acids CA and CDCA, because these are replaced by the more hydrophilic and less detergent UDCA.

CA pool size decreased, whereas fractional turnover rate and synthesis were increased after UDCA treatment.

A moderate decrease of DCA percentage molar was observed after UDCA administration. This result partially differs from our previous findings. The difference may be due to the characteristics of the patient groups. In this study the histological grading is different (four patients were stage III, only

Table 4 Biliary lipid secretion

Patients	Cholesterol (μmol/h)				Bile acids (μmol/h)				Phospholipids (μmol/h)			
	B	U	S	S + U	B	U	S	S + U	B	U	S	S + U
1	120	90	120	90	1400	1610	1420	1610	320	350	350	350
2	80	84	78	85	850	1365	800	1415	150	300	210	310
3	90	83	82	85	840	1275	780	1250	200	230	195	240
4	110	105	100	110	1180	1720	980	1780	249	380	300	410
5	100	98	90	95	1060	1650	870	1840	290	380	210	360
Mean	100	92	94	93	1066	1524	970	1579	242	328	253	334
± SE	7	4	8	5	105	86	118	111	30	29	31	28

B: Before; S: SAMe (1600 mg/day); U: UDCA (10 mg/kg per day); S + U: SAMe (1600 mg/day) + UDCA (10 mg/kg per day)
Bile acids: B vs U & S + U, U vs S, S vs S + U $p < 0.01$

Table 5 Cholic acid kinetics

Patients	Pool (mmol)				Turnover (day^{-1})				Synthesis (mmol/day)			
	B	U	S	S + U	B	U	S	S + U	B	U	S	S + U
1	1.9	1.5	1.9	2.1	0.22	1.05	0.47	0.70	0.42	1.57	0.89	1.52
2	2.5	1.8	2.3	2.6	0.38	0.87	0.37	0.69	0.95	1.56	0.85	1.87
3	2.0	1.3	2.0	1.9	0.21	0.91	0.18	0.50	0.42	1.18	0.36	0.95
4	2.4	1.8	2.2	2.5	0.37	0.61	0.35	0.72	0.89	1.09	0.77	1.81
5	2.2	1.6	2.3	2.4	0.20	0.73	0.21	0.70	0.44	1.16	0.48	1.68
Mean	2.2	1.6	2.1	2.3	0.28	0.83	0.32	0.66	0.62	1.31	0.67	1.57
± SE	0.11	0.09	0.08	0.13	0.04	0.08	0.05	0.04	0.12	0.10	0.11	0.17

B: Before; S: SAMe (1600 mg/day); U: UDCA (10 mg/kg per day); S + U: SAMe (1600 mg/day) + UDCA (10 mg/kg per day)
Pool: B vs U, U vs S & S + U $p < 0.01$; turnover: B vs U & S + U, U vs S, S vs S + U $p < 0.01$; synthesis: B vs U & S + U, U vs S, S vs S + U $p < 0.01$

one in stage II), three patients were overweight (BMI > 26), and basal DCA percentage molar was lower than previous study.

The association therapy UDCA + SAMe improved LFT, with a slight further reduction of γ-GT when compared to UDCA treatment alone.

A peculiar effect of UDCA + SAMe administration seems to be an increase of CA pool size and a moderate increase in CA synthesis with respect to UDCA alone. The mechanism of this effect is unknown. SAMe restores liver membrane fluidity in experimental models of intrahepatic cholestasis[16] and increases the bioavailability of sulphates[17] and glutathione[18]; these mechanisms may have a synergic effect with UDCA in CA metabolism and in the anticholestatic activity of the two molecules.

References

1. Poupon R, Chretien Y, Poupon RE et al. Is ursodeoxycholic acid an effective treatment for primary biliary cirrhosis? Lancet. 1987;1:834–6.
2. Roda E, Mazzella G, Bazzoli F et al. Effect of ursodeoxycholic acid administration on biliary lipid secretion in primary biliary cirrhosis. Dig Dis Sci. 1989;34(12):52S–58S.
3. Mazzella G, Parini P, Bazzoli F et al. UDCA administration on bile acid metabolism in patients with early stages of primary biliary cirrhosis. Dig Dis Sci. 1993;38(5):896–902.
4. Scholmerich J, Becher MS, Schmidt KH. Influence of hydroxylation and conjugation of bile salts on their membrane damaging properties – studies on isolated hepatocyte and lipid membrane vesicles. Hepatology. 1984;4:661–6.
5. Frezza M, Di Padova C and the Italian Study Group for SAMe in liver disease. Multicenter placebo controlled clinical trial of intravenous and oral S-adenosyl-L-methionine (SAMe) in cholestatic patients with liver disease. Hepatology. 1987;7:1105.
6. Frezza M, Surrenti C, Manzillo G et al. Oral SAMe in the symptomatic treatment of intrahepatic cholestasis. Gastroenterology. 1990;99:211–15.
7. Almasio P, Bortolini M, Pagliari L et al. Role of SAMe in the treatment of intrahepatic cholestasis. Drug. 1990;40(Suppl. 3):111–23.
8. Grundy SM, Metzger AL. A physiological method for estimation of hepatic secretion of biliary lipids in man. Gastroenterology. 1972;62:1200–17.
9. Roda A, Festi D, Sama C et al. Enzymatic determination of cholesterol in bile. Clin Chim Acta. 1975;64:377–81.
10. Fausa O, Skallhegg BA. Quantitative determination of bile acids and their conjugates using thin layer chromatography and a purified 3 alpha-hydroxysteroid-dehydrogenase. Scand J Gastroenterol. 1974;9:249–54.
11. Roda A, Festi D, Sama C et al. Enzymatic determination of phospholipids in bile. Lab J Res Med. 1975;2:119–22.
12. Hyden S. A turbidimetric method for determination of high polyethylene glycols in biological materials. Annu R Agric Coll Sved. 1955;22:139–49.
13. Abell LL, Levi BB, Brodie BB. Cholesterol in serum. In: Saligson D, editor. Standard methods of clinical chemistry, Vol. 2. New York: Academic Press; 1958:26–33.
14. Grundy SM. Effects of polyunsaturated fats on lipid metabolism in patients with hypertri-gliceridemia. J Clin Invest. 1975;55:269–82.
15. Van Berge-Henegouwen GP, Ruben A, Brandt K-H. Quantitative analysis of bile acids in serum and bile using gas–liquid chromatography. Chim Clin Acta. 1973;54:249–61.
16. Fricker G, Landmann L, Meier PJ. Ethynylestradiol (EE) induced structural and functional alterations of rat liver plasma membranes and their reversal by SAMe in vitro. Hepatology. 1988;8:122.
17. Pisi E, Marchesini G. Mechanisms and consequences of the impaired transsulfuration pathway in liver disease. Part II. Clinical consequences and potential for pharmacological intervention in cirrhosis. Drugs. 1990;40(Suppl. 3):65–72.
18. Vendemiale G, Altomare E, Trizio T et al. Effects of oral SAMe on hepatic glutathione in patients with liver disease. Scand J Gastroenterol. 1989;24:407–15.

31
Clinical use of S-adenosylmethionine and ursodeoxycholic acid in chronic cholestatic and inflammatory liver diseases

G. P. BRAY

INTRODUCTION

Many forms of treatment have been found to be unsuccessful in patients with the chronic cholestatic liver diseases primary biliary cirrhosis (PBC) and primary sclerosing cholangitis (PSC). Although liver transplantation has been shown to improve survival in patients with more advanced liver dysfunction, there is an urgent need for effective forms of treatment for those with milder disease to extend life and/or delay the time at which transplantation is required.

S-adenosylmethionine (SAMe) and ursodeoxycholic acid (UDCA) are promising therapeutic agents in this regard as they act quite differently from many of those which have been tested in the past (see Table 1). As PBC and PSC may be autoimmune in aetiology, the main group of agents assessed have been immunomodulators – these include prednisolone, azathioprine, chlorambucil and more recently cyclosporine and methotrexate. Although there have been some encouraging reports with this approach (particularly cyclosporine in PBC), results have generally been disappointing. Colchicine

Table 1 Classes of drugs used in the treatment of primary biliary cirrhosis

Disease-modifying	
Immunomodulatory	
Cupriuretic	Penicillamine
Antifibrotic	Colchicine, Hoe-077
Anticholestatic	UDCA, SAMe
Symptomatic	
Complications	

(acting as an antifibrotic) and penicillamine (a cupriuretic) are also largely ineffective.

Although with different pharmacological actions (as discussed elsewhere in this symposium), SAMe and UDCA are both anticholestatic with excellent toxicity profiles and few adverse effects. In this chapter the increasing experience with UDCA and SAMe in adults with chronic cholestatic and inflammatory liver diseases will be described, and the pharmacological mechanisms by which UDCA and SAMe may work will be discussed. Possible combined use of the two agents will also be considered as an avenue for future investigation.

URSODEOXYCHOLIC ACID IN CHRONIC LIVER DISEASE

Primary biliary cirrhosis

Primary biliary cirrhosis (PBC) is a cholestatic liver disease that predominantly affects middle-aged females and is the commonest indication for liver transplantation in most centres. Since the first descriptions of PBC[1,2], the discovery of effective treatment has been a major goal of research into the condition, although the exact aetiology of the disease remains uncertain. There is considerable evidence that autoimmune processes are involved in the aetiology of PBC[3], particularly in the early stages of the disease leading to granulomata and inflammation around small intrahepatic bile ducts. The principal features suggesting an autoimmune aetiology for PBC are the presence of: (1) antimitochondrial antibodies in over 95% of patients, (2) lymphocytic infiltrates around damaged bile ducts, (3) an association with HLA-DRw8 and C4B2[4,5] and (4) expression of MHC class II antigens on bile duct epithelium[6,7].

Subsequently fibrosis, increasing cholestasis and liver failure occur and eventually the patient will die or need liver transplantation. Not only is the clinical course of PBC before symptom development unpredictable, the autoimmune, fibrotic and cholestatic phases of PBC are not distinct. In fact many patients remain asymptomatic indefinitely or have only pruritus or fatigue without developing marked liver dysfunction.

Anticholestatic drugs such as UDCA and SAMe may act by reducing the harmful effects of cholestasis; there is increasing evidence that UDCA is an immunomodulator and that SAMe may be antifibrotic. In this way pharmacological effects may be exerted on each of the pathogenic processes involved in disease progression. To show that either UDCA or SAMe can delay disease progression, it is necessary to demonstrate either prolongation of survival, delay in the time at which transplantation becomes necessary or, at least, a reduction in histological deterioration. Surrogate markers of prognosis, such as serum bilirubin or the Mayo risk score[8], are useful, but may be inappropriate when a drug such as UDCA is being taken which affects the serum bilirubin. An improvement in symptoms, such as pruritus, is helpful for the patient but rarely correlates with an effect on disease progression.

Table 2 Randomized, double-blind placebo-controlled trials of ursodeoxycholic acid in primary biliary cirrhosis

			Effect on				
	n	Daily dose	Symptoms	Biliary enzymes	Bilirubin	Histology	Survival or transplant
Leuschner (1989)[10]	20	10 mg/kg	?	Yes	No*	?	—
Oka (1991)[11]	45	600 mg	Yes	Yes	No	—	—
Poupon (1991)[12]	146	13–15 mg/kg	?	Yes	Yes	Yes	—

*Mainly stage I and II disease

Evidence for a beneficial effect of UDCA in primary biliary cirrhosis

There have been numerous studies of the use of UDCA in PBC but very few randomized, placebo-controlled, double-blind trials which have been published in full. These are essential for evaluating a drug such as UDCA in PBC in which the clinical response is variable[9].

The results of the three randomized, placebo-controlled, double-blind trials which have been published in full are presented in Table 2[10-12]. Many other studies have confirmed the improvements in liver function and cholestasis seen in these trials, but it is less clear whether UDCA has an effect on either histology or survival. In the largest of the three studies (146 patients), Poupon et al.[12] found a significant improvement in mean histological score after 2 years treatment, as well as fewer treatment failures (defined as either (1) a doubling of the serum bilirubin to more than $70\,\mu$mol/l or a value of $200\,\mu$mol/l on two consecutive occasions; (2) a major complication such as a variceal bleed or (3) an adverse effect). Patients treated with UDCA had significantly fewer treatment failures than those in the placebo group (6 v 13, $p < 0.01$). These encouraging results are difficult to interpret as serum bilirubin is only a surrogate marker for survival, and the question remains as to whether UDCA prolongs life. It seems clear that UDCA does reduce biochemical features of cholestasis and possibly symptoms of PBC. However, we must wait for full publication of the other large studies being completed. A meta-analysis of these may also help to assess the efficacy of UDCA.

Pharmacological effects of UDCA in primary biliary cirrhosis

How does UDCA reduce cholestasis in patients with PBC? Various mechanisms have been proposed for the beneficial effects of UDCA. These include:

1. reduction in ileal absorption of toxic bile acids[13];
2. inhibition of secretion of toxic, hydrophobic bile acids into bile[14,15] with an increase in hydrophilicity;
3. promotion of bile flow (hypercholeresis);
4. alteration in the effects of toxic bile acids; and
5. stabilizing liver cell membranes against disruption by toxic bile acids (a form of cytoprotection)[16,17].

As well as aggravating cholestasis, toxic bile acids such as chenodeoxycholic

Table 3   Drugs with immunomodulatory activity used in primary
biliary cirrhosis

Mainly immunomodulatory	
Prednisolone	
Azathioprine	
Chlorambucil	
Cyclosporine	
Methotrexate	
Immunomodulatory effects also present	
Penicillamine	cupriuretic
Colchicine	antifibrotic
Ursodeoxycholic acid	

acid may impair cell-mediated immunity within the liver. UDCA may
therefore also act as an immunomodulator – hepatocellular and biliary
expression of both class I and II HLA antigens in PBC are reduced by
UDCA[18,19]. As class I expression, in particular, may be related to cholestasis,
its suppression may be secondary to the anticholestatic effects of UDCA.
Although the immunomodulatory effects of UDCA may be important, it is
unlikely that this is the main way that it is working in view of the relative
lack of efficacy of the other immunomodulatory drugs used in PBC (see
Table 3). The observation that UDCA can reduce cholestasis within 2–3
months of commencement is also inconsistent with experience with other
immunomodulatory drugs in PBC.

   In conclusion, the exact mechanisms of action of UDCA in PBC (and
other liver diseases) remain unclear, but increasing evidence suggests that it
may exert its effects by protecting liver cells from the effects of toxic bile
acids and by an effect on the immune system, perhaps also related to a
reduction in bile acid toxicity within the liver.

Clinical use of UDCA in primary biliary cirrhosis

How should the results of the clinical trials of UDCA affect management of
patients with PBC? The large European multicentre study of cyclosporine
treatment in PBC recently published[20] suggested that cyclosporine prolonged
the time from entry into the trial to death or transplantation (Cox analysis:
50–60% increase, $p < 0.05$) and resulted in significantly fewer liver-related
deaths than in the placebo group. The rise in serum bilirubin was also slower
in those patients given cyclosporine and histology tended to change less.
Cyclosporine also had beneficial effects on serum bilirubin and biliary
enzymes. The possible benefits of cyclosporine need to be balanced against
a 9% incidence of nephrotoxicity (serum creatinine $> 150\,\mu$mol/l) and 11%
who developed hypertension. There has also been interest in low-dose pulsed
methotrexate therapy in PBC[21], but there are insufficient controlled data to
assess its benefits in PBC at present. There are, however, significant worries
about its toxic effects on both the liver and bone marrow.

   There is no doubt that the safety profile of UDCA is preferable to that of
either cyclosporine or methotrexate. All these agents have been suggested to
be most helpful early in the natural history of the disease. In more advanced

disease (when jaundice is increasing and stage IV disease is present) neither cyclosporine nor methotrexate is likely to be of any help, as all the immunological damage has been done. Even at this stage of the disease, UDCA may still exert a beneficial anticholestatic effect. Ultimately the risk/benefit ratio needs to be assessed in individual patients before deciding which agent to choose, if any. In patients with advanced disease who are unsuitable for transplantation, UDCA seems to be the best option available. It should be remembered that, in those with advanced disease, liver transplantation can drastically improve their prognosis and quality of life to a degree that drug therapy has so far been unable to match.

The use of combinations of UDCA with immunomodulators such as cyclosporine or methotrexate is worthy of future study.

Primary sclerosing cholangitis

Whereas PBC is a disease of small intrahepatic bile ductules, primary sclerosing cholangitis (PSC) affects both intra- and extrahepatic ducts leading to fibrosis, stricturing and ultimately liver failure[22]. PSC is diagnosed in the presence of compatible cholangiographic and liver histological features. Although progress has recently been made in determining the prognosis of individual patients with PSC[23], liver transplantation remains the most successful therapeutic option for those with advanced disease. Drug therapies are clearly needed for patients with early disease in order to slow disease progression and delay the time at which transplantation becomes necessary.

Although UDCA is the most promising agent so far evaluated in PSC, there are few controlled studies published of its use in this condition. In 15 patients treated with 750–1250 mg/day of UDCA for 6 months, Chazouilleres et al.[24] reported improvements in both symptoms and serum levels of biliary enzymes. O'Brien et al.[25] performed a 30-month open study of 10 mg/kg per day in 12 patients with PSC (3 months pretreatment, six on UDCA, three after withdrawal and 18 back on UDCA). Treatment with UDCA resulted in a significant fall in serum cholesterol, bilirubin, biliary enzymes and transaminases. Symptoms of pruritus and fatigue were also thought to have improved with UDCA.

In the only double-blind study so far published in full, Beuers et al.[26] randomized 14 patients with PSC to either 13–15 mg/kg per day of UDCA or placebo for 1 year. In patients who received UDCA there was a significant reduction in serum bilirubin, biliary enzymes and transaminases compared to the placebo group. Changes in serum levels of hydrophobic bile acids did not reach statistical significance, but there did seem to be an improvement in histological features.

These results suggest that UDCA has a beneficial effect on biochemical features of PSC but larger placebo-controlled, double-blind, randomized trials are needed as the degree of improvement with UDCA is variable. The pharmacological actions of UDCA in PSC are likely to be similar to those thought to be important in PBC. Although not a cure for PSC, UDCA is safe and associated with few side-effects. Diarrhoea does not seem to be especially frequent, even though most patients with PSC have associated inflammatory bowel disease. Randomized studies should be able to determine whether UDCA has an effect on the liver histological changes and cholangiographic features of PSC[27] and ultimate survival.

In terms of routine clinical management of patients with PSC, UDCA can be used in symptomatic patients to attempt to delay transplantation and improve well-being. It is also suitable for patients in whom liver transplantation is not feasible. At present there are insufficient data to support its use in those who are asymptomatic or have very mild disease. Hopefully more information to guide its use in PSC will become available in the near future.

Cystic fibrosis

In patients with cystic fibrosis, focal biliary cirrhosis may develop probably due to plugging, sludging and obstruction of intrahepatic bile ducts by abnormally viscid bile. As in PBC and PSC, the presence of biliary cirrhosis can lead to portal hypertension and ultimately hepatocellular failure. Although liver transplantation has now been performed in many of these patients (in some cases as part of a triple heart/lung/liver transplant procedure), few drug therapies have been successfully used in those with less advanced disease.

UDCA is the most promising agent available for the treatment of cystic fibrosis-related liver disease. It appears to have a beneficial short-term effect on liver function, bile acid metabolism and nutritional status, probably by preventing accumulation of toxic, hydrophobic bile acids and improving the viscosity of bile. In a trial of 10–15 mg/kg per day of UDCA in nine patients given for 2–6 months, both serum transaminases and biliary enzymes fell during treatment[28]. Similar results were obtained in eight patients using a dose of 15–20 mg/kg per day[29] and 22 patients treated with 10–20 mg/kg per day for 1 year[30]. As well as improved liver function there were improvements in nutritional indices (body mass, nitrogen balance) which did not appear to be due to increased absorption of fat (as might have been expected). Improved hepatobiliary excretion of radioisotope has also been shown in cystic fibrosis-related liver disease after giving UDCA for 1 year[31].

It is reasonable to conclude, therefore, that UDCA can improve liver dysfunction in cystic fibrosis – larger studies are being carried out to clarify the effects of UDCA and determine if it has an effect on disease progression. The mechanisms of action of UDCA in cystic fibrosis may be similar to those acting in PBC and PSC, although a mucolytic effect may be more important in this situation in view of the viscid bile present in these patients.

It needs to be determined which patients with cystic fibrosis should receive UDCA, e.g. just those with abnormal liver function tests or all patients beyond a certain age. Until these uncertainties are addressed, UDCA should probably only be used in those with demonstrable liver disease or as part of a clinical trial.

Table 4 Randomized, double-blind, placebo-controlled trials of ursodeoxycholic acid in chronic viral hepatitis

	n	Fall in AST?	Fall in γ-GT?	Trial length (months)	Aetiology
Podda (1990)[35]	24	Yes	Yes	2–4	HCV/HBV
Floreani (1991)[36]	29	No	Yes	6	HCV
Rolandi (1991)[34]	26	Yes	Yes	3	HCV/HBV

Chronic hepatitis

Chronic viral hepatitis

There have been several reports of improved liver function (reduction in serum transaminases) with UDCA in patients with chronic viral hepatitis in which inflammation rather than cholestasis is the prominent feature. In almost all cases the patients have had hepatitis B and/or C.

Buzzelli et al.[32] randomized 40 patients to 6 months of 600 mg/day of UDCA or 400 mg/day of SAMe in an unblinded trial. Treatment with UDCA produced statistically significant falls in transaminases and γ-glutamyl transpeptidase compared to the rather low dose of SAMe used (half the 800 mg/day dose usually recommended). Similar results for UDCA were found by Ideo et al.[33] in an uncontrolled study of 24 patients.

Three double-blind studies have been performed of short-term administration of UDCA to patients with chronic viral hepatitis (see Table 4). Although both Rolandi et al.[34] and Podda et al.[35] observed a reduction in serum transaminase and γ-glutamyl transpeptidase levels in patients treated with UDCA, Floreani et al.[36] were unable to reproduce these results in 42 patients with predominantly hepatitis C-related liver disease.

If UDCA is effective in chronic viral hepatitis the pharmacological mechanisms could be similar to those mediating its anticholestatic effects, i.e. by reducing the effects of toxic bile acids and immunomodulation (as discussed earlier). A large randomized, placebo-controlled double-blind study is needed to confirm that UDCA is effective and determine whether it can improve histology[36]. It also needs to be clarified in which patients UDCA should be used (e.g. those in whom α-interferon therapy has been unsuccessful or is contraindicated) and the optimal dose to be given[37] (which may be as low as 4 mg/kg). Studies of its use in conjunction with α-interferon are being performed at present, and it may well prove that UDCA has greatest potential in chronic hepatitis C, a condition in which α-interferon can only suppress activity.

Autoimmune chronic active hepatitis

There is insufficient experience with UDCA to comment on its effects in autoimmune chronic active hepatitis, although it has been reported to be beneficial in isolated patients[38].

Table 5 Randomized, double-blind, placebo-controlled trials of S-adenosylmethionine in chronic liver disease associated with cholestasis

	n	Oral/i.v.	Daily dose	Duration (weeks)	Effect on		
					Symptoms	Biliary enzymes	Bilirubin
Frezza (1990)[39]	220	Oral	1600	2	Yes	Yes	Yes
Manzillo (1992)[40]	343	i.v.	800	2	Yes	Yes	Yes

*Followed by oral SAMe (1600 mg/day) or placebo in responders; oral SAMe led to a significant further reduction in biochemical cholestasis compared to placebo

S-ADENOSYLMETHIONINE IN CHRONIC LIVER DISEASE

The principal studies of S-adenosylmethionine (SAMe) in chronic liver disease have involved patients with intrahepatic cholestasis associated with conditions such as PBC, chronic viral hepatitis and alcoholic liver disease. The studies of the use of SAMe in chronic liver disease with cholestasis will now be assessed.

Evidence for a beneficial effect of SAMe in chronic liver disease with cholestasis

The two principal controlled studies of SAMe in cholestatic liver disease are shown in Table 5. Frezza et al.[39] randomized 220 patients with chronic liver disease and cholestasis to either 1600 mg/day of oral SAMe or placebo. Of these 220, 61 (27.8%) had chronic hepatitis B, 14 (6.4%) primary biliary cirrhosis, 55 (25%) alcoholic liver disease and 90 (40.9%) cryptogenic cirrhosis (many of which may have been related to hepatitis C which had not been identified at that time). Although the study was relatively short there were significant effects on serum bilirubin, biliary enzymes and symptoms (pruritus, fatigue, well-being).

Manzillo et al.[40] randomized 343 patients to either intravenous SAMe (800 mg/day) or placebo. Ninety-three (27.1%) had chronic hepatitis, 131 (38.2%) cirrhosis, 32 (9.3%) had primary biliary cirrhosis and 87 (25.4%) cholestasis post-acute hepatitis. Treatment with SAMe led to significant improvements in serum bilirubin, biliary enzymes and pruritus in patients with chronic liver disease and acute hepatitis compared to those on placebo. Patients with chronic liver disease who 'responded' to intravenous SAMe were continued on either oral SAMe (1600 mg/day) or placebo for a further 8 weeks. In patients who received oral SAMe, markers of cholestasis continued to improve compared to those given placebo. Analysis of the 32 patients with PBC in that study[40] confirms that they responded in a similar way to the total group (see Table 6).

The findings in these two studies are consistent with other uncontrolled studies in patients with chronic liver disease and cholestasis[41,42] and preliminary data in patients with PBC that we have studied in London[43].

From these studies it is reasonable to conclude that, like UDCA, SAMe is well tolerated with very few side-effects. Although treatment with SAMe

Table 6 Analysis of the 32 patients with primary biliary cirrhosis given S-adenosylmethionine (SAMe) in Manzillo et al. 1992[40]

				Effect on		
	n	Daily dose	Duration (weeks)	Symptoms	γ-GT	Bilirubin
IV phase	32:16/16	800	2	?Yes	Yes	Yes

reduces cholestasis (whether given orally or intravenously), longer studies are needed to determine the duration of these effects and whether SAMe can alter the natural history of PBC or other liver diseases. In order to investigate the possible antifibrotic activity of SAMe, serial studies including liver histology are needed.

Pharmacological effects of SAMe in chronic liver disease with cholestasis

The pharmacological actions of SAMe have been reviewed elsewhere in this symposium.

S-adenosylmethionine is the principal methyl group donor in humans. Availability and turnover of SAMe in the liver are impaired in cirrhosis (and presumably other forms of liver disease) due to reduced activity of the enzyme SAMe-synthetase[44]. This results in impairment of the two main metabolic pathways of SAMe, transmethylation and trans-sulphuration. The stable salt of SAMe used clinically may act by overcoming the reduced activity of the enzyme, restoring both methylation and trans-sulphuration. In the former case, improved SAMe-dependent methylation of phospholipid may lead to an improvement in membrane fluidity[45], sodium pump and Na^+/H^+ antiport activity and bile flow.

By acting on the trans-sulphuration pathway, SAMe may promote the synthesis of cysteine, glutathione, taurine and sulphates[46-48]. These are involved in conjugation reactions with endogenous and exogenous toxic substances with cholestatic activity (including bile acids) thus protecting liver cells against damage by free radicals and toxic bile acids[49]. Work using animal models of the development of cirrhosis, suggests that SAMe may also reduce the development of fibrosis[50].

Clinical use of SAMe in chronic liver disease with cholestasis

Trials are needed to determine whether SAMe can alter the natural history of common cholestatic disorders such as PBC and PSC. Organization of these trials is facilitated by the lack of side-effects that have been observed with SAMe. Apart from its use in other conditions such as benign recurrent intrahepatic cholestasis and drug-induced cholestasis (which are outside the scope of this review), SAMe is useful in conditions such as PBC as a way of improving symptoms in those with marked pruritus.

Combination therapy with SAMe and UDCA

There are no data as yet on the combined use of SAMe and UDCA, but as they are thought to act on cholestasis in different ways this may be a promising approach in the future. A combination of the improvements in membrane fluidity and cholestatic bile acid excretion with SAMe combined with beneficial alterations in the bile acid pool, hypercholeresis and perhaps immunomodulation produced by UDCA may be particularly effective in relieving cholestasis.

CONCLUSIONS

UDCA is increasingly used in PBC, PSC, chronic viral hepatitis and cystic fibrosis. Although there is little doubt that UDCA improves cholestasis, larger clinical trials are needed to determine if it can improve survival in patients with these conditions. SAMe is another anticholestatic agent with considerable potential and, like UDCA, is associated with very few side-effects. The role of SAMe in chronic cholestatic liver disease remains to be clarified, but its indications are likely to increase as more is understood about its pharmacological effects.

References

1. Sherlock S. Primary biliary cirrhosis (chronic intrahepatic obstructive jaundice). Gastroenterology. 1959;37:574–86.
2. Ahrens EH, Pater MA, Kunkel HG et al. Primary biliary cirrhosis. Medicine. 1950;29:299–364.
3. Gershwin ME, Mackay IR. Primary biliary cirrhosis: paradigm or paradox for autoimmunity. Gastroenterology. 1991;100:822–33.
4. Underhill J, Donaldson P, Bray G et al. Susceptibility to primary biliary cirrhosis is associated with the HLA DR8-DQB1*0402 haplotype. Hepatology. 1992;16:1404–8.
5. Briggs D, Donaldson PT, Hayes P et al. A major histocompatibility complex class III allotype (C4B 2) associated with primary biliary cirrhosis (PBC). Tissue Antigens. 1987;29:141–5.
6. Spengler U, Pape GR, Hoffmann RM et al. Differential expression of MHC class II subregion products on bile duct epithelial cells and hepatocytes in patients with primary biliary cirrhosis. Hepatology. 1988;8:459–62.
7. Ballardini G, Bianchi FB, Mirakian R et al. HLA-A, B, C, HLA-D/DR and HLA-D/DQ expression on unfixed liver biopsy sections from patients with chronic liver disease. Clin Exp Immunol. 1987;70:35–46.
8. Dickson ER, Grambsch PM, Fleming TR et al. Prognosis in primary biliary cirrhosis: model for decision making. Hepatology. 1989;10:1–7.
9. Perdigoto R, Wiesner RH. Progression of primary biliary cirrhosis with ursodeoxycholic acid. Gastroenterology. 1992;102:1389–91.
10. Leuschner U, Fischer H, Kurtz W et al. Ursodeoxycholic acid in primary biliary cirrhosis: results of a controlled double-blind trial. Gastroenterology. 1989;97:1268–74.
11. Oka H, Toda G, Ikeda Y et al. A multi-center double-blind controlled trial of ursodeoxycholic acid for primary biliary cirrhosis. Gastroenterol Jpn. 1990;25:774–80.
12. Poupon RE, Balkau B, Eschwege E et al. and the UDCA-PBC study group. A multicenter, controlled trial of ursodiol for the treatment of primary biliary cirrhosis. N Engl J Med. 1991;324:1548–54.
13. Eusufzai S, Ericsson S, Cederlund T et al. Effect of ursodeoxycholic acid treatment on ileal absorption of bile acids in man as determined by the SeHCAT test. Gut. 1991;32:1044–8.

14. Crosignani A, Podda M, Battezzati PM et al. Changes in bile acid composition in patients with primary biliary cirrhosis induced by ursodeoxycholic acid administration. Hepatology. 1991;14:1000–7.
15. Calmus Y, Weill B, Ozier Y et al. Immunosuppressive properties of chenodeoxycholic acid and ursodeoxycholic acid in the mouse. Gastroenterology. 1990;103:617–21.
16. Guldutana S, Zimmer G, Imhof M et al. Molecular aspects of membrane stabilisation by ursodeoxycholic acid. Gastroenterology. 1993;104:1736–44.
17. Heuman DM. Hepatoprotective properties of ursodeoxycholic acid. Gastroenterology. 1993;104:1865–70.
18. Calmus Y, Gane P, Rouger P et al. Hepatic expression of class I and class II major histocompatibility complex molecules in primary biliary cirrhosis: effect of ursodeoxycholic acid. Hepatology. 1990;11:12–15.
19. Terasaki S, Nakanuma Y, Ogino H et al. Hepatocellular and biliary expression of HLA antigens in primary biliary cirrhosis before and after ursodeoxycholic acid therapy. Am J Gastroenterol. 1991;86:1194–9.
20. Lombard M, Portmann B, Neuberger J et al. Cyclosporin A treatment in primary biliary cirrhosis: results of a long-term placebo controlled trial. Gastroenterology. 1993;104: 519–26.
21. Kaplan MM, Knox TA. Treatment of primary biliary cirrhosis with low-dose weekly methotrexate. Gastroenterology. 1991;101:1332–8.
22. LaRusso NF, Wiesner RH, Ludwig J et al. Primary sclerosing cholangitis. N Engl J Med. 1984;310:899–903.
23. Dickson ER, Murtaugh PA, Wiesner RH et al. Primary sclerosing cholangitis: refinement and validation of survival models. Gastroenterology. 1992;103:1893–901.
24. Chazouilleres O, Poupon R, Capron JP et al. Ursodeoxycholic acid for primary sclerosing cholangitis. J Hepatol. 1990;11:120–3.
25. O'Brien CB, Senior JR, Arora-Mirchandani R et al. Ursodeoxycholic acid for the treatment of primary sclerosing cholangitis: a 30 month pilot study. Hepatology. 1991;14:838–47.
26. Beuers U, Spengler U, Kruis W et al. Ursodeoxycholic acid for treatment of primary sclerosing cholangitis: a placebo-controlled trial. Hepatology. 1992;16:707–14.
27. Lebovics E, Salama M, Elhosseiny A et al. Resolution of radiographic abnormalities with ursodeoxycholic acid therapy of primary sclerosing cholangitis. Gastroenterology. 1992;102:2143–7.
28. Colombo C, Setchell KDR, Podda M et al. Effects of ursodeoxycholic acid therapy for liver disease associated with cystic fibrosis. J Pediatr. 1990;117:482–9.
29. Cotting J, Lentze MJ, Reichen J. Effects of ursodeoxycholic acid treatment on nutrition and liver function in patients with cystic fibrosis and longstanding cholestasis. Gut. 1990;31:918–21.
30. Galabert C, Montet JC, Lengrand D et al. Effects of ursodeoxycholic acid on liver function in patients with cystic fibrosis and chronic cholestasis. J Pediatr. 1992;121:138–41.
31. Colombo C, Castellani MR, Balistreri WF et al. Scintigraphic documentation of an improvement in hepatobiliary excretory function after treatment with ursodeoxycholic acid in patients with cystic fibrosis and associated liver disease. Hepatology. 1992;15:677–84.
32. Buzzelli G, Moscarella S, Focardi G et al. Long-term treatment with ursodeoxycholic acid in patients with chronic active hepatitis. Curr Ther Res. 1991;50:635–42.
33. Ideo G, Bellati G, Pedraglio E et al. Efficacy of ursodeoxycholic acid in lowering alanine aminotransferase and gamma-glutamyl transpeptidase serum levels in patients with chronic active hepatitis and primary biliary cirrhosis. Curr Ther Res. 1990;47:62–6.
34. Rolandi E, Franchescini R, Cataldi A et al. Effects of ursodeoxycholic acid (UDCA) on serum liver damage indices in patients with chronic active hepatitis. A double-blind controlled study. Eur J Clin Pharmacol. 1991;40:473–5.
35. Podda M, Ghezzi C, Battezzatti PM et al. Effects of ursodeoxycholic acid and taurine on serum liver enzymes and bile acids in chronic hepatitis. Gastroenterology. 1990;98:1044–50.
36. Floreani A, Chiaramonte M, Fabris P et al. Poor effect of ursodeoxycholic acid in anti-hepatitis C virus-positive chronic liver disease. Curr Ther Res. 1991;50:579–85.
37. Crosignani A, Battezzatti PM, Setchell KDR et al. Effects of ursodeoxycholic acid on serum liver enzymes and bile acid metabolism in chronic active hepatitis: a dose–response study. Hepatology. 1991;13:339–4.

38. Bateson MC. Ursodeoxycholic acid therapy in chronic active hepatitis. Postgrad Med J. 1990;66:781–3.
39. Frezza M, Surrenti C, Manzillo G et al. Oral S-adenosylmethionine in the asymptomatic treatment of intrahepatic cholestasis. Gastroenterology. 1990;99:211–15.
40. Manzillo G, Piccinino F, Surrenti C et al. Multicentre double-blind placebo-controlled study of intravenous and oral S-adenosyl-L-methionine (SAMe) in cholestatic patients with liver disease. Drug Invest. 1992;4(Suppl. 4):90–100.
41. Adachi Y, Nanno T, Kanbe A et al. The effects of S-adenosylmethionine on intrahepatic cholestasis. Jpn Arch Intern Med. 1986;33:185–92.
42. Cacciatore L, Varriale A, Cozzolino G et al. S-adenosylmethionine (SAMe) in the treatment of pruritus in chronic liver disease. Acta Therapeutica. 1989;15:363–71.
43. Bray GP, Di Padova C, Tredger JM et al. A comparison of S-adenosylmethionine (SAMe), rifampicin (R) and ursodeoxycholic acid (UDCA) in primary biliary cirrhosis (PBC); interim results. J Hepatol. 1991;13:S101.
44. Duce AM, Ortiz P, Cabrero C et al. S-adenosyl-L-methionine synthetase and phospholipid methyltransferase are inhibited in human cirrhosis. Hepatology. 1988;8:65–8.
45. Almasio P, Bortoloini M, Pagliaro L et al. Role of S-adenosyl-L-methionine in the treatment of intrahepatic cholestasis. Drugs. 1990;40(Suppl. 3):111–23.
46. Marchesini G, Bugianesi E, Bianchi G et al. Effects of S-adenosyl-L-methionine administration on plasma levels of sulphur containing amino-acids in patients with liver cirrhosis. Clin Nutr. 1992;11:303–8.
47. Vendemiale G, Altomare E, Trizio T et al. Effects of oral S-adenosyl-L-methionine on hepatic glutathione in patients with liver disease. Scand J Gastroenterol. 1989;24:407–15.
48. Bray GP, Tredger JM, Williams R. S-adenosylmethionine protects against acetaminophen hepatotoxicity in two mouse models. Hepatology. 1992;15:297–301.
49. Villanova N, Mazzella M, Roda A et al. Effects of oral S-adenosyl-L-methionine (SAMe) on bile acid metabolism in primary biliary cirrhosis. Eur J Clin Invest. 1992;22:A19.
50. Corrales F, Gimenez A, Alvarez et al. S-adenosylmethionine treatment prevents carbon tetrachloride-induced S-adenosylmethionine synthetase inactivation and attenuates liver injury. Hepatology. 1992;16:1022–7.

Index